Don't forget to check out the additional online content!

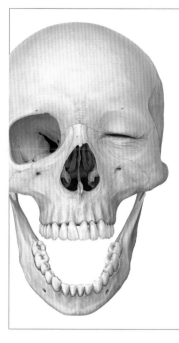

WinkingSkull.com *PLUS*

Quiz yourself with nearly 100 online questions and answers with your WinkingSkull.com *PLUS* access

Simply visit WinkingSkull.com and follow these instructions to get started today.

If you do not already have a free WinkingSkull.com account, visit www.winkingskull.com, click on "Register" and complete the registration form. Enter the scratch-off code below.

If you already have a WinkingSkull.com account, go to the "Manage Account" page and click on the "Register a Code" link. Enter the scratch-off code below.

This product cannot be returned if either of the access code panels are scratched off.

Some functionalities on WinkingSkull.com require support for advanced web technologies. A major browser (IE, Chrome, Firefox, Safari) within the last three major versions is suggested for use on the site.

Practice your technique using 160 invaluable videos through MediaCenter.Thieme.com

Simply visit MediaCenter.thieme.com and, when prompted during the registration process, enter the code to the right to get started today.

D1294633

	WINDOWS & MAC	**TABLET**
Recommended Browser(s)	Recent browser versions on all major platforms and any mobile operating system that supports HTML5 video playback. *All browsers should have JavaScript enabled.*	
Flash Player Plug-in	Flash Player 9 or higher. *For Mac users, ATI Rage 128 GPU doesn't support full-screen mode with hardware scaling.*	Tablet PCs with Android OS support Flash 10.1.
Recommended for optimal usage experience	Monitor resolutions: • Normal (4:3) 1024×768 or higher • Widescreen (16:9) 1280×720 or higher • Widescreen (16:10) 1440×900 or higher A high-speed internet connection (minimum 384 Kps) is suggested.	WiFi or cellular data connection is required.

Connect with us on social media

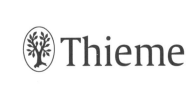

Osteopathic Techniques

The Learner's Guide

Sharon Gustowski, DO, MPH
Chair and Associate Professor
Department of Osteopathic Principles, Practices, and Integration
University of the Incarnate Word School of Osteopathic Medicine
San Antonio, Texas

Maria Budner-Gentry, DO
Osteopathy Matters PLLC
Ithaca, New York

Ryan Seals, DO
Assistant Professor
OMM Department
Texas College of Osteopathic Medicine
University of North Texas Health Science Center
Fort Worth, Texas

Illustrations by
Markus Voll
Karl Wesker

153 illustrations

Thieme
New York • Stuttgart • Delhi • Rio de Janeiro

Acquisitions Editor: Delia K. DeTurris
Developmental Editor: Julie Montalbano
Managing Editor: J. Owen Zurhellen IV
Editorial Director, Educational Products: Anne M. Sydor, PhD
Director, Editorial Services: Mary Jo Casey
Production Editor: Kenny Chumbley
International Production Director: Andreas Schabert
International Marketing Director: Fiona Henderson
International Sales Director: Louisa Turrell
Director of Sales, North America: Mike Roseman
Senior Vice President and Chief Operating Officer: Sarah
    Vanderbilt
President: Brian D. Scanlan
Medical Illustrators: Markus Voll and Karl Wesker

Library of Congress Cataloging-in-Publication Data

Names: Gustowski, Sharon, author. | Budner-Gentry, Maria,
    author. | Seals, Ryan, author.
Title: Osteopathic techniques : the learner's guide /
    Sharon Gustowski, Maria Budner-Gentry, Ryan Seals.
Description: New York : Thieme, [2017] | Includes
    bibliographical references and index.
Identifiers: LCCN 2016051877| ISBN 9781626234253
    (hardcover : alk. paper) | ISBN 9781626234260 (eISBN)
Subjects: | MESH: Manipulation, Osteopathic
Classification: LCC RZ342.9 | NLM WB 940 | DDC 615.5/33—
    dc23LC record available at https://lccn.loc.gov/2016051877

© 2017 Thieme Medical Publishers, Inc.
Thieme Publishers New York
333 Seventh Avenue, New York, NY 10001 USA
+1 800 782 3488, customerservice@thieme.com

Thieme Publishers Stuttgart
Rüdigerstrasse 14, 70469 Stuttgart, Germany
+49 [0]711 8931 421, customerservice@thieme.de

Thieme Publishers Delhi
A-12, Second Floor, Sector-2, Noida-201301
Uttar Pradesh, India
+91 120 45 566 00, customerservice@thieme.in

Thieme Publishers Rio de Janeiro, Thieme Publicações Ltda.
Edifício Rodolpho de Paoli, 25º andar
Av. Nilo Peçanha, 50 – Sala 2508
Rio de Janeiro 20020-906, Brasil
+55 21 3172 2297

Cover design: Thieme Publishing Group
Typesetting by Prairie Papers

Printed in China by Everbest Printing Co. Ltd.   5 4 3 2 1

ISBN 978-1-62623-425-3

Also available as an e-book:
eISBN 978-1-62623-426-0

Important note: Medicine is an ever-changing science undergoing continual development. Research and clinical experience are continually expanding our knowledge, in particular our knowledge of proper treatment and drug therapy. Insofar as this book mentions any dosage or application, readers may rest assured that the authors, editors, and publishers have made every effort to ensure that such references are in accordance with **the state of knowledge at the time of production of the book.**

Nevertheless, this does not involve, imply, or express any guarantee or responsibility on the part of the publishers in respect to any dosage instructions and forms of applications stated in the book. **Every user is requested to examine carefully** the manufacturers' leaflets accompanying each drug and to check, if necessary in consultation with a physician or specialist, whether the dosage schedules mentioned therein or the contraindications stated by the manufacturers differ from the statements made in the present book. Such examination is particularly important with drugs that are either rarely used or have been newly released on the market. Every dosage schedule or every form of application used is entirely at the user's own risk and responsibility. The authors and publishers request every user to report to the publishers any discrepancies or inaccuracies noticed. If errors in this work are found after publication, errata will be posted at www.thieme.com on the product description page.

Some of the product names, patents, and registered designs referred to in this book are in fact registered trademarks or proprietary names even though specific reference to this fact is not always made in the text. Therefore, the appearance of a name without designation as proprietary is not to be construed as a representation by the publisher that it is in the public domain.

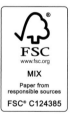

Contents

Menu of Accompanying Videos

About the Authors

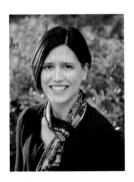

Sharon Gustowski, DO, MPH, is a 2001 graduate of the University of North Texas Health Science Center, Texas College of Osteopathic Medicine (UNTH-SC-TCOM) and the School of Public Health. She completed a traditional rotating internship at Bay Area Corpus Christi Medical Center and residency training at the UNTHSC-TCOM in Neuromusculoskeletal Medicine and Osteopathic Manipulative Medicine, where Jerry Dickey, DO, FAAO was the program director. She began a career in academic medicine immediately after residency as a founding faculty member of the Touro University Nevada College of Osteopathic Medicine. She returned to Texas after seven years in Nevada, serving as Course Director for the Year 2 Osteopathic Manipulative Medicine Courses at UNTHSC-TCOM. In 2014, Dr. Gustowski returned to her hometown of San Antonio, Texas, to serve as the Chair of the Osteopathic Principles, Practices, and Integration Department at the University of the Incarnate Word School of Osteopathic Medicine. Her osteopathic teaching focus is to preserve osteopathic history and to encourage more integration of OMT into clinical practice. She is also active in state and national osteopathic organizations. She has a particular interest in providing osteopathic care to children and their families.

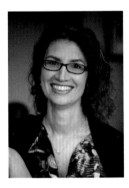

Maria Budner-Gentry, DO, is a 1999 graduate of A. T. Still University-Kirksville College of Osteopathic Medicine. After internship training at Riverside Osteopathic Hospital (Trenton, MI) and Henry Ford Hospital (Detroit, MI), she completed Family Medicine residency at Bay Area Corpus Christi Medical Center in Corpus Christi, Texas. Her hospital-based residency included a specific emphasis in osteopathic manipulative medicine under the direction of Ronald Bowen, DO. Dr. Budner-Gentry practiced Family Practice/OMM and ER medicine in Arizona before settling near Ithaca, New York. In Ithaca, Dr. Budner-Gentry has an OMM practice serving newborns to nonagenarians. Dr. Budner-Gentry is especially passionate about trauma strains as well as early care for babies and new mothers.

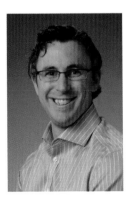

Ryan Seals, DO, is a 2008 graduate of Oklahoma State University Center for Health Sciences, College of Osteopathic Medicine. He completed his residency training at an integrated Family Practice/Neuromusculoskeletal Medicine residency at Florida Hospital East in Orlando, Florida. He has worked at the University of North Texas Health Sciences Center, Texas College of Osteopathic Medicine since finishing residency and is currently the year 2 OMM curriculum director. He enjoys applying the osteopathic approach to a wide variety of patients and conditions, and training students and residents at various levels.

Foreword

With the international growth of osteopathy worldwide, the osteopathic profession needs textbooks to train all levels of osteopathic learners. Dr. Sharon Gustowski's *Osteopathic Techniques: The Learner's Guide* focuses on training the beginning student in osteopathic history, principles, and practice of osteopathic manipulative techniques (OMT). This book is easy to read and understand and includes online access to videos of techniques that will help the learner develop competence in osteopathic principles and practice (OPP) and osteopathic manipulative medicine (OMM).

Osteopathic students must develop competency in OPP and OMM knowledge and skills before entering clinical practice. Dr. Gustowski's textbook is designed as a teaching aid with these competencies at the core of its design. Internationally, OPP and OMM competencies have been defined in the World Health Organization's (WHO) publication *Benchmark for Training in Osteopathy*. These competencies include knowledge and skill in osteopathic history, philosophy, basic science, physical examination, and OMT. Within the United States, OPP and OMM competencies, which should be obtained during predoctoral training, have been defined by the American Association of Colleges of Osteopathic Medicine (AACOM) in their publication *Osteopathic Core Competencies for Medical Students*. These competencies include approaching diagnosis and treatment of the patient holistically with consideration of their entire spiritual, mental, and physical well-being; understanding the body's structure, function, and physiological mechanisms within the context of health and disease; communicating osteopathic principles to the patient and the healthcare team; and manual skills of somatic diagnosis and osteopathic manipulative treatment. For licensure in the United States, the National Board of Osteopathic Medical Examiners (NBOME) assesses these OPP and OMM competencies as defined in their publication *Fundamental Osteopathic Medical Competency Domains: Guidelines for Osteopathic Medical Licensure and the Practice of Osteopathic Medicine*. Each osteopathic physician entering into unsupervised clinical practice must demonstrate minimally competency in OPP and OMM knowledge and skills by passing the COMLEX-USA licensure examination series. Therefore, all formal osteopathic education must include training and assessment in these competencies and this textbook can contribute to the development of OPP and OMM competencies in the osteopathic student.

Dr. Gustowski's textbook goes beyond just educating the learner in the OPP and OMM competencies, but also includes information on how to study and the milestones to indicate the progression of skills from beginner to expert. This information is translatable to the American Council on Graduate Medical Education (ACGME) *Osteopathic Recognition Milestones* for the newly established *Osteopathic Recognition Requirements* for residency programs. Dr. Gustowski's textbook also includes self-assessment questions at the end of each chapter for the learner to use to prepare for their competency assessments. With the scope of the textbook to include osteopathic history, philosophy, diagnosis of somatic dysfunction within all ten body regions and treatment with the required OMT techniques as defined by the competencies documents from the AACOM, NBOME, ACGME, and the WHO, this textbook will be valuable for training osteopathic students worldwide.

References

American Association of Colleges of Osteopathic Medicine (AACOM). Osteopathic Core Competencies for Medical Students. August 2012 (https://www.aacom.org/docs/default-source/core-competencies/corecompetencyreport2012.pdf?sfvrsn=4)

American Council for Graduate Medical Education. Osteopathic Recognition Requirements. July 2015 (http://www.acgme.org/Portals/0/PFAssets/ProgramRequirements/Osteopathic_Recogniton_Requirements.pdf)

American Council for Graduate Medical Education. The Osteopathic Recognition milestone Project. December 2015 (http://www.acgme.org/Portals/0/PDFs/Milestones/OsteopathicRecognitionMilestones.pdf)

National Board of Osteopathic Medical Examiners. Fundamental Osteopathic Medical Competency Domains: Guidelines for Osteopathic Medical Licensure and the Practice of Osteopathic Medicine. September 2016 (https://www.nbome.org/docs/Flipbooks/FOMCD/index.html#p=1)

World Health Organization. Benchmark for Training in Osteopathy. 2010 (http://apps.who.int/medicinedocs/documents/s17555en/s17555en.pdf)

Karen T. Snider, DO, FAAO
Professor
Neuromusculoskeletal Medicine and
Osteopathic Manipulative Medicine
Assistant Dean for Osteopathic
Principles and Practice Integration
A. T. Still University
Kirksville College of Osteopathic Medicine
Kirksville, Missouri

Preface

As I learned, practiced, and taught osteopathic techniques, I found that neither I nor my students could always replicate treatment steps as they were communicated in textbooks. I needed to make modifications to the steps to suit not only my own and my students' skills and abilities, but to adapt the steps to the needs and optimal care of each patient. After all, my hands are not the hands of my students or of the technique authors, and no two patients' bodies are exactly alike.

But modifications to techniques are not always so easy to make, especially in the context of trying to teach large numbers of students. Typically, techniques are written in an ordered, temporal fashion, often without identification of principles or sufficient background information. With colleagues at Touro University Nevada College of Osteopathic Medicine, I began identifying the core principles and end-goal focus of each style of technique. Then, the steps of a technique could be linked back to the principles. This exercise enabled me to identify which steps were modifiable and which were critically essential. It also enabled me to develop a universal assessment rubric for measuring students' skill levels. This manual represents the evolution of those efforts, and it is their culmination.

Two of my osteopathic colleagues were gracious enough to offer their assistance in this endeavor. I cannot say why they agreed to it, but I am forever thankful for the many hours of work and ideas that propelled this project forward in just a little over a year.

I hope that all physicians who perform OMT do so in accord with the best of their own unique talents and in concord with the body, mind, and spirit of the patient. Each patient encounter is a new exploration in the intimate act of human healing and care. It is thus, in some ways, an experiment performed by an unblinded physician-scientist with an "n of one." I offer this manual as one strategy to undertake that noble experiment well.

Sharon Gustowski, DO, MPH

Acknowledgments

Gratitude is expressed to Victoria Chang for assistance with the manuscript.

Gratitude is expressed to the following individuals for their assistance in the video production:

- John Miller, Tom Mohr
- Videographers: Meagan Piña, Megan Gaitan, Joel Nevarez
- Models: The Dang, Jaylen Dawson, Mary Griffin, Matthew Hansen, Patricia Lew, Maggie Meigs, Sara Mohr, Samuel Piña, Jeff Wood

Finally, gratitude is expressed to all of the authors' friends and family for their love and commitment to this project.

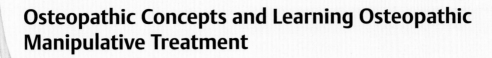

Osteopathic Concepts and Learning Osteopathic Manipulative Treatment

LEARNING OBJECTIVES

1. Outline the general history of the evolution of osteopathic techniques.
2. Identify major figures in osteopathic manipulative medicine.
3. Recall the tenets of osteopathic medicine and relate them to basic patient care.
4. Identify the general indications for performing osteopathic manipulative treatment.
5. Compare and contrast the use of osteopathic manipulative treatment as a primary and an adjunct treatment.
6. Use clear communication with patients.
7. Relate the common effects patients experience after receiving osteopathic manipulative treatment.
8. Recognize the differences between novices and experts in the performance of clinical (psychomotor) skills.
9. Construct study and practice strategies for learning osteopathic manipulative techniques.

Brief History of Osteopathic Techniques

We want and must have all Osteopaths who, when they find pneumonia, flux, scarlet fever, diphtheria, know the exact location and cause of the trouble, and how to remove it. He must not be like a blacksmith, only able to hit large bones and muscles with a heavy hammer, but he must be able to use the most delicate instruments of the silversmith in adjusting the deranged, displaced bones, nerves, muscles, and remove all obstructions, and thereby restore the machinery of life to its normal movement. To do this is to be an Osteopath.[1]

Osteopathic medicine was and remains today largely a philosophy. Osteopathic manipulative techniques are its hallmark treatment. Andrew Taylor Still, DO (1828–1917) founded the Ameri-can School of Osteopathy in 1892, having invented a new form of medical care that he coined osteopathy (**Fig. 1.1**). Today, *osteopathy* has been broadened to *osteopathic medicine* in the United States, distinguishing it as one of two systems of medical care. Osteopathic physicians have complete medical training and an unlimited scope of medical practice.

Dr. Still mostly used and taught three types of manual techniques: articulatory, indirect, and challenge the barrier, which are classified as exaggeration techniques in this manual. Although Dr. Still documented some of his techniques in his four books, he never authored a complete technique manual. This was probably to reinforce the core concepts of osteopathy—that the osteopath should find the cause of a disease in each individual patient, looking specifically in the musculoskeletal system and related vascular structures. Then the osteopath should use anatomical knowledge to correct any structural abnormalities and thereby enable the body to heal itself. The osteopath was not to use

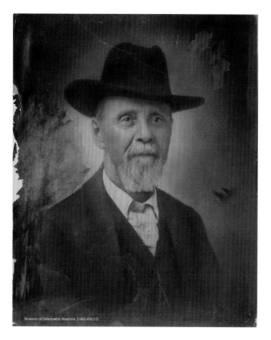

Fig. 1.1 Andrew Taylor Still, Founder of Osteopathy. Museum of Osteopathic Medicine SM, Kirksville, MO [1980.406.01] ca. 1905.

Major Osteopathic Techniques Timeline

1885	Indirect and Articulatory techniques, Andrew Taylor Still, D.O.
1889	Challenge the barrier techniques, Andrew Taylor Still, DO
1898	Lymphatic techniques, Andrew Taylor Still, DO, described in *Osteopathy Complete* by Elmer Barber, DO
1921	Low table with speed (high velocity low amplitude [HVLA] techniques), Earle Willer, DO
1929	Neurolymphatic Reflexes (Chapman Points) (visceral: neurolymphatic reflex technique), Frank Chapman, DO
1950s	Muscle energy technique, Fred Mitchell Sr, DO
1950s	Functional technique, Harold Hoover, DO
1950s	Osteopathic Cranial Manipulative Medicine (Osteopathy In The Cranial Field), William Sutherland, DO
1955	Counterstrain technique, Lawrence H. Jones, DO
1980s	Facilitated positional release technique, Stanley Schiowitz, DO
1980s	Myofascial release techniques, various styles, John Peckham, DO, Anthony Chila, DO, and Robert Ward, DO
1990s	Myofascial release technique (bioenergetics model), Judith O'Connell, DO
1996	Still techniques, Richard Van Buskirk, DO
2000	Progressive inhibition of neuromuscular structures, Dennis Dowling, DO

techniques arbitrarily. Students, however, yearned to emulate Dr. Still's techniques, owing to their remarkable results, so technique manuals were naturally created. Some of the first manuals were written by Charles Hazzard, DO and Carl McConnell, DO. The original techniques, however, were apparently difficult to teach and replicate. As the schools of osteopathy grew, and as newer methods of technique were developed, some of the newer techniques replaced the exaggeration techniques. This trend continues today, as technique methodologies come into and out of favor with academic institutions and professional groups.

Although the evolution and sheer number of techniques may seem overwhelming, the diversity has, no doubt, led to the successes of the profession. Today, as at no other time, osteopathic physicians have a vast array of techniques with which to address their patients' needs, and new techniques are always being developed. As Dr. Still said, "Dig on!" This technique manual is but one iteration among many other manuals designed specifically for those new to osteopathic medicine.

A timeline of the development of some of the major osteopathic techniques is presented here.[2] Additional, historical information on techniques included in this manual can be found in each chapter.

Osteopathic Philosophy, Osteopathic Manipulative Treatment, and Patient Care

The philosophy of osteopathy is expansive and holistic, focused on the patient, with specific attention to the cause of a disease. Although not directly spoken by Dr. Still, the osteopathic tenets are substantive, but not comprehensive, extrapolations of the core osteopathic concepts, such as identifying the cause of a disease. An early first version of the tenets, as taught by osteopathic medical colleges, was developed in 1952.[3] The ones presented here are the most modern version published by Felix Rogers, DO, in 2005.[4] The tenets serve as a framework that guides and distinguishes osteopathic clinical reasoning and patient care. All learners are encouraged to adopt and integrate the osteopathic tenets into their own clinical practices.

Osteopathic Tenet

A person is the product of dynamic interaction between body, mind, and spirit.

Each patient is a person with a unique life history, social relationships, and cultural framework. Each patient has his or her own spiritual, religious, moral, and value belief systems. The role that each of these components plays in each patient's health and recovery from illness should be recognized and respected by the physician.

Osteopathic Tenet

An inherent property of this dynamic interaction is the capacity of the individual for the maintenance of health and recovery from disease.

When a patient's health is compromised, the person's homeostatic, self-healing mechanisms are functioning but have been overwhelmed by the disease process. Conservative measures, such as physical and mental rest, adequate hydration, appropriate nutrition, and time can often assist in a patient's recovery. Osteopathic manipulative treatment (OMT), should also be considered as a conservative treatment in the spectrum of medical treatments. When higher-risk medical treatments are necessary, however, the patient's capacity to adjust and respond to the interventions should be assessed and the patient prepared mentally, physically, and spiritually for the challenges ahead.

Osteopathic Tenet

Many forces, both intrinsic and extrinsic to the person, can challenge this inherent capacity and contribute to the onset of illness.

Constantly faced with challenges to survival, the human being is an amazingly adaptive organism. But emotional, physical, and cognitive stressors, acute or chronic, can overwhelm a person's system, and mental and physical disease or injury can occur.

Osteopathic Tenet

The musculoskeletal system significantly influences the individual's ability to restore this inherent capacity and therefore to resist disease processes.

If the musculoskeletal system truly is a significant factor in health maintenance and prevention of disease, then physician and patient efforts toward restoring optimal health of the musculoskeletal system are indeed important. Osteopathic techniques are specifically designed to treat the musculoskeletal system by restoring structural integrity, which improves bodily function for healing and maintenance of wellness.

Osteopathic Manipulative Treatment

OMT is the use of one or more osteopathic techniques as a patient treatment. OMT is performed after somatic dysfunction is identified by physical examination. A formal definition of somatic dysfunction is presented here to orient the learner for further discussions in this and subsequent chapters.

Somatic Dysfunction

"Impaired or altered function of related components of the somatic (body framework) system: skeletal, arthrodial and myofascial structures, and their related vascular, lymphatic, and neural elements. Somatic dysfunction is treatable using osteopathic manipulative treatment. The positional and motion aspects of somatic dysfunction are best described using at least one of three parameters: (1) The position of a body part as determined by palpation and referenced to its adjacent defined structure, (2) The directions in which motion is freer, and (3) The directions in which motion is restricted."[5]

Effects of Performing Osteopathic Manipulative Treatment

OMT has many beneficial effects for patients. The Five Models of Osteopathic Medicine represent a useful categorization of healthy and diseased patient states, as well as the effects of OMT for patient recovery.[4] The Five Models are: Biomechanical, Neurologic, Respiratory Circulatory, Metabolic-Energy, and Behavioral. This manual highlights the more relevant effects of each technique in each chapter's Technique Introduction section. A summary of those effects is found in Table 1.1.

Table 1.1 Effects of performing osteopathic manipulative treatment based on the five models of osteopathic medicine

Biomechanical Model	– Improves structural alignment – Restores normal muscle and fascial tone and tension – Improves regional and joint range of motion
Neurologic Model	– Balances autonomic nervous system functioning – Decreases pain
Respiratory Circulatory Model	– Improves arterial, venous, and lymphatic circulation – Improves gas exchange
Metabolic-Energy Model	– Improves cellular functioning – Contributes to efficient use of energy (calories)
Behavioral Model	– Supports general mental well-being of the patient

Incorporating Osteopathic Manipulative Treatment into Patient Care

OMT is performed after an appropriate medical history, physical examination, and diagnostic tests are performed and the physician has a working diagnosis. An exam for, and subsequent diagnosis of, somatic dysfunction is also required to perform OMT, although selected techniques may be performed empirically. Oftentimes, the use of only one technique during one patient visit is not sufficient to fully address a patient's complaint, as somatic dysfunction isolated to one joint, muscle, visceral organ, or piece of fascia is rare (because the body is interconnected). So each patient requires an individualized overall treatment approach or systematic method for diagnosing the somatic dysfunction and then choosing techniques and technique order.

OMT as Primary Treatment

OMT can be used as a primary treatment when somatic dysfunction is the most significant contributing factor causing the patient's condition, such as painful lumbar and pelvic somatic dysfunction resulting from lifting a heavy object. In these cases, OMT may be the only treatment necessary, although supplemental home exercises, nutritional recommendations (e.g., hydration), or prevention strategies (e.g., proper lifting technique), and may be added to support the patient's complete recovery and wellness.

OMT as an Adjunct Treatment

OMT can be used as an adjunct treatment, along with other standard medical therapies when somatic dysfunction is impeding the body's self-healing homeostatic mechanisms but is not the primary cause of a patient's complaint. For example, a hospitalized patient with pneumonia can benefit from OMT to the rib cage and lymphatic system to improve chest wall biomechanics (gas exchange), arterial blood flow (to bring nutrients and medications to lung tissue), and lymphatic drainage of the lungs (**Fig. 1.2**). In this case, OMT is performed in addition to standard medical treatments and therapies.

Clinical Considerations

Before using OMT, be sure to keep in mind the clinical indications, contraindications, and precautions. Some general guidelines are found in Table 1.2, and more specific recommendations are in each technique chapter.

An OMT Treatment Session

The number of techniques per treatment, the time spent per treatment, and the frequency of OMT are dependent on the patient's body, the type of technique chosen, and the skill of the physician. In general, diagnosing somatic dysfunction and performing OMT can take as few as 3 minutes or as many as 45 minutes, with 10–20 minutes being an average time. Patient follow-up visits are recommended, spaced 1–2 weeks apart, for acute and subacute conditions, and subsequent visits may be spread out in 4- to 6-week intervals. The exact frequency, duration, and number of techniques performed at each visit are based on clinical judgment. It should be remembered that the body requires time to heal and adjust after each application of OMT.

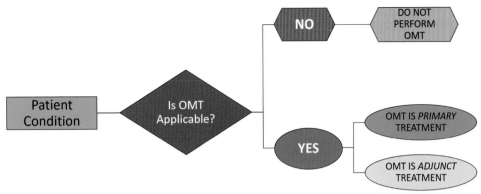

Fig. 1.2 Using osteopathic manipulative treatment in patient care. OMT, osteopathic manipulative treatment.

Patient Participation in the Delivery of OMT

Clear and specific communication is necessary to safely and successfully perform OMT and provide patient care. The patient must move, breathe, and relax at the appropriate times, in the designated magnitude and direction. Before any osteopathic technique is performed, verbal consent should be obtained and the patient informed of possible outcomes, which include any possible tissue responses (see OMT Aftercare section). The basic steps of the technique should also be explained. Sometimes it is helpful if the physician demonstrates any actions that the patient will be asked to perform. Patients should also be given permission to communicate about any concerns or tender areas throughout the technique performance.

OMT Aftercare

Patients who receive OMT should be informed of possible side effects and given aftercare instructions. Efficacy and side effects of manual techniques performed on the body will in part be determined by the patient's physical state (metabolic, hydration, and nutritional status), the patient's state of mind (emotional mood, affect, mental health), and the patient's spirit (vision of health and ability to achieve health). However, it is impossible to predict each patient's response to OMT, so offering a range of responses, as listed here, is recommended.

- Advise patients that they may experience improvement, muscle soreness, or no change after receiving OMT.
    - Soreness is attributed to the liberation of lactic acid and other built-up metabolic waste products, as well as the increase in cellular activity required for healing.
        - If soreness is severe or persists for more than 2 days, the patient should be thoroughly re-examined for additional pathology.
            - In the case of uncertainty, it is preferable to perform fewer techniques at each visit rather than to overtreat a patient.

Table 1.2	General osteopathic manipulative treatment indications, contraindications, and precautions	
Indications	**Contraindications**	**Precautions**
OMT is indicated when somatic dysfunction is present.	Do not use OMT in cases of unstable life- or limb-threatening emergencies. Do not use OMT when somatic dysfunction is not identified on a physical exam or is absent in the patient's condition.	Use OMT on a limited basis when the musculoskeletal system is in a frail condition or when the patient is unable to cooperate.

- Advise patients to drink plenty of water if not contraindicated due to medical conditions.
- Advise patients to perform gentle movements in the 24 hours following OMT, such as walking, to facilitate circulation of fluids and cellular waste products. Strenuous physical activity should be avoided, and concurrent physical therapy may need to be lessened or suspended for a few days to allow the biomechanical and physiological changes to occur.
- Advise parents that pediatric patients may express altered behaviors instead of soreness, such as fussiness, irritability, changes in appetite, or sleepiness. If such behaviors persist for more than 2 days the patient should be re-examined.

Osteopathic Manipulative Treatment Skills Learning Strategies

Physicians use hands-on skills as a part of their diagnostic and treatment process. These psychomotor skills are distinct from the intellectual skills of obtaining and applying knowledge in patient care. Therefore, learners should apply different strategies for acquiring psychomotor skills, such as osteopathic techniques. Proficiency in psychomotor skills advances in a predictable fashion, but the amount of time a learner spends at each area may vary based on past experiences, inherent abilities, and practice efforts (Table 1.3).

This manual helps learners advance from a novice to an intermediate stage of proficiency in performing OMT. Intermediate proficiency enables an osteopathic medical student to safely perform OMT while supervised by an attending or faculty physician. In general, physicians become experts when they are capable of performing clinical skills independently, fluidly, and without many, if any, errors. Some evidence-based strategies can enable learners to advance their skills from the level of a novice to that of an expert.[6]

- Conceptualize and visualize.
  - Preview the videos and skim through the technique instructions to get a general sense of what performing the technique looks like.
    - Observe and take notes during live faculty demonstrations and summarize key concepts.
- Focus on the end goal.
  - Identify an end goal for each technique. One is listed in most techniques, exams, and tests in this manual as a reference and reminder.
  - An end goal is the intended effect of performing a technique. It is an external focus, in contrast with an internal focus, where you focus on your own body mechanics that are needed to perform the skill. The external focus shifts your mental concentration away from your own body

Table 1.3 Stages and development of psychomotor skills

	Novice	Intermediate	Expert
Stages	**Cognitive**	**Associative**	**Autonomous**
What is being learned?	Verbal information and procedural rule	Initial errors corrected; psychomotor connections; deeper understanding of procedural rule	Fine tuning
How easy is knowledge retrieval?	Labor intensive and effortful	Still have to think before retrieval	Effortless; no conscious retrieval
How good is performance?	Trial and error; erratic	More fluid with fewer interruptions	Smooth, with accuracy and speed

Source: Table adapted with permission from Collins V. Psychomotor Learning—Osteopathic Manipulative Medicine, Kun Huang, Center for Innovative Learning, University of North Texas Health Science Center, June 2013.

mechanics, or what you are doing, onto the intended effect and yields best results.

- For example, in baseball, when a pitch is thrown, the batter must focus on hitting the ball, instead of focusing on his own grip and stance.

- Verbalize the steps.
  - Recite the steps of the technique out loud or mentally just prior to practicing. Do this by reading directly out of the manual or summarizing the steps in your own words.
    - Eventually, this step will no longer be necessary. However, it becomes invaluable later in practice when techniques must be explained to patients.
- Practice consistently.
  - "Perfect practice makes perfect." Practice the same way every time for the first few attempts, then refine your process if necessary.
  - Practice regularly both inside and outside of classroom time.
  - Observe others practicing to enhance your own practice.
  - If you find yourself struggling with some skills, ask peers and faculty about their practice habits.
- Use feedback.
  - Seek out and be open to receiving feedback from peers and faculty.
    - Sometimes learners are hesitant to receive feedback about performing skills unsuccessfully. However, it is easier to catch an error early on and make an adjustment, rather than try to identify and change a formed habit.

Using these strategies, learners should find that practicing psychomotor skills becomes efficient and ultimately rewarding, when proficiency is reached and OMT can be applied to patient care.

Osteopathic Manipulative Treatment Assessment Strategies

Assessment for skills proficiency, or a practical examination, can be a daunting idea for both learners and faculty graders. Learners often encounter performance anxiety, lack of confidence, and fear of judgment when preparing for and performing practical examinations. This is partly due to the nature of taking an exam but is worsened by the fact that most learners, up to this point, have been in highly competitive academic environments and were heavily judged on course grades and standardized test scores. Recent reforms in medical education encourage substituting grade-focused assessments for competency-based ones. A competency-based assessment rubric describes and quantifies skills performance, enabling learners and graders to shift away from numerical, pass/fail scoring systems. Rubrics also engage faculty and learners in identifying learner areas of strengths and weakness, promoting the development of competent osteopathic physicians.

Assessing for competency in OMT performance, however, can be challenging. Generous liberties must be given to permit learners to make adjustments and refinements, such as accommodating for body size/shape disparities or the patient's health status. Nevertheless, there are some identified overarching concepts and steps that should be employed across the spectrum of examinations for somatic dysfunction and osteopathic techniques. These concepts and steps have been mapped onto competency-based assessment rubrics. Two different sample rubrics are presented for faculty members and learners. Faculty members can customize the rubrics, as the steps or concepts can be assessed in any order and combination, and the words can be adjusted to best suit faculty teaching and assessment objectives and goals. Faculty members are also encouraged to validate their chosen assessment rubric to reach consensus for consistent grading. Several published research bibliographies on this topic are listed at the end of this chapter.

Sample Rubric A

Author: Ryan Seals, DO

The sample rubric in Table 1.4, Table 1.5, Table 1.6, and Table 1.7 has been validated and is used at the University of North Texas Health Science Center, Texas College of Osteopathic Medicine.

Milestone Templates

The following rubrics have been created in an effort to assess learner competence in various skills. Table 1.4 lists all of the diagnostic and treatment skills that specifically apply to osteopathic manipulative medicine and neuromusculoskeletal medicine.

The subsequent rubrics can be used to assess these various skills as they relate to performing a screening exam, making a specific osteopathic diagnosis, performing OMT, and explaining the technique performed. Each rubric lists the skills that can be assessed by that particular rubric, thus allowing the same rubric to be applied to a variety of procedural skills.

To obtain a particular level, the student/resident must be able to fully complete all of the described elements of that level. The learner who performs all qualities of level 2 and some qualities of level 3 will be assessed at a level 2. As a general rule, at the first assessment of skill performance, learners are expected to achieve a level 2. By the time students finish the second year of osteopathic medical school, they should have achieved a level 3 in the items that the teacher deems critical or fundamental in the curriculum.

Table 1.4 Osteopathic technique and diagnostic skills

Technique skills in OMM/NMM	Diagnostic skills in OMM/NMM
Soft tissue	General medical exam
Muscle energy	Orthopedic
High-velocity low-amplitude	Neurologic
Articulatory	Standing postural exam
Counterstrain	Respiratory circulatory exam
Myofascial release	TART assessment
Visceral	Vertebral segmental diagnosis
Facilitated positional release	Sacrum
Still technique	Muscle energy/structural model
Balanced ligamentous tension	Cranial
Ligamentous articular strain	Pelvis
Cranial osteopathic manipulative medicine	Structural
Prolotherapy	Fascial
Trigger point injections	Ribs
Ultrasound-guided injections	Respiratory
Postural balancing	Structural
	Upper extremity
	Shoulder, elbow, wrist, hand
	Muscles and fascia
	Lower extremity
	Hip, knee, fibula, ankle, foot
	Cranium
	CRI, strain patterns, sutures
	Abdomen/visceral
	Chapman's reflexes
	Postural/leg length evaluation
	Area of greatest restriction/key lesion

Abbreviations: CRI, cranial rhythmic impulse; NMM, neuromusculoskeletal medicine; OMM, osteopathic manipulative medicine; TART, *t*issue texture changes, *a*symmetry, *r*estriction of motion, *t*enderness.

Table 1.5   Screening exams

Year 1 screening	Year 2 screening
Standing postural	Respiratory circulatory
Area of greatest restriction (AGR)	Cardiac
Key lesion	Pulmonary
Local osteopathic exam	Abdominal
Cervical spine	HEENT
Thoracic spine	Cranial
Lumbar spine	Musculoskeletal
	Shoulder
	Knee
	Neck
	Back

Screening exam milestones	
Level 0	– Has not acquired the skill.
Level 1 (beginner)	– This relates to the very beginning stages of acquiring a new skill. Is able to perform skill at very basic level. – *Steps are forgotten* and may require prompting. – The motions are not fluid and hand placement may be *significantly off* from the proper structure. – Forces and contacts *significantly prevent* obtaining correct diagnostic information.
Level 2	– Is able to perform skill at beginner level. The *steps have been memorized* and can be reproduced correctly *without prompting*. – Hand placement and motions are mostly correct but may *lack precision/accuracy*. – Motions and forces are used that do not inhibit obtaining correct diagnostic information.
Level 3	– Can perform the skill fluidly and precisely *without hesitation or awkwardness*. – *Contacts correct anatomical structure and tissue layer* and uses correct *motion and amount of force* to perform diagnosis to the structure.
Level 4	– Can perform skill fluidly and precisely as in level 3. – Can apply diagnostic skills to various structures in the same area simultaneously. – *Can correctly identify dysfunction at various tissue layers*.
Level 5 (expert)	– Can perform skill fluidly and precisely to multiple tissue layers as in level 4. – Is able to *distinguish subtleties in various tissue layers* quickly without hesitation.

Abbreviation: HEENT, head, eyes, ears, nose, throat.

Table 1.6 Palpatory diagnosis	
Year 1 skills	**Year 2 skills**
Standing postural exam Respiratory circulatory exam Tissue texture assessment Vertebral segmental diagnosis Sacrum Pelvis Ribs Upper extremities Lower extremities	All skills from year 1 Cranial palpation/diagnosis Abdomen/visceral Chapman's reflexes Area of greatest restriction
Palpatory diagnosis milestones	
Level 0	– Has not acquired the skill.
Level 1 (beginner)	– This relates to the very beginning stages of acquiring a new skill. The motions are *not fluid*; the steps may be forgotten and *prompting* may be required. – Hand placement may be significantly off from the structure. – Forces, contacts, and movements *significantly prevent* proper technique performance and may worsen dysfunction or cause pain.
Level 2	– Is able to perform the skill at beginner level. The *steps have been memorized and can be reproduced/explained correctly without prompting*. – Hand placement, tissue layer, and motions are mostly correct but may *lack precision*; however, imprecise motions and forces do not overly inhibit therapeutic response.
Level 3	– Can perform the skill *fluidly and precisely* without hesitation or awkwardness. – Contacts correct *anatomical structure and tissue layer* and uses correct *motion and amount of force* to perform technique comfortably and safely.
Level 4	– Can perform the skill fluidly and precisely without hesitation as in level 3. – Can *adapt and adjust* technique to unique situations with some effort. – Amount and direction of force are *precise to optimize therapeutic response*.
Level 5 (expert)	– Can perform the skill fluidly and precisely as in level 4 with *little to no mental effort*. – Can quickly adapt and adjust technique appropriately for various patients or circumstances. – Achieves *precise and efficient results*.

Table 1.7 Explanation

Year 1 skills	Year 2 skills
Explain the steps of each technique Explain the mechanism of action of the techniques	Explain the rationale for performing a variety of osteopathic manipulative techniques in the following conditions: 　Gastrointestinal 　Cardiovascular 　Respiratory 　Neurologic 　Musculoskeletal 　Genitourinary 　Obstetric

Explanation milestones	
Level 0	– Has not acquired the skill.
Level 1 (beginner)	– Is able to explain a few steps of the technique/rationale but is *unorganized and incomplete* in the response.
Level 2	– Is able to explain the steps of the technique *completely* in the proper order with some hesitation or simplification. – Explains the rationale using accurate anatomy and physiology *but lacks detail* in description. Is too "broad" or "vague" in the description.
Level 3	– Is able to explain the steps of the technique completely and in the proper order. – Explains the rationale using accurate anatomy and physiology with *good specificity and accuracy.*
Level 4	– Can explain osteopathic techniques and philosophy clearly to *patients, attending physicians, and students* with clarity and accuracy.
Level 5 (expert)	– Can explain osteopathic techniques and philosophy clearly to *any subtype* of person using *examples that are relevant* to that person or group.

Sample Rubric B

Author: Sharon Gustowski, DO, MPH

The headings used in the exams for somatic dysfunction technique descriptions in this manual are the same ones used in the corresponding rubrics (Table 1.8, Table 1.9, Table 1.10, and Table 1.11). This helps learners and faculty maintain consistency from classroom teaching to assessment. The sample rubrics shared here will be reviewed, revised, and validated by new faculty for use at the University of the Incarnate Word School of Osteopathic Medicine.

Table 1.8 Humanistic domain grading rubric

Humanistic domain	Distinguished	Proficient	Essential	Developing	Unsatisfactory
Overall verbal communication	Uses communication that supports and enhances performance of exams and techniques	Uses communication that supports performance of exams and techniques	Uses communication that minimally supports performance of exams and techniques	Uses communication that does not support performance of exams and techniques	Communication unclear or disrespectful
Overall professional nonverbal communication	Demonstrates respectful, thoughtful, precise touch and mannerisms with confidence	Touch and mannerisms express average confidence with minimal awkwardness	Touch and mannerisms express below-average confidence and awkwardness	Touch and mannerisms express little to no self-confidence and/or are generally awkward	Any unprofessional touch or mannerism
Overall tissue handling	Uses gentle interaction and maneuvers tissues thoughtfully with care	Interacts with and maneuvers tissues appropriately	Maneuvers tissues safely	Interacts with and maneuvers tissues which may lead to harm of self or partner	Causes any degree of harm to practice patient or self

Table 1.9 Cognitive domain grading rubric

Cognitive domain	Distinguished	Proficient	Essential	Developing	Unsatisfactory
Verbal description of goal(s) of technique (principles and/or end goal)	Organizes and synthesizes evidence to reveal insightful application of technique	Organizes evidence to reveal important aspects of technique application	Organizes evidence but is not effective in revealing important aspects application of technique	Lists evidence but is not organized and is unfocused	Unable to describe

Table 1.10 Exam for somatic dysfunction grading rubric

Exam for somatic dysfunction	Distinguished	Proficient	Essential	Developing	Unsatisfactory
Observational assessment	Assembles exam fluidly with accuracy and precision	Designs and performs exam correctly	Performs exam adequately without demonstrating insight	Performs exam without accuracy or precision	Exam not performed
Tissue texture changes assessment	Assembles exam fluidly with accuracy and precision	Designs and performs exam correctly	Performs exam adequately without demonstrating insight	Performs exam without accuracy or precision	Exam not performed or performed without safe tissue handling
Active range of motion testing	Organizes and performs testing fluidly with accuracy and precision with clear instructions	Designs and performs testing correctly with mostly clear instructions	Performs testing adequately without demonstrating insight and without clear instructions	Performs testing without accuracy or precision and without clear instructions	Exam not performed or inappropriate instructions given
Positional asymmetry assessment	Location and findings accurately and correctly described	Location or findings off by one level or one direction	Location or findings off by two levels or two directions	Location or findings off by three levels or three directions	Exam not performed or performed without safe tissue handling
Passive range of motion testing	Organizes and performs testing fluidly with accuracy and precision	Designs and performs testing correctly	Performs testing adequately without demonstrating insight	Performs testing without accuracy or precision	Exam not performed or performed without safe tissue handling
Synthesis of exam findings	Somatic dysfunction diagnosis correctly synthesized	Somatic dysfunction diagnosis synthesized but one element is incorrectly identified	Somatic dysfunction diagnosis synthesized but two elements are incorrectly identified	Somatic dysfunction diagnosis synthesized, but more than two elements are incorrectly identified	Unable to synthesize findings

Table 1.11 Technique performance grading rubric

Technique performance	Distinguished	Proficient	Essential	Developing	Unsatisfactory
Positioning and preparation	Arranges self, partner, and equipment for ergonomic and safe performance with insight	Arranges self, partner, and equipment for safe performance but requires some adjustment	Arranges self, partner, and equipment after technique has started and requires adjustment (lacks insight)	Performs technique without arranging self, partner, and/or equipment	Potentially harmful setup for self or partner or misuse of equipment
Tissue contact	Contacts appropriate structure(s) and appropriate layer for fluid performance of technique	Contacts appropriate structure(s) and is able to perform technique	Contacts tissues in such a way that performing the technique is awkward	Contacts tissues without regard to structures or layers	Does not contact appropriate structure, is not able to appropriately perform technique due to contacts
Movements	Maneuvers self and partner fluidly and accurately in correct direction(s) throughout entire technique	Maneuvers self and partner in direction(s) adequately but not precisely throughout entire technique	Maneuvers self and partner appropriately throughout most of the technique	Has difficulty maneuvering self and partner throughout most of the technique	Unsafe maneuvers or performed incorrectly
Barriers	Localizes tissues precisely in appropriate relationship to barrier	Identifies barriers and is closely localized to barrier but not precisely	Tissues are generally near an appropriate barrier	Has difficulty localizing tissues to barrier and/or in appropriate relationship	Tissues are not localized and not in appropriate relationship to barrier
Forces	Both applies and instructs partner to use a precise amount and duration of force(s)	Both applies and instructs partner to use an amount or duration of force(s) which is not precise but sufficient	Applies or instructs partner to use force(s) in a general amount or general direction(s) but not both	Performs technique without focused attention to operator and patient force(s)	Inappropriate application of force or instruction to partner regarding use of force(s)
Retest for effectiveness	Somatic dysfunction resolved	Demonstrates improvement in original diagnosis by more than 50%	Demonstrates improvement in original diagnosis by less than 50%	Diagnosis is unchanged	Retesting not performed

Chapter Summary

This chapter offers a timeline of osteopathic history and development. Modern osteopathic tenets are explained to allow learners to begin to incorporate osteopathic medical philosophy into their own medical educational approach. The fundamentals of psychomotor skills learning are outlined, including some suggested steps learners can take to advance their proficiency in performing osteopathic manipulative techniques. Finally, assessment rubrics are provided to give learners insight into evaluation goals.

Review Questions

Q1. Which of the following statements is true regarding the philosophy of osteopathic medicine?

A. Healing is determined by the osteopathic physician's intervention.

B. Host influences do not play a role in the development of a disease.

C. It is the object of the osteopathic physician to find the cause of a disease.

D. The disease is the focus of health care delivery.

E. The use of pharmaceutical drugs and surgery are its hallmarks.

Q2. A 70-year-old man presents with low back pain. Which of the following, if detected, is an indication that OMT may be used to treat this patient's condition?

A. Inability to move the great toe.

B. Loss of sensation over the lateral side of the foot.

C. Pulsatile mass in the abdomen.

D. Somatic dysfunction in the sacrum.

E. Vertebral compression fracture.

Q3. A 25-year-old man presents with neck pain. After a thorough history and physical exam, you determine that osteopathic manipulative treatment is indicated. To perform OMT, you

A. Explain to the patient that the risk of OMT includes death.

B. Find a nurse or medical assistant chaperone to be present in the room.

C. Obtain consent from the patient or patient's guardian.

D. Order imaging studies.

E. Put on gloves and a mask.

Answers to Review Questions

Q1. The correct answer is **C**.

Q2. The correct answer is **D**. Somatic dysfunction is the indication for OMT. The other answers are often relative contraindications to OMT.

Q3. The correct answer is **C**.

References

1. Still AT. Autobiography of Andrew T. Still. A.T. Still; 1908: 289–290
2. Chila A; American Osteopathic Association. Foundations of Osteopathic Medicine. 3rd ed. Baltimore, MD: Lippincott Williams & Wilkins; 2010
3. Thompson M. Interpretation of osteopathic concept prepared by committee at Kirskville. Designed for use toward more effective teaching throughout curriculum. Report to board of trustees for Kirksville College of Osteopathy and Surgery, Morris Thompson, President (1952)
4. Rogers FJ. Advancing a traditional view of osteopathic medicine through clinical practice. J Am Osteopath Assoc 2005;105(5):255–259
5. Glossary Review Committee of the Educational Council on Osteopathic Principles and the American Association of Colleges of Osteopathic Medicine. Glossary of Osteopathic Terminology. 2011. http://www.aacom.org/news-and-events/publications/glossary-of-osteopathic-terminology. Accessed July 27, 2016
6. Wulf G, Shea C, Lewthwaite R. Motor skill learning and performance: a review of influential factors. Med Educ 2010;44(1):75–84 doi: 10.1111/j.1365-2923.2009.03421.x

OMT Skills Assessment Research Bibliography

Beal MC, Spraflka SA. Precepts and Practice: Practical Examinations in Osteopathic Skills. American Academy of Osteopathy; n.d.

Boulet JR, Gimpel JR, Dowling DJ, Finley M. Assessing the ability of medical students to perform osteopathic manipulative treatment techniques. J Am Osteopath Assoc 2004;104(5):203–211

Degenhardt BF, Snider KT, Snider EJ, Johnson JC. Interobserver reliability of osteopathic palpatory diagnostic tests of the lumbar spine: improvements from consensus training. J Am Osteopath Assoc 2005;105(10):465–473

Rapacciuolo J, Channell MK, Cooley D. Standardizing the osteopathic practical. Int J Osteopath Med 2013;16(4):220–225. http://www.journalofosteopathicmedicine.com/article/S1746-0689(13)00055-2/abstract?cc=y=

Sandella JM, Smith LA, Dowling DJ. Consistency of interrater scoring of student performances of osteopathic manipulative treatment on COMLEX-USA Level 2-PE. J Am Osteopath Assoc 2014;114(4):253–258

Osteopathic Manipulative Treatment Overview

LEARNING OBJECTIVES

1. Define somatic dysfunction and the barrier concept.
2. Define the TART criteria for diagnosing somatic dysfunction.
3. Define anatomical barrier, physiological barrier, restrictive barrier.
4. Identify the direct, indirect, and combined methods of performing osteopathic techniques.
5. Develop strategies to effectively communicate with patients so that they may assist in performing osteopathic techniques.
6. Describe and use proper ergonomics to safely perform osteopathic manipulative techniques.
7. Describe normal motion of the thoracoabdominal diaphragm.
8. Describe and explain motion in other areas of the body in response to thoracoabdominal diaphragm motion.
9. Compare and contrast the various types of thoracoabdominal breathing technique enhancements that can be used when performing osteopathic manipulative techniques.

Introduction

This chapter prepares the learner to perform osteopathic manipulative treatment (OMT), beginning with two essential topics: somatic dysfunction and the barrier concept. Specific details for examinations to diagnose somatic dysfunction, separated by body region, are found in chapter 4. The Osteopathic Technique Descriptions section acquaints the learner with the format applied in this manual. Special attention is given to physician and patient ergonomics, which are emphasized to ensure accuracy in technique performance and also patient and physician safety. The chapter concludes with a description of respiratory cooperation, a patient-performed technique enhancement that can be incorporated into almost any osteopathic technique and is included in the steps of many of the techniques in this manual.

Somatic Dysfunction and the Barrier Concept

Somatic dysfunction is the term that describes the physical effects of minor strain on the physical body: the muscles, bones, ligaments, tendons, fascia, and everything in between. Minor strain can be generated from a variety of conditions, including, but not limited to, trauma, lack of body movement, and aberrant nervous system activity, such as increased autonomic tone. In all cases of somatic dysfunction, the qualities of body structures change slightly, including body symmetry, tissue qualities, and permitted motions. It is critical that the osteopathic physician first recognize what is "normal" before identifying what is "abnormal." Achieving the normal state is, after all, the intended goal of performing osteopathic techniques, and some characteristic normal findings of the somatic system include:

- Body symmetry: the musculoskeletal system is a fairly symmetrical structure. Significant deviations from symmetry indicate that structure–function relationships are altered and that somatic dysfunction is likely present.
- Tissue qualities: tissues have normal qualities, including temperature, texture, and tone. Regions of tissues that have increased or decreased temperatures as well as changes in texture or tone are indicative of underlying somatic dysfunction. Tissues with these changes may also be tender.
- Permitted motions: joints, fascia, and visceral organs have intact, or full, normal ranges of permitted motion. Limitations of normal motions impair optimal body functions. As such, limited active, and especially limited passive, range of motion indicates the presence of somatic dysfunction.

It is important to remember that somatic dysfunction is not gross tissue damage, such as fractures, dislocations, muscle, fascial, or ligamentous tears. The tissues affected with somatic dysfunction, while altered, still retain functional capacity. Therefore, rather than an image-based (ultrasonography, magnetic resonance imaging, radiography) or biochemistry-based (bloodwork) diagnostic process, somatic dysfunction remains a physician-performed, observational, manual diagnosis.

To aid in remembering the criteria for somatic dysfunction diagnosis, the mnemonic TART was developed.[1] TART describes the abnormalities found upon examination of body symmetry, tissue qualities, and permitted motion. In most cases of somatic dysfunction, more than one TART finding is identified.

TART Criteria

T = Tissue texture changes
A = Asymmetry
R = Restriction of motion
T = Tenderness

Descriptions regarding performance of examinations for somatic dysfunction are found in chapter 4.

Barrier Concept and Somatic Dysfunction

Understanding the barrier concept is key for diagnosing somatic dysfunction and performing osteopathic manipulative techniques. Technique instructions in this manual use the barrier concept to identify the corrective positions needed for osteopathic techniques. This section highlights only those concepts most essential for somatic dysfunction examination and techniques. A bar figure is traditionally used to illustrate the barrier concept and has been re-created in **Fig. 2.1**. The barrier concept depicts the association between somatic dysfunction, normal range of motion, and positional asymmetry of body structures. Somatic dysfunction and techniques that specifically address muscle tone require a slightly varied interpretation, which is outlined in chapter 4.

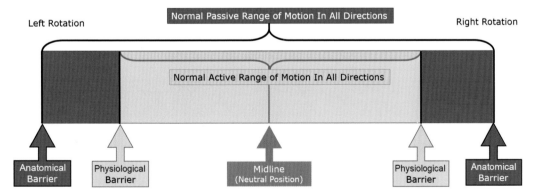

Fig. 2.1 Barrier concept: ranges of motion. The bar figure is a tool and does not depict actual ranges of motion. The distances between anatomical, physiological, and restrictive barriers are suggested only. Most structures do not have uniplanar, or linear, motion. Rotational motion to the right and left (in a transverse plane) was chosen as an example for explanatory purposes.

Anatomical Barriers

Anatomical barriers define the ultimate limit, or end range of motion, of a body structure. The anatomical range of motion is the total distance a joint can move before the structure tears, dislocates, or fractures. Anatomical barriers are rarely approached during normal, everyday movements. The forces used when performing OMT should not challenge or broach the anatomical barrier.

Physiological Barriers

The physiological barriers identify the permitted motion of a body structure, usually considered to be active range of motion. The range of motion between physiologic barriers is less than that of the anatomical range of motion. One end goal of performing OMT is to restore physiological range of motion, which is limited when somatic dysfunction is present.

Restrictive Barriers

When the physiological range of motion becomes impaired, a restrictive barrier is created. A restrictive barrier occurs in each plane of permitted body motion and is found during both active and passive range of motion testing. Restrictive barriers can occur in any tissue with permitted motion, such as joints, fascia, and visceral organs.

Fig. 2.2 depicts the restrictive barrier in one direction in the simple plane of rotational motion. For example, a patient may acquire somatic dys-

function in the L1 vertebra from excessive bending, twisting, and lifting such that L1 is now rotated to the left and has restricted motion in right rotation. The restrictive barrier depicts this loss of right rotation, and it can be identified with both static palpation and passive motion testing.

The somatic dysfunction is named for the direction of motion that is largely unaffected. This is also called the position of ease, or motion preference. Therefore, in this example, L1 has somatic dysfunction in left rotation. The named somatic dysfunction *implies* the restricted motion of right rotation. This example is not the complete diagnosis of L1, because it has three planes of motion—rotation, side bending, and flexion/extension. Chapter 4 provides further details regarding vertebral motion.

In joints and fascia that have multiple planes of motion, such as the vertebrae, often all planes of motion are restricted. This is one application of the third principle of physiological motion, which is that motion in one plane affects motion in all others.

Osteopathic techniques are generally categorized into three methods, based on the barrier concept: direct, indirect, and combined (**Fig. 2.3**, Table 2.1). Direct method techniques are those that move tissues in the direction of the restrictive barrier; they usually require physician force to move the tissues and correct the somatic dysfunction. Indirect method techniques are those that position tissues in the direction of the physiological barrier(s) that are opposite those of the restrictive barrier(s). This way, the patient's inherent healing forces can resolve the somatic dysfunction, and the physician generally holds tissues still, at ease, instead of applying force. Combined techniques both move and position a patient in the

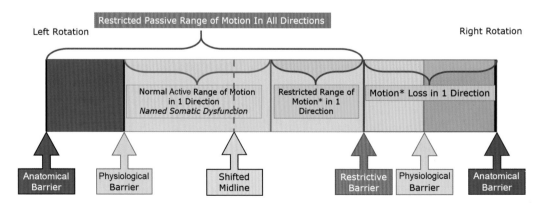

Fig. 2.2 Barrier concept—restricted range of motion and somatic dysfunction.

Table 2.1	Common osteopathic technique methods	
Direct method techniques	**Indirect method techniques**	**Combined method techniques**
Challenge the barrier	Balanced ligamentous tension	Articulatory
High velocity low amplitude	Counterstrain	Myofascial release
Lymphatic	Facilitated positional release	Osteopathic cranial manipulative
Muscle energy	Functional	medicine
Neurolymphatic reflex	Indirect	Still
Soft tissue		Visceral

direction of the restrictive and physiological barriers, usually sequenced at different times. Although not every osteopathic manipulative technique is included in this manual, the most commonly performed techniques are presented. The term *indirect* can be used to describe both the method of a technique and a specific type of procedure (e.g., indirect [IND] technique).

Osteopathic techniques are also categorized as active or passive. Active techniques are those that require patient movements (e.g., muscle energy techniques), whereas passive techniques are those during which the patient remains relaxed (e.g., counterstrain techniques).

Osteopathic Technique Descriptions

This section outlines the method and format used in this instructional manual and includes some recommendations in preparation for performing

techniques. The text and video demonstrations correlate, and both should be used for learning and practicing techniques.

Technique Introduction Sections: Goals, Background, Clinical Considerations

Unique to the first section of each technique category is relevant contextual information. Historical accounts and relevant research are presented along with clinical considerations. Clinical considerations include indications, contraindications, and precautions as guidelines. Detailed explanations are given under the subheadings for Somatic Dysfunction Corrected; Positioning and Preparation; Tissue Contact; and Movements, Barriers, and Forces. Those same subheadings are also replicated in each technique section with information specific to that technique. At the end of each technique introduction is a Retest for Effectiveness section

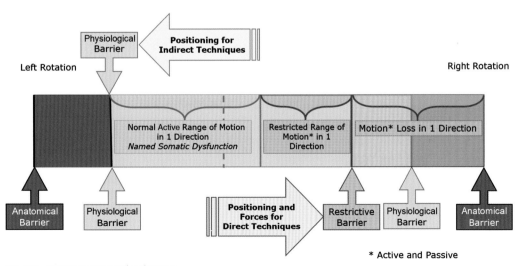

Fig. 2.3 Barrier concept and techniques.

that offers some suggestions in the event that the somatic dysfunction did not correct after the technique performance.

Technique Title

Each technique is titled by the chapter category (type of technique), followed by a body region. After the body region, specific joints or structures are identified. Below the title are a few sentences that offer some perspectives about the technique, such as historical context, clinical applications, or author experiences.

Somatic Dysfunction Corrected

Somatic dysfunctions best corrected and diagnostically required for performing the technique are listed here.

End Goal

This is a statement in each specific technique that describes the external focus the physician should keep in mind when performing the technique.

Positioning and Preparation

- This section describes the specific patient and physician starting positions.
- Patient Preparation
  - The physician asks the patient to begin in one of the following positions: standing, supine, prone, sitting, or laterally recumbent. Patient positions may change throughout the performance of a technique.
- Physician Preparation
  - The physician is instructed as to the starting location and position to assume relative to the patient and/or the treatment table.
  - Unless otherwise indicated in this manual, the OMT table should also be positioned at "customary" table height, based on the position of the physician, as follows:
    - Standing: the top of the table should reach the tips of the physician's fingertips when the physician is standing beside it.
    - Sitting: the top of the table should permit the physician's forearms to rest on the table with the elbows bent at 90 degrees.

Tissue Contact

- This section first informs the learner as to the designation and primary goal of each hand and body contact. It then instructs the physician as to where and how to make initial tissue contact. One or both hands are used, and sometimes tissue contact is made additionally with the abdomen or torso. Each hand may perform multiple roles. The accompanying video narrations may not include detailed suggestions, especially when the details are well visualized.
- Tissue contacts are generally named as follows, but other names may be used:
  - Performing contact: primarily creates the correcting force(s).
  - Assisting contact: moves, stabilizes, or creates additional corrective forces, or performs in some other capacity.
  - Monitoring contact: monitors the tissues and does not create forces.
  - Fulcrum contact: used in some high velocity, low amplitude (HVLA) techniques to indicate when the corrective force requires the use of a fulcrum.
- Keep in mind that each time the physician touches a patient, compassion, confidence, and skill are wordlessly communicated.

Movements, Barriers, and Forces

- This section outlines the steps required to perform each technique and includes a retest for effectiveness reminder. These steps are narrated in the videos, although some of the bulleted items are omitted for brevity.
- Movements: outlines how and why to move a patient. All movements are referenced from the anatomical position of the patient.
- Barriers: describes the movements in relationship to restrictive and/or physiological barriers and includes strategies for barrier localization as well as palpatory characteristics.
- Forces: describes the corrective force or forces that the physician creates.
- Retest for effectiveness: serves as a reminder to retest the original somatic dysfunction and to assess for changes.

When performing OMT, physician movements and forces are performed with the intention of supporting the patient's structure within the laws of basic biomechanics. Thus it is important to know the physical properties of the various body tissues and how the tissues respond and react to changes. This way, the physician can precisely create the correct amount of force in the appropriate directions so that the body responds positively and is able to shift or return to neutral body position and function. Remember that the body heals itself; the osteopathic physician simply helps to support and guide the body. If physician-created forces are excessive, the body responds with guarding, such as withdrawal, tightening of musculature, increased sympathetic tone, to avoid injury or tissue damage. Physicians should start with smaller movements and use gentle forces at first to approach barriers, not overcome them. The specifics of force—how much, what type, the directions—take some time and concentrated study to discover.

Osteopathic Techniques: Preparation, Ergonomics, Physician and Patient Safety

"First, do no harm."

Safe, precise performance of osteopathic manipulative techniques requires mindfulness and awareness. Attention to personal hygiene, posture, movements, and equipment setup are all important aspects of performing osteopathic techniques. Following ergonomic principles during technique preparation and performance ensures patient safety and prevents physician work-related injuries, repetitive use injuries, muscle strain, and arthritis.

Preparation: Equipment

- OMT table: an OMT table is different from other examination tables because it is flat, is long enough for a patient to lie upon, and has firm foam padding that doesn't give way under forces. Patients should be asked to remove shoes and all items from pockets prior to positioning on the table to prevent excessive table wear.
- Pillows: sometimes a pillow under the head or knees increases patient comfort, especially when the patient is supine. However, it may become a barrier when performing some techniques. So, if necessary, remove the pillow temporarily. A pillow may also be used by the physician as a cushion between the physician's and the patient's bodies. Techniques in this manual are demonstrated without a pillow.

Preparation: Physician Personal Hygiene

- Performing osteopathic techniques requires close contact with patients. Therefore, perfume or cologne should be avoided, as patients can be sensitive or allergic.
- Hands must be kept clean and fingernails neatly groomed. Clothing should be modest and permit movement. A cleanly appearance with minimized personal body and breath odors is also recommended.

Preparation: Patients

- Patients may be asked ahead of time to wear thin, loose-fitting clothing that permits movement.
- Jewelry that could potentially harm the physician or the patient during technique performance should be removed, such as large earrings or necklaces.

Ergonomics: Patients

- When using an adjustable-height table, it would be helpful to lower the table for patients to get on and off. Some patients may not be able to comfortably change positions, and this should be considered before the request is made. Patients may be assisted by guidance and direction of their movements, ensuring that they are not in danger of falling or slipping off.
- When patients rise from a supine position on the table, the preferred and safest way is to instruct the patient as follows: "Roll onto one side and bend your knees. Swing your legs off of the table and push yourself up with your hands, using your arms and core musculature."
- Sometimes sudden changes in positioning can cause lightheadedness, so the patient should be asked to remain seated for a few seconds.

> **WATCH ▷ ▶ ▷**
>
> ▶ *Video 2.1 Demonstration of a Patient Rising from Table*

Ergonomics: Physician

- Proper posture ensures that a physician can generate the appropriate amount, direction, and duration of forces. It is important to be continually mindful of body posture.

- The spine should be kept in a neutral position, with the core engaged and without slouching.
  - Bending should occur at the waist.
  - When standing, a broad-based stance should be used and, if necessary, one or both thighs may lean up against the table edge, using it as a fulcrum. Hyperextension of the knees should be avoided.
  - When seated, both ischial tuberosities should contact the stool, with hips and knees bent to 90 degrees and feet flat on the floor.
  - Standing or kneeling upon the table should be avoided.
- Developing fluid, efficient, and safe movements requires perfect practice, mindfulness of ergonomics, and physician and patient safety.
  - Larger, rather than smaller, muscles, should be used as much as possible. For example, biceps should be used for lifting instead of wrist flexors.
  - Joints may be minimally flexed at all times to avoid hyperextension; this is particularly important for the knees.
  - It is important to rest, which includes sitting, because OMT can constitute a large physical exertion on the part of the physician.
  - Fulcrums and levers should be employed to decrease the amount of work required to create or hold forces.
- Increased forces that could extend beyond the patient's anatomical barriers, in distance or magnitude, should never be used.
- The patient should never be lifted without proper training and assistance, nor should the patient be allowed to pull on the physician or use the physician as a brace for getting up.

Ergonomics: Physician–Patient Size and Strength Differentials

- This manual is written for an average-sized, able-bodied adult physician to perform techniques on an average-sized, abled-bodied adult patient. Physicians should make adjustments in tissue contacts, movements, barriers, and forces based on their own body size, shape, and abilities. Likewise, physicians should make adjustments to accommodate patients of different sizes, shapes, and abilities, including pediatric patients.

- Adjustments should be made for patients who are unable to maintain a stable posture on an OMT table. Sometimes a physician has to sit on the ground with a pediatric patient, or work through a wheelchair of a patient with limited mobility.
- A physician–patient size differential should *never* be accommodated with use of excessive force. It is better to fail to correct a somatic dysfunction on the first attempt than to risk injury. A biomechanical advantage may be created by employing fulcrums and levers, focusing on hand contacts, body positions, and equipment adjustments.

Technique Enhancement: Respiratory Cooperation

Thoracoabdominal breathing is a necessary life function. Far more than a means of gas exchange at a cellular level, the biomechanical motions of breathing are transmitted throughout the entire body. Therefore, when any part of the body has somatic dysfunction, the motion transmitted by thoracoabdominal breathing becomes restricted. Conversely, when breathing is impaired, the transmitted motion is diminished. The palpable transmitted motion is more subtle in distant areas of the body.

Normal thoracoabdominal inspiration effort produces the following general effects:

- The thoracic and abdominal cavities expand in all directions.
- The thoracoabdominal diaphragm flattens and moves inferiorly.
- The pelvic diaphragm flattens and moves inferiorly.
- The anterior shafts of the ribs move superiorly while the posterior angle moves inferiorly (pump-handle motion).
- The lateral margin of the ribs moves superiorly, and the transverse diameter increases (bucket-handle motion).
- The spinal curves flatten slightly.
- The extremities externally rotate very slightly.
  - In the upper extremities, this is transmission of motion through the upper ribs and clavicles. In the lower extremities, this is transmission of motion through the iliopsoas and pelvic diaphragm musculature.
- During the expiration phase, the structures recoil in the opposite directions of the inspiration phase.

Respiratory Cooperation

Respiratory cooperation is a patient-performed assistive force, whereby the patient breathes in a certain fashion or holds the breath. It is written in as an option in the steps in many myofascial release (MFR), indirect (IND), and high velocity low amplitude (HVLA) techniques. The physician can therefore choose to instruct the patient to use respiratory cooperation. There are two types of respiratory cooperation outlined in this manual: breathing for relaxation and breath retention.

Respiratory Cooperation: Breathing for Relaxation

This option may be chosen when patients are challenged with relaxing the body, or when body relaxation is essential to the technique performance. To perform this type of respiratory cooperation, ask the patient to take three to five slow and full deep breaths. As the patient relaxes, technique performance often becomes easier.

Respiratory Cooperation: Breath Retention

Clinically, it is noted that when patients hold their breath, tissue releases are faster and more easily palpated. To add optional breath retention, the patient is first asked to take a couple of slow, deep breaths. While the patient is breathing, the physician palpates the tissues for changes in tension, noting which phase, inspiration or expiration, tightens or loosens the tissues more. When performing indirect method MFR, or IND techniques, the physician asks the patient to hold his breath in the inspiration/expiration phase, which further loosens the tissues. When performing direct method MFR, the physician asks the patient to hold his breath in the inspiration/expiration phase, which tightens the tissues. Tissue release often occurs when the patient needs to breathe again. To maximize release potential, the physician may ask the patient to mentally count to five after he first feels the need to breathe, and then to resume breathing. For patients who can hold their breath for longer than 2 minutes, ask the patient to resume normal breathing after 2 minutes.

Chapter Summary

This chapter summarizes both the utility of this manual for the purposes of learning basic OMT, as well as the utility of OMT in assisting a patient to transition beyond restrictive barriers into physiological health. Somatic dysfunction is defined in contrast to normal health, and the barrier concept is explained. This chapter also serves as a reference for the basics of performing OMT, including equipment positioning, hygiene, and ergonomics. Finally, a technique enhancement that can be incorporated into most osteopathic techniques, called respiratory cooperation, is explained.

Review Questions

Q1. Somatic dysfunction affects the somatic system, which includes
   A. Central nervous system structures.
   B. Myofascial structures.
   C. Special sensory structures.
   D. Vascular structures.
   E. Visceral structures.

Q2. Which of the following osteopathic techniques is classified as an indirect technique?
   A. Articulatory.
   B. Challenge the barrier.
   C. Counterstrain.
   D. Muscle energy.
   E. Soft tissue.

Q3. A 47-year-old woman presents with neck pain following a minor motor vehicle accident. After performing a history and physical exam, multiple somatic dysfunctions are diagnosed. You decide to start by performing a cervical inhibition technique on a supine patient. Which most accurately describes the proper positioning of the physician when performing this technique?
   A. Standing with back bent to 90 degrees.
   B. Seated, back straight, with arms at 90 degrees and resting forearms on the table.
   C. Seated, leaning forward with back bent to 45 degrees, with upper arms on the table.
   D. Seated with legs straight and back slightly arched.
   E. Standing, knees and back slightly bent, with wrists on the table.

Q4. What is the proper way to ask patients to get up from the supine position?

    A. Roll to the side, bend the knees, then swing the knees off the table while pushing themselves up.

    B. Perform a situp to strengthen their core.

    C. Gently rock back and forth repeatedly until the momentum allows them to sit up.

    D. Pull the patient up by one arm swiftly to help them sit up.

    E. Cross one leg underneath the other and use a twisting motion.

Q5. In a healthy individual, thoracoabdominal respiratory inspiration effort will induce slight

    A. Anterior rotation of the innominate.

    B. Depression of the anterior aspect of the first rib.

    C. External rotation of the humerus.

    D. Increased curvature of the cervical spine.

    E. Superior tightening of the pelvic diaphragm.

Answers to Review Questions

Q1. The correct answer is **B**. Somatic dysfunction is defined as "Impaired or altered function of related components of the somatic (body framework) system: skeletal, arthrodial, and myofascial structures, and their related vascular, lymphatic, and neural elements."

Q2. The correct answer is **C**. Indirect techniques include balanced ligamentous tension, counterstrain, facilitated positional release, and functional.

Q3. The correct answer is **B**. The proper positioning is seated, back straight, with arms at 90 degrees and forearms resting on the table.

A is incorrect. Standing with back bent to 90 degrees puts stress on the physician's back.

C is incorrect. The back should be straight when at all possible, and the lower arms, not the upper arms, should be on the table.

D is incorrect. Legs should be at 90 degrees and the back straight.

E is incorrect. Forearms should be on the table and the technique should be performed seated.

Q4. The correct answer is **A**. Patients should roll to the side, bend the knees, then swing the knees off the table while pushing themselves up.

B is incorrect. Performing a situp to strengthen their core may put strain on the neck and low back.

C is incorrect. Gently rocking back and forth repeatedly until the momentum allows them to sit up may be challenging for some patients and involves excessive movement.

D is incorrect. Pulling patients up by one arm swiftly to help them sit up does not give them control of their movements and may involve harsh movements or forces.

E is incorrect. Crossing one leg underneath the other and using a twisting motion is awkward and excessive.

Q5. The correct answer is **C**. Normal thoracoabdominal inspiration effort produces the following general effects:

- The thoracic and abdominal cavities expand in all directions.
- The thoracoabdominal diaphragm flattens and moves inferiorly.
- The pelvic diaphragm flattens and moves inferiorly.
- The anterior shafts of the ribs move superiorly while the posterior angle moves inferiorly (pump-handle motion).
- The lateral margin of the ribs moves laterally and the anterior-posterior diameter increases (bucket-handle motion).
- The spinal curves flatten slightly.
- The extremities externally rotate very slightly.

References

1. Glossary Review Committee of the Educational Council on Osteopathic Principles and the American Association of Colleges of Osteopathic Medicine. Glossary of Osteopathic Terminology. 2011. http://www.aacom.org/news-and-events/publications/glossary-of-osteopathic-terminology. Accessed July 27, 2016

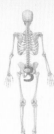

3 Osteopathic Screening Exams

LEARNING OBJECTIVES

1. Explain the relevance of performing an osteopathic screening exam.
2. Relate the background and clinical application of each osteopathic screening exam.
3. Distinguish the three views used when performing a standing postural exam.
4. Distinguish the three parts of the respiratory/circulatory exam, including identification of a compensated or an uncompensated fascial pattern.
5. Compare and contrast the standing postural and respiratory/circulatory exams.
6. Perform the standing postural and respiratory/circulatory exams using appropriate positioning, contacts, and documentation.

Osteopathic Screening Exams

Future osteopathic physicians train their hands and eyes to observe differences that may be important in the overall context of health. Osteopathic screening exams (OSEs) provide a framework within which to "see" a patient. Performing screening exams repetitively in training enables one to develop a critical eye so that gross deformities become obvious, and subtle inequities become the basis for further examination. The exams are intended to be performed expeditiously to direct the physician to areas in need of more focused attention. One OSE should be performed in every comprehensive exam and before a focused musculoskeletal exam.

In general, OSEs are used to

- identify abnormal structural and/or functional patterns.

- serve as a place of focus for a more specific musculoskeletal diagnosis, such as somatic dysfunction.
- aid in the development of comprehensive diagnostic and treatment strategies.
- provide an indicator of the progression or effectiveness of treatment.

Background: Standing Postural Exam

There are many variations of the standing postural exam (SPE), and the one presented here is abbreviated for high-yield observations. The SPE is useful for identifying gross postural abnormalities and visualizing the influence of lower extremity, pelvis, and spinal alignment on overall posture. When posture and joint alignment are impaired, decreased range of motion, pain with movement, muscle soreness, muscle imbalance, and movement inefficiency may result.

The SPE is sensitive for the detection of static muscular and bony asymmetries in the standing patient through both observation and static palpation.[1] Visual observations alone can be made, but the addition of light palpation can increase both reliability and confidence in the observation.

Studies of interexaminer reliability for detecting various body asymmetries have yielded slight to modest agreement in findings.[2,3,4] To minimize interexaminer disagreement, a minimum deviation is suggested for the reporting of positional findings.

A forward-bending test to screen for scoliotic curves is useful to perform in conjunction with the SPE, as a scoliotic curve may be related to identified asymmetries (**Fig. 3.1**). Scoliotic curves can be functional (treatable) or congenital (permanent). In cases of lower body postural asymmetry, the head and neck will rotate and side-bend to keep the eyes level with the horizon. Using the postural balance model, the physician would identify and correct somatic dysfunctions found in the pelvis and lower extremities first. If postural asymmetry does not resolve with osteopathic manipulative treatment (OMT) or becomes more pronounced, exercise therapy or use of a heel or full foot lift to level the pelvis must be considered. Detailed information can be found in Irvin's article "The Origin and Relief of Common Pain."[5]

Clinical Correlation

The standing postural exam can be performed on any patient who can stand unassisted. It is well suited for outpatient settings and for patients with primary musculoskeletal complaints.

Background: Respiratory/Circulatory Exam

This respiratory/circulatory exam (RCE) is based on the work of G. Gordon Zink, DO.[6] As the name implies, the RCE involves an evaluation of the relationships between somatic dysfunction, the low pressure venous and lymphatic systems, and thoracoabdominal breathing. This abbreviated RCE therefore offers a functional view of the patient and the impact somatic dysfunction has on fluid circulation. Recall that lymphatic and venous fluids return to the heart through pressure differentials created by breathing and muscle contraction. Easily compromised due to the thin structure and passive function of the vessels, somatic dysfunction can impair fluid circulation, leading to a variety of symptoms, including malaise, muscle soreness, headache, nonrestful sleep, and bloating/puffiness. Patients presenting with these symptoms should receive a full medical workup, including an exam for somatic dysfunction.

This RCE has three parts:

1. Evaluation of respiration.
2. Examination of the junctional regions for passive range of motion restrictions and ease.
3. Identification of passive fluid congestion.

When abnormalities are found, a more detailed exam for somatic dysfunction and subsequent OMT should be performed. Special attention is paid to the passive range of motion restrictions at the junctional regions or vertebral transition zones. The pattern detected through motion testing these junctional regions and associated diaphragms is either compensated or uncompensated. The expected compensatory mechanism in the body is to balance rotation in one region by creating rotation in the opposite direction above and below the rotated segment. Any disruption in this alternating sequence would deem the entire pattern "uncompensated." The arrows in **Fig. 3.2** indicate the rotation of each vertebral transition zone. Adjacent junctional regions rotating in opposite directions are considered compensated. Adjacent regions rotating in the same direction are uncompensated. An uncompensated pattern suggests that somatic dysfunction has adversely affected venous and lymphatic fluid circulation, so it is recommended that the uncompensated regions should be prioritized in an OMT treatment session.

Clinical Correlation

The respiratory/circulatory exam can be performed on any patient who can lie supine. It is well suited for hospitalized patients, newborns and infants, and patients with infectious or inflammatory processes.

Retest for Effectiveness

A screening exam can be repeated after an OMT session to assess changes from the initial abnormal findings. Screening exams can be used to track the progress of a series of treatments. All findings should be documented.

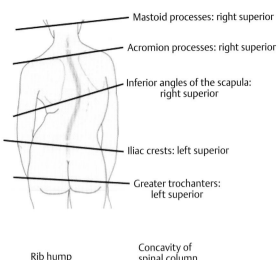

Mastoid processes: right superior

Acromion processes: right superior

Inferior angles of the scapula: right superior

Iliac crests: left superior

Greater trochanters: left superior

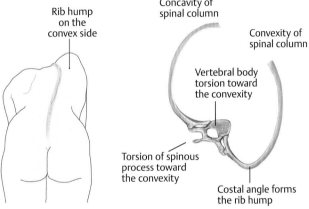

Rib hump on the convex side

Concavity of spinal column

Convexity of spinal column

Vertebral body torsion toward the convexity

Torsion of spinous process toward the convexity

Costal angle forms the rib hump

Fig. 3.1 Postural imbalance, right convex thoracic scoliosis with forward-bending test.

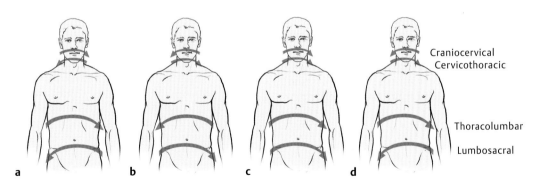

Craniocervical
Cervicothoracic

Thoracolumbar

Lumbosacral

a   b   c   d

Fig. 3.2 Compensated and uncompensated junctional pattern. **(a,b)** Images demonstrate a compensated junctional pattern; **(c,d)** images demonstrate an uncompensated junctional pattern.

Standing Postural Screening Exam

This exam has three views to create a three-dimensional picture of the patient: posterior, lateral, and anterior. In a clinical setting, one view may be performed, but at least two views are preferred. Also, the order and content of each exam can be altered to best apply to the patient.

The end goal is to identify (Table 3.1) global body posture and landmark symmetry/asymmetry.

Positioning and Preparation

▶ Patient: standing comfortably with bare feet. The feet should be separated naturally, without aligning them in any particular way.

▶ Physician: standing directly behind the patient for the posterior view, to one side for the lateral view, in front of the patient for the anterior view.

Posterior View

- Observe and, with finger pads, lightly palpate landmarks and body regions. When observing, use both eyes, but if in doubt, close your nondominant eye.
- Identify bilateral bony landmarks for levelness in a horizontal plane. Describe as superior those landmarks deviated 0.5 cm superiorly or more from the counterpart on the opposite side: head–mastoid process, shoulder–acromion process, shoulder–inferior scapular angle, pelvis–iliac crest, thighs–greater trochanter (Fig. 3.3).
- Identify joint angulations as within normal limits or, if deviated, as follows:
  - Knee: tibia/femur angulation increased (genu valgum) or decreased (genu varum).[7]
  - Ankle: calcaneal angulation inverted or everted.

Lateral View

- The mid–gravity line is a vertical line that bisects the listed landmarks, in the lateral view, when body alignment is neutral/normal. Describe as "in alignment" those landmarks that fall on the mid–gravity line. Describe as anterior or posterior those landmarks deviated 0.5 cm or more away from the mid–gravity line: external auditory meatus, head of the humerus, greater trochanter of the femur, lateral condyle of the femur, and lateral malleolus.
- Roughly estimate each spinal curve for deviation from normal (Fig. 3.4). Palpation is often required, especially in the thoracic spine where the scapula can interfere with observation. Describe as increased those curves that appear grossly accentuated from normal, and decreased those curves that appear flattened.[8]
  - Cervical spine curve: normal is 20 to 40 degrees, convex anterior.
  - Thoracic spine curve: normal is 25 to 45 degrees, convex posterior.
  - Lumbar spine curve: normal is 40 to 60 degrees, convex anterior.

Anterior View

- Facial features: compare eyes, nose, chin, cheek bones, and ears for symmetry, shape, and position in horizontal and vertical planes. This is subjective, but if there are no obvious asymmetries, describe as a high degree of symmetry. If a majority of the facial features are deviated and different sizes and shapes, then describe as a low degree of symmetry.
- Anterior view, body positions: determine if the body region is facing forward or deviated in either the coronal or transverse planes (side bent and/or rotated). Evaluate the head and neck, thoracic cage, and lumbopelvic regions. Body regions are not tested for active or passive range of motion (Fig. 3.5).
- Identify joint angulations as within normal limits or, if deviated, as follows:
  - Foot, medial arch: describe as increased (pes cavus) an arch that is elevated more than ~ 1 cm and decreased if an arch is absent or minimal (pes planus).
  - Carrying angle: evaluate with arms in the anatomical position. Describe as increased when the forearm is laterally deviated (cubitus valgus), and decreased when the forearm is medially deviated (cubitus varus).[7]

WATCH ▷ ▶ ▷

▶ *Video 3.1 Complete Standing Postural Exam—Narrated*

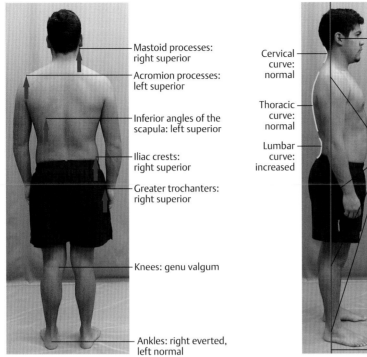

Mastoid processes:
right superior

Acromion processes:
left superior

Inferior angles of the
scapula: left superior

Iliac crests:
right superior

Greater trochanters:
right superior

Knees: genu valgum

Ankles: right everted,
left normal

Fig. 3.3   Posterior view with assessments.

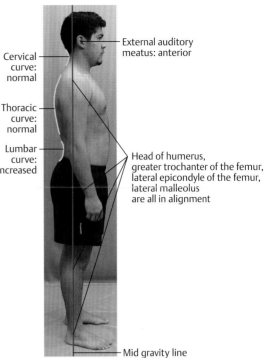

External auditory
meatus: anterior

Cervical
curve:
normal

Thoracic
curve:
normal

Lumbar
curve:
increased

Head of humerus,
greater trochanter of the femur,
lateral epicondyle of the femur,
lateral malleolus
are all in alignment

Mid gravity line

Fig. 3.4   Lateral view with assessments.

Facial features:
moderate degree
of symmetry

Head and neck position:
rotated: left
side bent: left

Thoracic cage position:
rotated: right
side bent: right

Lumbopelvic position:
rotated: right
side bent: right

Right medial foot arch:
decreased

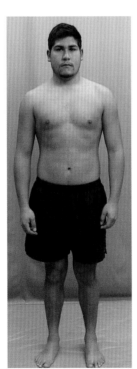

Fig. 3.5   Anterior view with assessments.

Table 3.1 Complete standing postural exam form

Posterior View	
Head: mastoid process	☐ heights level superior: ☐ R ☐ L
Shoulder: acromion process	☐ heights level superior: ☐ R ☐ L
Shoulder: inferior scapular angle	☐ heights level superior: ☐ R ☐ L
Pelvis: iliac crest	☐ heights level superior: ☐ R ☐ L
Thighs: greater trochanter	☐ heights level superior: ☐ R ☐ L
Knee: tibia/femur angulation	☐ WNL ☐ increased (genu valgum) ☐ decreased (genu varum)
Ankle: calcaneal angulation	R: ☐ WNL ☐ inverted ☐ everted L: ☐ WNL ☐ inverted ☐ everted
Lateral View	
Cervical spine curve	☐ WNL ☐ increased ☐ decreased
Thoracic spine curve	☐ WNL ☐ increased ☐ decreased
Lumbar spine curve	☐ WNL ☐ increased ☐ decreased
External auditory meatus	☐ in alignment ☐ anterior ☐ posterior
Head of the humerus	☐ in alignment ☐ anterior ☐ posterior
Greater trochanter of femur	☐ in alignment ☐ anterior ☐ posterior
Lateral condyle of the femur	☐ in alignment ☐ anterior ☐ posterior
Lateral malleolus	☐ in alignment ☐ anterior ☐ posterior
Anterior View	
Facial features	degree of symmetry: ☐ high ☐ medium ☐ low
Head and neck position	☐ neutral rotated: ☐ R ☐ L side bent: ☐ R ☐ L
Thoracic cage position	☐ neutral rotated: ☐ R ☐ L side bent: ☐ R ☐ L
Lumbopelvic position	☐ neutral rotated: ☐ R ☐ L side bent: ☐ R ☐ L
Foot: medial arch	R: ☐ WNL ☐ increased (pes cavus) ☐ decreased (pes planus) L: ☐ WNL ☐ increased (pes cavus) ☐ decreased (pes planus)

Abbreviations: L, left; R, right; WNL, within normal limits.

Respiratory/Circulatory Screening Exam

This RCE provides a quick snapshot of the influence of somatic dysfunction on the venous and lymphatic circulation in the body. The end goals are to identify the patient's breathing patterns, passive range of motion at the junctional regions, and areas of passive fluid congestion (Table 3.2).

Positioning and Preparation

▶ Patient: supine.
▶ Physician: stand on one side of the patient, near the region being evaluated.

Part 1: Evaluation of Respiration (Observational Only)

• Respiratory excursion: observe thoracic and abdominal motion. Normal inhalation is obvious to the pubic symphysis. If impaired, indicate the most inferior level of expansion: upper rib cage, xiphoid process, or umbilicus.
• Respiratory ratio of inhalation to exhalation: estimate the ratio of time spent inhaling versus exhaling. Ideal breathing is a ratio of 1:2 or 1:3 (inhalation: exhalation). Impaired breathing is a ratio of 1:1 (inhalation: exhalation).

Part 2: Junctional Regions

Tissue Contact

• With the fingertips, contact each junctional region posteriorly and laterally with the fingertips a few inches from midline. Wrap hands to follow the contour of the patient to lift each region into rotation.

Movements, Barriers, and Forces

Test the entire region. This is not an isolated test for fascial or joint motion.

• Rotate each junctional region to the right and left, noting the quality and quantity of motion using slow and deliberate movements. Identify motion as symmetric (no rotation) or left/right if one side rotates farther than the other. Note that the rotation in the craniocervical region tends to be greater than that of the other regions due to the flexibility of the cervical spine.
• Identification of junctional pattern: after testing all regions, determine if the pattern of rotation is compensated or uncompensated.

Part 3: Sites of Passive Congestion

• In some areas, arteries and lymph nodes can be palpated. In these cases, it is appropriate to integrate general physical examination for pulses and lymphadenopathy with this exam for passive fluid congestion.

Tissue Contact

• With the fingertips of one or two fingers, gently palpate to the layer just beneath the skin. Avoid excessive force, so as not to displace extracellular fluid.

Movements, Barriers, and Forces

• Use light forces and either a slight rubbing or crawling motion with your fingertips, similar to an exam for lymphadenopathy.
• Identify the presence or absence of increased extracellular fluid.

> **WATCH** ▷ ▶ ▷
> ───────────────
> ▶ *Video 3.2 Complete Respiratory Circulatory Exam—Narrated*

Table 3.2 Respiratory/circulatory exam form	
Respiratory excursion	Normal: ☐ abdominal to the pubic symphysis Impaired: ☐ upper rib cage ☐ xiphoid ☐ umbilicus
Respiratory ratio of inhalation to exhalation	☐ 1:2 or 1:3 ☐ 1:1
Craniocervical junction	☐ no rotation rotated: ☐ R ☐ L
Cervicothoracic junction	☐ no rotation rotated: ☐ R ☐ L
Thoracolumbar junction	☐ no rotation rotated: ☐ R ☐ L
Lumbosacral junction	☐ no rotation rotated: ☐ R ☐ L
Junctional pattern	☐ compensated ☐ uncompensated
Sites of passive congestion	Suboccipital regions: ☐ none ☐ R ☐ L Supraclavicular regions: ☐ none ☐ R ☐ L Axillary regions: ☐ none ☐ R ☐ L Inguinal regions: ☐ none ☐ R ☐ L Popliteal spaces: ☐ none ☐ R ☐ L Achilles tendons: ☐ none ☐ R ☐ L

Abbreviations: L, left; R, right; WNL, within normal limits.

Chapter Summary

OSEs are basic, holistic, global assessments using observations of static positioning and passive motion. In this chapter, two screening exams are presented in detail. The SPE is an assessment of structural asymmetries and abnormal curvatures. The RCE provides a functional assessment of breathing and fluid circulation. These comprehensive osteopathic exams suggest pathology, orient the physician toward OMT plans, and provide a means of objective reassessment.

Clinical Cases and Review Questions

Case 1

History/subjective: A-34-year-old man presents to the clinic with diffuse neck pain that he describes as achy and worsening with turning and tilting his head to the right. He is a navigator for the U.S. Air Force and has to reach and look toward his right repetitively during flights. His pain is scaled as low to moderate, comes and goes, but is worse after a long flight.

Physical Examination/Objective: Positive Findings

- Musculoskeletal
  - SPE reveals the right mastoid process superior, right acromion process superior, left iliac crest superior, increased thoracic curvature (kyphosis), decreased lumbar lordosis, and external auditory meatus anterior to the mid–gravity line.
  - Forward-bending test reveals prominent right ribs in the midthoracic region.
  - Cervical spine active range of motion is restricted in right rotation, right side bending, and flexion.

In this patient, global body asymmetries have been identified through the SPE, including iliac crest, acromion and mastoid process asymmetries, and a scoliotic curve. These findings indicate that his head and neck somatic dysfunction may be compensatory, and that the primary cause of his neck pain may not be an isolated, local muscular strain. Therefore, a more detailed exam for somatic dysfunction that includes the head, neck, thorax, pelvis, and lower extremities is warranted. OMT to the neck alone may provide only temporary or incomplete relief. Additionally, a home exercise program can be beneficial to counter his repetitive asymmetrical occupational movements and to maintain his overall postural balance.

Case 2

History/subjective: A 65-year-old woman is hospitalized with an exacerbation of congestive heart failure after eating avocados with salt. She was admitted 2 days ago with worsening shortness of breath and lower extremity edema. She has a history of congestive heart failure for 3 years, and a recent echocardiogram revealed an ejection fraction of 35%. Her treatment includes fluid and sodium restrictions, intravenous diuretics, and an angiotensin-converting enzyme inhibitor. Although her shortness of breath is significantly improved, her lower extremity edema has only mildly improved.

Physical Examination/Objective

- Lungs: few mild rales in the bilateral lung bases.
- Heart: S3 heart sound.
- Lower extremities: bilateral 3+ edema.
- Musculoskeletal: RCE reveals a costal breathing pattern with a ratio of 1:1 (inhalation: exhalation), craniocervical region rotated left, cervicothoracic region rotated left, thoracolumbar region rotated left, and lumbosacral region rotated left. Sites of passive congestion are left supraclavicular region, bilateral inguinal popliteal, and Achilles regions.

In this patient, an uncompensated pattern and decreased thoracoabdominal excursion have been identified. Beyond heart failure, the musculoskeletal restrictions can also be contributing to her fluid retention. Further exam for somatic dysfunction with subsequent performance of OMT can improve the patient's ability to breathe and circulate fluids. From a lymphatic perspective, OMT first to the thoracic outlet is recommended, followed by treatment of the junctional regions. Minimal use of OMT should be performed in this patient, as her ability to incorporate treatment changes is compromised by her clinical condition. Consider performing OMT in short sessions over a few days.

Review Questions

Q1. An 80-year-old woman presents with neck pain. During a standing postural exam, which of the following is considered a normal finding of her lumbar spine curvature?
   A. 25 degrees posterior convexity.
   B. 35 degrees anterior convexity.
   C. 45 degrees posterior convexity.
   D. 55 degrees anterior convexity.
   E. 65 degrees anterior convexity.

Q2. A 15-year-old girl presents for a pre-sports physical. While performing a standing postural exam, you notice her right acromion is superior by 1 cm and the left iliac crest is superior by 1 cm. What additional test should you perform to assess her thoracic spine alignment?
   A. Compensation pattern of transition zones.
   B. Lateral view for mid–gravity line.
   C. Sites of passive congestion.
   D. Diaphragmatic excursion.
   E. Forward-bending test.

Q3. Which of the following accurately describes the standing postural exam (SPE) and the respiratory/circulatory exam (RCE)?
   A. The RCE offers a more functional view of the patient, whereas the SPE offers a more structural view of the patient.
   B. The RCE focuses on symmetry of landmarks, whereas the SPE focuses on the venous and lymphatic systems.
   C. The RCE is more helpful for musculoskeletal complaints, whereas the SPE analyzes respiratory mechanics.
   D. The RCE and SPE both examine for passive range of motion.
   E. Both the RCE and SPE focus on individual regions of somatic dysfunction and do not assess abnormal patterns in the body.

Q4. Which of the following respiratory/ circulatory exam findings indicates a compensated pattern?
   A. Craniocervical junction rotated right, cervicothoracic junction rotated left, thoracolumbar junction rotated right, lumbosacral junction rotated left.
   B. Craniocervical junction rotated left, cervicothoracic junction rotated left, thoracolumbar junction rotated right, lumbosacral junction rotated left.
   C. Craniocervical junction rotated right, cervicothoracic junction rotated left, thoracolumbar junction rotated right, lumbosacral junction rotated right.
   D. Craniocervical junction rotated left, cervicothoracic junction rotated right, thoracolumbar junction rotated right, lumbosacral junction rotated right.

Q5. The respiratory/circulatory exam evaluates the
   A. Effects of poor posture on muscle function.
   B. Venous and lymphatic systems.
   C. Impact of viscerosomatic reflexes on overall health.
   D. Arterial vascular system.
   E. Positional symmetry of bony landmarks.

Answers to Review Questions

Q1. The correct answer is **D**. The normal curve of the lumbar spine is 40–60 degrees anterior convexity (lordotic).

Q2. The correct answer is **E**. The forward-bending test is performed to look for a rib hump when scoliosis is suspected. None of the other tests are directly indicated as an assessment of scoliosis.

Q3. The correct answer is **A**. The RCE offers a more functional view of the patient, whereas the SPE offers a more structural view of the patient. **B** is incorrect because the SPE focuses on symmetry of landmarks, whereas the RCE focuses on the venous and lymphatic systems. **C** is incorrect because the SPE is more helpful for musculoskeletal complaints, whereas the RCE analyzes respiratory mechanics. **D** is incorrect due to the fact that the RCE examines junctional areas for passive range of motion (PROM), whereas the SPE assesses for static asymmetry. **E** is incorrect because both the RCE and the SPE identify global patterns in the body that then warrant closer evaluation and diagnosis for somatic dysfunction.

Q4. The correct answer is **A**. A compensated pattern has alternating rotation at each transition zone. None of the other answer choices demonstrate alternating rotation at adjacent junctional regions, thus making them uncompensated patterns.

Q5. The correct answer is **B**. The RCE evaluates the venous and lymphatic systems. **A** and **C** are incorrect because the RCE does not evaluate muscle function or viscerosomatic reflexes. **D** is incorrect because the RCE emphasizes the importance of costal and abdominal breathing. **E** is incorrect due to the fact that the RCE, as described here, does not evaluate specific body landmark asymmetries; however, the SPE does.

References

1. Chila AG; American Osteopathic Association. Foundations of Osteopathic Medicine. 3rd ed. Baltimore, MD: Lippincott Williams & Wilkins; 2010
2. Holmgren U, Waling K. Inter-examiner reliability of four static palpation tests used for assessing pelvic dysfunction. Man Ther 2008;13(1):50–56
3. Bengaard K, Bogue RJ, Crow WT. Reliability of diagnosis of somatic dysfunction among osteopathic physicians and medical students. Osteopathic Family Physician 2012;4(1):2 7. doi: 10.1016/j.osfp.2011.08.003
4. Pattyn E, Rajendran D. Anatomical landmark position—can we trust what we see? Results from an online reliability and validity study of osteopaths. Man Ther 2014;19(2):158–164
5. Irvin RE. The origin and relief of common pain. J Back Musculoskeletal Rehabil 1998;11(2):89–130
6. Zink JG, Lawson WB. An osteopathic structural examination and functional interpretation of the soma. Osteopathic Annals 1979;7(12):433–440
7. LeBlond RF, Brown DD, Suneja M, Szot JF. The spine, pelvis, and extremities. In: LeBlond RF, Brown DD, Suneja M, Szot JF, eds. DeGowin's Diagnostic Examination, 10th ed. New York, NY: McGraw-Hill; 2015. http://accessmedicine.mhmedical.com.uiwtx.idm.oclc.org/content.aspx?bookid=1192&Sectionid=68669600.
8. Tay BB, Freedman BA, Rhee JM, Boden SD, Skinner HB. Chapter 4. Disorders, diseases, and injuries of the spine. In: Skinner HB, McMahon PJ, eds. Current Diagnosis & Treatment in Orthopedics, 5th ed. New York, NY: McGraw-Hill; 2014. http://accessmedicine.mhmedical.com.uiwtx.idm.oclc.org/content.aspx?bookid=675&Sectionid=45451710.

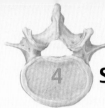

LEARNING OBJECTIVES

1. Identify the TART criteria for diagnosing somatic dysfunction.
2. Assess each body region for somatic dysfunction.
3. Name somatic dysfunction.
4. Diagnose somatic dysfunction in the head, cervical spine, thoracic spine, lumbar spine, costal cage, pelvis, sacrum, upper extremity, lower extremity, and abdomen.

Somatic Dysfunction Diagnosis Introduction

A somatic dysfunction diagnosis is made by synthesizing the patient's history, general physical, and specific osteopathic structural exams. The osteopathic structural exam is performed in order to identify body structures, such as muscles, fascia, bones, and joints, which are altered from normal healthy textures, shapes, and motions. These changes are categorized by the acronym TART.

TART Criteria

T = Tissue texture changes (TTCs)
A = Asymmetry
R = Restriction of motion
T = Tenderness

Tissue alterations are subtle palpatory findings so diagnostic imaging, measurements with instruments, and laboratory tests are not used to make a somatic dysfunction diagnosis. Therefore it becomes necessary that a physician fully develops sensitive physical examination skills to distinguish "normal" exam findings from "abnormal" ones in order to diagnose somatic dysfunction.

Somatic dysfunctions, however, do not always "follow the book," and somatic dysfunctions not described in this manual can occur. It is prudent, therefore, that physicians ultimately examine, "diagnose, and treat what they find," using anatomical knowledge and applying the principles of techniques.

This chapter identifies the key steps needed to examine a patient for somatic dysfunction in one body region at a time. It is intended to be used in a skills laboratory setting with faculty guidance and supplemental resources that explain anatomy, biomechanics, and clinical integration for complete learning.

Types and Severity of Somatic Dysfunction

Once identified, somatic dysfunction can be categorized by severity and chronicity in the following ways, based on onset and mechanism:

- Primary and secondary.
- Physiological and nonphysiological.
- Acute and chronic.
- Autonomic reflexes (viscerosomatic, somatovisceral, viscerovisceral, somatosomatic).

These categories are not mutually exclusive; a primary somatic dysfunction can be acute and nonphysiological.

Primary and Secondary Somatic Dysfunction

Primary somatic dysfunction is the somatic dysfunction that occurs first and is sometimes colloquially called the key lesion. Often the primary somatic dysfunction manifests as the one dysfunction with the most significant TTCs, positional asymmetry, and motion testing restrictions of all of the patient's somatic dysfunctions. When the primary somatic dysfunction is corrected, secondary (compensatory) somatic dysfunctions may resolve. However, differentiating primary and secondary somatic dysfunctions remains more of an art, and correlation with the patient's history and other exam findings is warranted. There are some methods to distinguish primary from secondary somatic dysfunctions, but this topic is beyond the scope of this manual.

Physiological and Nonphysiological Somatic Dysfunction

Physiological and nonphysiological somatic dysfunctions are defined by mechanism of injury and also suggest severity. Physiological somatic dysfunctions are those that occur within normal structural biomechanics, such as muscle tightness from prolonged sitting at a desk and using a computer. Osteopathic structural examination reveals slight positional asymmetries and modest motion-testing restrictions. Nonphysiological somatic dysfunctions are those that are more significant deviations from normal, and may be traumatically induced, such as by a fall. Osteopathic structural examination reveals easily identifiable positional asymmetries and significant motion testing restrictions may often be reported by patients. Osteopathic manipulative treatment (OMT) is often the only primary treatment available to correct nonphysiological somatic dysfunctions.

Acute and Chronic Somatic Dysfunction

Acute and chronic somatic dysfunctions may be identified on physical exam based on the tissue manifestations (Table 4.1). Tissues more recently

| Table 4.1 General tissue manifestations correlated to acute and chronic somatic dysfunction ||
Acute somatic dysfunction	Chronic somatic dysfunction
Tissue warmth	Tissue coolness
Moist skin	Dry skin
Tissue edema/bogginess	Thickened/fibrotic subcutaneous tissues
Muscle tenderness	Muscle tenderness
Tissue contraction	Muscle hypertonicity/firmness
Local pain	Stiff joint motion
Acne	Local itching
Skin provocation test[a] (red reflex): prolonged erythema	Acne
	Skin provocation test[a] (red reflex): rapidly fading erythema and blanching

[a]The skin provocation test is customarily performed in the thoracolumbar region.

injured exhibit signs and symptoms of local inflammation. However, the categories of acute and chronic often overlap, so correlation with a patient's history is essential. Acute changes can occur in chronically affected tissues, and those are called acute-on-chronic changes. Acute changes are usually identified in the more superficial tissues, whereas the chronic changes are identified in the deeper tissues.

Autonomic Reflexes

All somatic dysfunctions have related reflex nervous system activity called autonomic reflexes (viscerosomatic, somatovisceral, viscerovisceral, and somatosomatic). Autonomic reflexes manifest as nonspecific, palpable TTC and tenderness in the areas where the sympathetic (T1–L2) or parasympathetic (suboccipital region and sacrum) nerves exit the head and spine. Because these findings are nonspecific, correlation with the patient's symptoms, medical history, and additional standard physical exam findings is warranted.

Naming Somatic Dysfunction

Somatic dysfunction is named by distinct muscular, fascial, bone, or joint TART findings. A patient is examined for each TART element. Findings are synthesized to name somatic dysfunction, which should be documented in a medical record. The named somatic dysfunction also guides technique performance because techniques are performed based on the somatic dysfunction.

Somatic dysfunction is documented in a medical record and coded by the following body regions, per the World Health Organization's International Classification of Diseases–10: head, cervical, thoracic, lumbar, sacrum, pelvis, costal, upper extremity, lower extremity, and abdomen/other. Structures that span more than one region, such as the occipitoatlantal joint, can be categorized into either the head or the cervical region. Commonly accepted abbreviations for documentation, and those used in this manual, are listed in Table 4.2.

Somatic Dysfunction Diagnosis: Musculature and Fascia

Muscles (individually and in groups) and fascias are generally examined by palpating for TTC and tenderness in a sequential fashion from superficial to deep using tissue layer palpation. The novice physician should incrementally increase forces slightly to reach the deeper levels. A crawling or sliding type motion is often used to palpate the length of a muscle, a group or region of muscles, or fascia. Findings of altered tone or texture include,

Table 4.2 Common abbreviations used to name somatic dysfunction	
Abbreviation	**Description**
SD	Somatic dysfunction
Dx	Diagnosis
IR	Internally rotated
ER	Externally rotated
R	Right
L	Left
N	Neutral
NN	Non-neutral
F	Flexed
E	Extended
S_x	Side bent to one side, x. (x = right or left)
R_x	Rotated to one side, x. (x = right or left)
N S_xR_y	Neutral, Side bent to one side, $_x$, and Rotation to the opposite side, $_y$ Example: NS_RR_L= Neutral, side bent right, rotated left. In the thoracic and lumbar spines, this is Type I or Neutral Mechanics.
F or E S_xR_x also NNS_xR_x	Side bent and rotated to one side, $_x.$ Example: FS_RR_R= Flexed, Side bent right, Rotated right. In the thoracic and lumbar spines, this is type II or non-neutral mechanics.

but are not limited to, hypertonicity, tightness, firmness, ropiness, and bogginess. Related temperature changes can also be documented as a TTC. Patients should be asked to identify all areas that are tender when palpated. Tenderness and TTC findings, however, do not always correlate.

The term *restriction* is often used to name somatic dysfunction identified in a muscle or region of fascia. *Restriction* in this context is nonspecific and refers to the tissue's altered tone or texture, not to range of motion (or the barrier concept).

Somatic Dysfunction Diagnosis: Joints

Joint somatic dysfunction is named by the position and direction(s) of permitted motion (also called motion ease) based on the barrier concept. A full description of the barrier concept is presented in chapter 2. A joint with somatic dysfunction has both static positional asymmetry and active and passive motion restrictions that correlate. Passive motion restrictions are either tested by moving a joint through a range of motion, called passive range of motion (PROM) testing, or by moving the joint in one direction, called passive motion (PM) testing.

PROM testing is performed on larger joints because they are easier to assess. The physician moves a joint through all of its physiological ranges of motion and determines if the motions tested are full and symmetrical. For example, a vertebral joint is tested for right and left rotational motion. The joint is found to have intact left rotation but restricted right rotation. The rotational component of the vertebral somatic dysfunction is left rotated. Learners should be able to identify both directions of intact motion (or motion ease) and of restriction.

PM testing is performed on joints with limited motion, or when full range of motion testing is challenging to assess. Instead of determining the directions of permitted motion, joints are assessed for compliance, or spring. A joint with good compliance/spring yields slightly and quickly returns to neutral when sprung upon. A joint with poor compliance/spring exhibits stiff and very slight motion and is restricted. Findings of poor compliance/spring should be correlated with positional asymmetry in order to determine and name somatic dysfunction.

The term *restricted* may be used as an alternate name for somatic dysfunction. Restricted motion is always the opposite of motion ease (the way somatic dysfunction is named). Learners should become familiar and comfortable using the multiple ways somatic dysfunction can be named.

Finally, occasionally a bone such as a carpal or a tarsal may have somatic dysfunction identified only by positional asymmetry, rather than by motion ease and should be correlated with TTC or tenderness. Somatic dysfunction is named by the asymmetrical position.

Osteopathic Structural Examination

Structural examinations are performed to identify somatic dysfunction and best learned and performed in an orderly fashion, in one body region at a time. The structural examination should begin with observation, which is a complete or regional/problem-focused osteopathic screening exam (standing postural or respiratory circulatory). This whole-body view is designed to alert the physician as to global patterns and areas of possible somatic dysfunction.

Each regional structural examination description begins with a short summary and identifies TART as an end goal focus. The steps of each exam are written for an outpatient setting and intended to be performed on patients who are mobile and can change positions. However, patient and physician positioning must be adapted to accommodate patient and physician abilities. Chapter 2 provides tips for making those adjustments (see Osteopathic Techniques: Preparation, Ergonomics, Physician and Patient Safety).

Clinical reasoning points, or times when physicians must make determinations about exam findings, are indicated by the ✓ symbol. For example, when motion testing, the physician should determine if motion is limited and identify the direction of limited motion. Finally, at the end of the complete exam, findings should be combined to synthesize a somatic dysfunction diagnosis. Findings should be documented appropriately in a medical record.

Osteopathic Structural Exam Steps: Exam for Somatic Dysfunction

Observational Assessment

Key regional screening exam elements have been integrated into the steps; however, a complete exam can be substituted, and is recommended to be performed during all new patient encounters.

- Visually inspect the patient for signs of somatic dysfunction, such as body regions and landmarks for symmetry, skin changes, and muscular hypertrophy/atrophy.
    - ✓ Identify asymmetries and correlate them with the patient's presentation and additional physical exam findings, and proceed with the next step.

Active Range of Motion Testing

- Visually assess the patient's own ability to move a body region or joint through a range of motion.
  - ✓ Determine if the motions are full and symmetrical or limited and restricted.
    - If restricted, somatic dysfunction is likely present, and further examination for TART changes is warranted.

Palpation

Tissue Texture Changes and Tenderness Assessment

- Prior to tissue contact, ask the patient to identify areas that are tender when palpated. Tenderness may indicate somatic dysfunction.
- Palpate the skin and underlying soft tissues (muscles and fascia) for changes in textural qualities.
  - ✓ Identify areas of TTC or tenderness.
    - If identified, further examination for TART changes is warranted.
      - ▫ Somatic dysfunction of the musculature can be diagnosed if desired/appropriate.

Asymmetrical Position Assessment

- Examine bones and joints for position and alignment.
  - – Asymmetries may be identified by comparing paired structures (e.g., right and left upper extremities), as well as deviations from normal position, such as prominence or flatness.
  - ✓ Determine if the structure has positional asymmetry.
    - If identified, further examination for TART changes is warranted.

Passive Range of Motion Testing or Passive Motion Testing

- PROM testing: slowly and deliberately move a joint through its passive range of motion.
  - ✓ Determine if the motions are full and symmetrical, or limited/restricted.
- PM testing: apply a gentle springing motion, usually in one direction.
  - ✓ Determine if the tissues exhibit good or poor/restricted compliance/spring.
    - Correlate PROM/PM ease (and restrictions) with TTC, tenderness, and positional asymmetry findings.

Somatic Dysfunction Diagnosis

- ✓ Synthesize findings (TART) to diagnose somatic dysfunction. Use appropriate terminology to name the somatic dysfunction.

Summary Steps: Exam for Somatic Dysfunction

- Steps may be performed in an alternate order, and some steps are combined, depending on the body region being examined and/or physician preference.
- Observational assessment.
- Active range of motion (AROM) testing.
- Palpation: tissue texture changes (TTCs) and tenderness assessment.
- Palpation: positional asymmetry assessment.
- Passive range of motion (PROM) or passive motion (PM) testing.
- Somatic dysfunction diagnosis (SD Dx)
  - – Correlate and synthesize all findings to appropriately name the somatic dysfunction.

Tissue Layer Palpation

This activity develops a learner's proprioceptive and fine motor skills that are required for palpating various soft tissues and bones. When palpating, learners should pay attention to the temperature and texture of each tissue layer and pause at each layer before proceeding to the next. The amount of force to apply depends on the structure being palpated. Start with gentle forces and gradually increase forces as necessary for palpation. When motion testing the vertebra, observe both the quality and quantity of motion. Quality includes ease of motion, such as gliding or stickiness. Quantity of motion involves discrimination and comparison of tissue movements in opposite directions. Avoid sliding motions over the skin.

In general, the tissue layers of the back are as follows, from superficial to deep: skin → adipose → superficial fascia → muscle → deep fascia → bone (**Fig. 4.1**).

> **WATCH** ▷ ▶ ▷
> ───────────────────────
> ▶ *Video 4.1 Tissue Layer Palpation—Narrated*

Positioning

▶ Patient: prone.

▶ Physician: standing on one side of the patient at the level of the pelvis, facing the head of the table, preferably such that your dominate eye is closer to the patient.

Tissue Contact

• Performing hands: contact the skin of the thoracolumbar region on either side of the spine with the entire palmar surface of both hands and thumbs. The thumbs should be about 1–2 inches lateral to the spinous processes, pointed superiorly.

Movements, Barriers, and Forces

Use both hands throughout this activity. The tissue layers are named sequentially from superficial to deep.

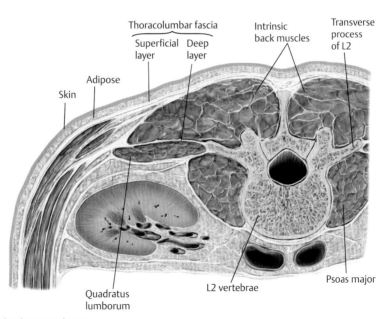

Fig. 4.1   Thoracolumbar tissue layers.

Skin

- Layer palpate to the skin.
- Do this by releasing all tension in your arms and hands, allowing them to gently rest upon the skin. This will be referred to as the neutral position.
  - ✓ Note the texture and moisture of the skin.
- Gently move the skin in superior and inferior directions, and from right to left a few millimeters to a centimeter.
  - ✓ Note quality and quantity of motion in the different directions, identifying motion ease and restrictions.
- Release forces but not contacts, allowing tissues to return to the neutral position.

Adipose Tissue

- Layer palpate to the adipose tissue: skin → adipose tissue.
  - ✓ Note the softness of the adipose tissue (compared to the skin).
- Release forces and return tissues to the neutral position.

Superficial Fascia

- Layer palpate to the superficial fascial layer: skin → adipose tissue → superficial fascia.
  - ✓ Note the firmness and stiffness of fascia compared to skin and adipose tissue.
- Gently move the fascia in superior and inferior directions, and from right to left.
  - ✓ Note the quality and quantity of motion in the different directions, identifying motion ease and restrictions.
- Release forces but not contacts, allowing tissues to return to the neutral position.

Musculature

- Layer palpate to the musculature: skin → adipose tissue → superficial fascia → muscle.
- Create a gentle springing motion into the muscle with the finger pads.
  - ✓ Note the thickness and texture of the muscle. Muscle is more firm than adipose tissue, more elastic than fascia, but softer than bone.
- Release forces but not contacts, allowing tissues to return to the neutral position.

Deep Fascia

- Layer palpate to the deep fascial layer: skin → adipose tissue → superficial fascia → muscle → deep fascia.
- Move the fascia superiorly and inferiorly, and from right to left.
  - ✓ Note quality and quantity of motion in the different directions, identifying motion ease and restrictions.
- Release forces and allow tissues to return to the neutral position.

Bone

- Layer palpate to the bony layer with your thumbs: skin → adipose tissue → superficial fascia → muscle → deep fascia → bone.
  - – When resistance is felt, this should be a transverse process. If not felt, reposition the thumb pads upon the transverse processes of L1.
- Apply additional anteriorly directed force with the pad of one thumb to rotate the vertebra. Note that force applied with the right thumb rotates the vertebra to the left, and force applied with the left thumb rotates the vertebra to the right.
  - ✓ Determine if the motions are full and symmetrical or restricted in one direction.
- Reverse layer palpation with both hands, moving from bone to skin: bone → deep fascia → muscle → superficial fascia → adipose tissue → skin.

Head

This manual details the examination for somatic dysfunction for three major articulations in the head: the temporomandibular joint, the sphenobasilar synchondrosis, and the occipitoatlantal (OA) joint. The exam for OA joint somatic dysfunction is included in this section, the cervical section, and the exam for cranial somatic dysfunction is found in chapter 13. The exam for occipitoatlantal joint (OA) somatic dysfunction is included in the cervical spine section, and the exam for cranial somatic dysfunction is in Chapter 13.

TART Criteria: Temporomandibular Joint Somatic Dysfunction

T = TTC: temporomandibular ligaments or muscles of mastication

A = Asymmetry of facial features: mandibular deviation, mastoid process levelness

R = Restriction of AROM: temporomandibular joint

T = Tenderness: muscles of mastication

Temporomandibular Joint Exam for Somatic Dysfunction

The following exam is used to identify somatic dysfunction of the temporomandibular joint (TMJ), and does not specifically diagnose temporomandibular joint disorder (TMD) (**Fig. 4.2**). Findings of TMJ somatic dysfunction are suspicious for TMD, and patients with TMD likely have TMJ somatic dysfunction.

PROM testing is not commonly performed and has been omitted from this exam. The TMJ may also be assessed in the context of osteopathic cranial manipulative medicine, which is beyond the scope of this manual.

> **WATCH** ▷ ▶ ▷
>
> ▶ *Video 4.2 Exam for Temporomandibular Joint Somatic Dysfunction*

Positioning and Preparation

▶ Patient: supine or sitting.

▶ Physician: sitting or standing, facing the patient.

Observational Assessment

• Visually inspect the face for symmetry as described in the Standing Postural Exam.

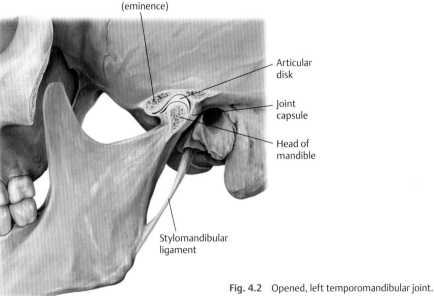

Articular tubercle (eminence)

Articular disk

Joint capsule

Head of mandible

Stylomandibular ligament

Fig. 4.2   Opened, left temporomandibular joint.

AROM Testing

- Ask the patient to open the jaw slowly and as widely as possible.
  - ✓ Determine if there are any deviations with opening, if opening is full or limited, and listen for audible pops or clicks.
- Ask the patient to close the jaw and move it from side to side.
  - ✓ Identify if motions are full and symmetrical or limited.
- Contact both TMJs with the pads of both the second and third fingers.
- Ask the patient to again open and close the jaw.
  - ✓ Determine if one or both mandibular articulations have full motion, and if the motion is symmetric or displaced toward one side. Note any audible pops/clicks.

Palpation: TTC and Tenderness Assessment

- Contact both TMJs with the finger pads.
- Layer palpate to the musculature.
  - ✓ Identify tissue texture changes in the associated musculature.

Somatic Dysfunction Diagnosis: Temporomandibular Joint

- Name somatic dysfunction by deviation of the jaw with opening.
  - – TMJ: right/left deviation, with or without crepitis.
  - – TMJ: bilateral restriction/decreased jaw opening.

Cervical Spine

Although categorized as a technique for the head in this manual, the OA joint is more easily assessed with the cervical spine because active and passive range of motion exams of the OA, atlantoaxial (AA), and C2–C7 facet joints can be performed together sequentially. Keep in mind that the cervical vertebrae are small and mobile. It is recommended that learners spend time examining the cervical spine as Dr. Still did, saying, "I've palpated miles and miles of necks" (**Fig. 4.3**, **Fig. 4.4**, **Fig. 4.5**, **Fig. 4.6**, and **Fig. 4.7**).

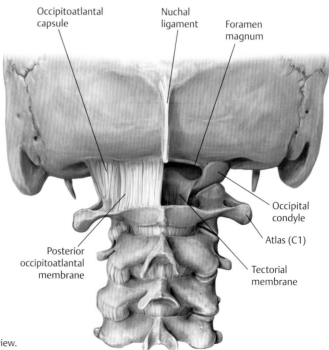

Occipitoatlantal capsule

Nuchal ligament

Foramen magnum

Posterior occipitoatlantal membrane

Occipital condyle

Atlas (C1)

Tectorial membrane

Fig. 4.3 Occipitoatlantal joint, posterior view.

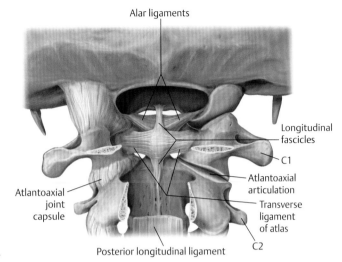

Fig. 4.4   Atlantoaxial joint, posterior view.

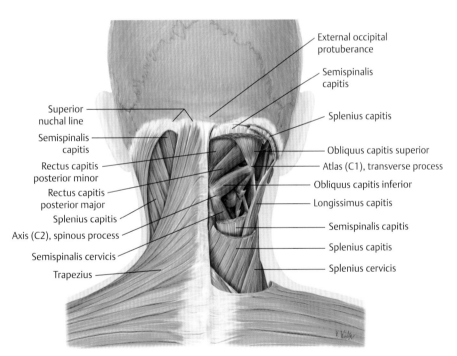

Fig. 4.5   Muscles of the posterior cervical region.

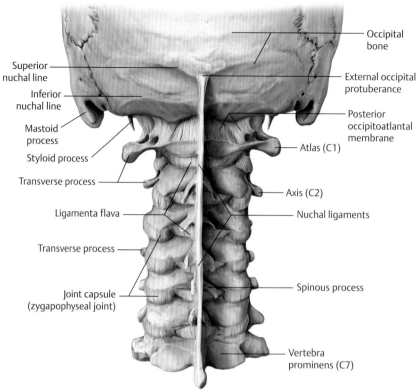

Fig. 4.6 Ligaments of the posterior cervical spine.

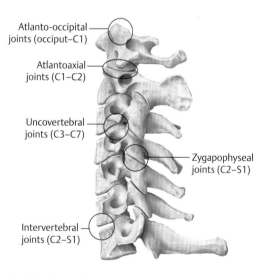

Fig. 4.7 Joints of the cervical spine.

TART Criteria: Cervical Spine

T = TTC: suboccipital and/or paraspinal musculature

A = Asymmetrical position: occipital condyles, vertebral arches

R = Restriction of AROM and PROM: regional and segmental (OA, AA, C2-C7 facet joints)

T = Tenderness: suboccipital and/or paraspinal musculature

OA, AA, C2–C7 Exam for Joint Somatic Dysfunction

Passive range of motion testing is performed on the cervical segments using translation to test for side bending, and rotation motion is inferred. Recall that rotation and side bending are coupled motions in the C2–C7 vertebral segments and occur in the same direction.

> **WATCH** ▷ ▶ ▷
>
> ▶ *Video 4.3 Exam for OA, AA, C2–C7 Joint Somatic Dysfunction*

Positioning and Preparation

▶ Patient: the positions shift based on the exam being performed. The patient begins sitting, then transitions to supine for passive range of motion testing.

▶ Physician: the positions shift based on the exam being performed. The physician begins standing or sitting, then ends sitting at the head of the table for passive range of motion testing.

Observational Assessment

- Visually inspect the face for symmetry, the mastoid process levelness, and head and neck position as described in the Standing Postural Exam.
- Visually inspect the skin of the neck.
    ✓ Identify rashes or muscular asymmetry.

Regional AROM Testing

- Ask the patient to move the head in all planes of motion: right/left rotation, right/left side bending, flexion, extension. Observe motion.
    ✓ Determine if all motions are full and symmetrical, or limited in one or more directions.

Regional PROM Testing

- Ask the patient to allow you to move the head and neck.
- Gently grasp the sides of the head around the ear.

- Slowly move the head and neck in all planes of motion: right/left rotation, right/left side bending, flexion, extension.
    ✓ Determine if all motions are full and symmetrical, or limited in one or more directions.

Palpation: TTC and Tenderness Assessment

- Ask the patient to identify areas that are tender when palpated.
- For the duration of the exam, use your right hand to contact the right side of the neck and the left hand to contact the left side.
- Contact the skin of the suboccipital region with the pads of the second, third, and fourth fingers.
- Gently press into the tissues, noting the textural qualities and tone of the skin, superficial fascia, muscle, and deep fascia.
- Move the fingers inferiorly one vertebral level at a time and palpate all musculature down to C7.
    ✓ Identify areas of TTC and tenderness.

Cervical Musculature Somatic Dysfunction Diagnosis

- Somatic dysfunction is named by the location, muscle group, or specific muscles and identified TTC.
    – Example: right/left/bilateral suboccipital/paraspinal musculature hypertonicity.

Palpation: Position Assessment

Occipitoatlantal (OA) Joint

- Contact the posterolateral aspects of the occiput.
    ✓ Identify if one or both sides of the occiput are anterior or posterior.
        ▪ The side that is posterior indicates that the occiput is rotated toward that side.
        ▪ If both sides are equally posterior or anterior compared to anticipated normal findings, it indicates that the occiput is bilaterally flexed (more posterior) or extended (more anterior).

Atlantoaxial Joint (C1)

- The C1 vertebra can be challenging to palpate so it is omitted here. If desired, however, the tips of the transverse processes can be palpated, noting the position of each in relationship to the mastoid process and jaw angle on the same side.

Cervical Facet Joints: C2–C7

- Move fingers inferiorly and laterally to contact the vertebral arches of C2.
- Layer palpate to the vertebral arches of C2.
  - ✓ Identify if one vertebral arch is posterior compared to the other.
- Move the fingers inferiorly, one vertebra at a time, to assess all vertebral arches for asymmetry.

Vertebral (Segmental) PROM Testing: OA Joint

- Contact the posterior lateral aspects of the occiput with the second and third fingertips of both hands.
- Side bending motion testing.
  - Apply anteromedially directed force to translate the occiput along its curved articulation with the atlas. Translation from right to left with your right hand tests for right side bending. Translation from left to right with your left hand tests for left side bending.
    - ✓ Determine if all motions are full and symmetrical or limited in one direction.
      - If limited, identify the sagittal plane component.
      - If both right and left translation motion testing reveal restrictions, it is likely that both condyles may be flexed or extended (bilaterally flexed/extended), without a side bending component. Correlate with positional findings and flexion/extension motion testing.
- Flexion/extension motion testing.
  - Repeat side bending motion testing with the occiput in flexed and extended positions.
  - Flexion: lift the head slightly to flex the occiput and perform side bending motion testing.

- Extension: extend the occiput slightly by applying anterior pressure with the fingers and perform side bending motion testing.
  - ✓ Determine if side bending motion improves when flexed or extended, or does not change.
    - If range of motion does not change with flexion or extension, the sagittal plane component is neutral.
    - If range of motion improves with flexion, the sagittal plane component is flexion.
    - If range of motion improves with extension, the sagittal plane component is extended.

OA Joint Somatic Dysfunction Diagnosis

- Somatic dysfunction is named by the position and direction of motion ease of the occipital condyles in relationship to the atlas. There are two types: (1) sagittal plane only; (2) triplanar; or affecting all three planes of motion.
  - Sagittal plane: OA: bilateral flexion/extension.
  - Triplanar: there are three components: sagittal plane, side bending, and rotation. Side bending and rotation motions are coupled and occur in opposite directions.
    - OA: N/F/E $S_X R_Y$.

Vertebral (Segmental) PROM Testing: AA Joint

- AA joint motion is inferred by using the head as a lever to rotate C1.
- Contact the vertebral arches of C1 with the finger pads of the second fingers of both hands. Use your right hand to contact the right side and the left hand to contact the left side.
- Wrap the hands and fingers around the contour of the head to cradle it.
- Flex the neck until the tissues just begin to tighten to limit movement of the typical cervical vertebrae. Hold this position.
- Rotate the head to the right, then return to midline. Then rotate the head to the left.
  - ✓ Determine if rotation is full and symmetrical, or limited in one direction.

AA Joint Somatic Dysfunction Diagnosis

- Somatic dysfunction is named for the direction of ease of rotation of C1 (atlas) in relationship to C2 (axis).
  - AA R_x.

Vertebral (Segmental) PROM Testing: C2–C7 Vertebrae

- Contact the posterior lateral aspect of both vertebral arches of C2 with the sides and/or pads of the second (and third) fingers. Use your right finger to contact the patient's right vertebral arch and left finger to contact the left.
- Layer palpate to the vertebral arch.
- Side bending motion testing.
  - Note: Perform on all vertebrae or only those with identified asymmetries and/or TTCs.
- Apply an anteromedially directed force along the plane of the articular surfaces in one direction to translate the vertebra. Use your right hand to translate from right to left to test right side bending. Use your left hand to translate from left to right to test left side bending.
  - ✓ Determine if all motions are full and symmetrical, or limited in one direction. If limited, the sagittal plane component must be identified.
- Sagittal plane motion testing.
  - Flexion: lift the patient's head and flex the neck at the level of the vertebra. Hold this position and repeat side bending motion testing.
  - Apply a slight anterior force to extend the neck at the level of the vertebra. Hold this position and repeat side bending motion testing.
  - ✓ Determine if side bending motion improves with flexion or extension or remains unchanged.
    - If range of motion does not change with flexion or extension, the sagittal plane component is neutral.
    - If range of motion improves with flexion, the vertebra is flexed.
    - If range of motion improves with extension, the vertebra is extended.

C2–C7 Vertebra Somatic Dysfunction Diagnosis

- Somatic dysfunction is named by the positions and directions of motion of the inferior articular facets of one vertebra as they are oriented and move upon the superior vertical facets of the vertebra below.
  - There are three components: sagittal plane, side bending, and rotation. Side bending and rotation are coupled motions and occur in the same directions.
  - C2–C7: N/F/E S_xR_x.

Thoracic and Lumbar Spines

The thoracic and lumbar spines are easily examined for somatic dysfunction at the same time because they have similar anatomy and biomechanics. The exam may be localized to a region if clinically indicated. The thoracic and lumbar spinal regions are also key areas for osteopathic physicians to examine and treat with OMT, in part due to the sympathetic nervous system innervation levels (**Fig. 4.8** and **Fig. 4.9**).

Patients with visceral diseases should be examined for corresponding viscerosomatic reflexes in the T1–L2 region. Conversely, when somatic dysfunctions are found in the T1–L2 region without a corresponding mechanism of physical injury, or if OMT performed in the T1–L2 region is ineffective, a high index of suspicion for underlying visceral pathology is warranted. In addition, because of the sympathetic innervation, the skin provocation test (also called an erythematous friction rub or red reflex test) is a good screening exam to help identify vertebral levels of somatic dysfunction and may also differentiate acute from chronic changes. It can be performed after palpation for warmth but before palpation of the skin.

TART Criteria: Thoracic and Lumbar Spines

T = TTC: superficial or deep paraspinal musculature or fascia

A = Asymmetrical position: transverse processes, spinous processes

R = Restriction of AROM and PROM: T1–L5 facet joints

T = Tenderness: paraspinal musculature

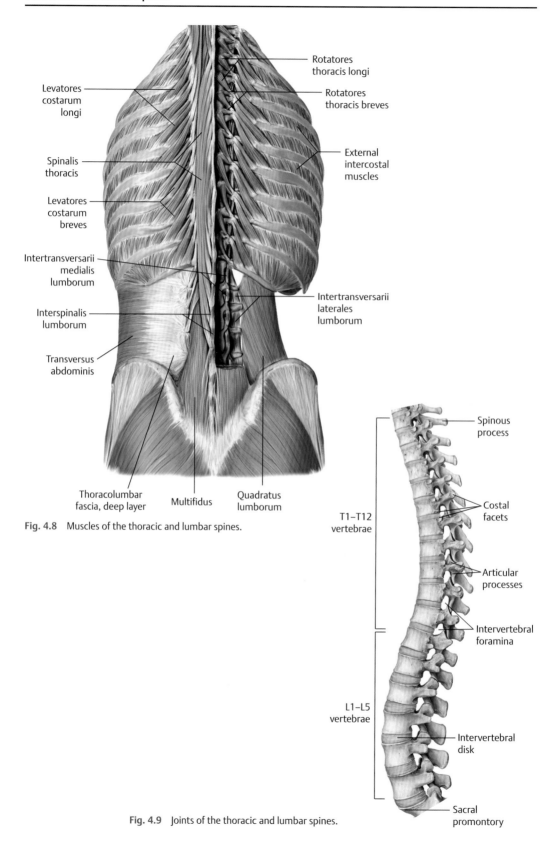

Rotatores
thoracis longi

Rotatores
thoracis breves

Levatores
costarum
longi

External
intercostal
muscles

Spinalis
thoracis

Levatores
costarum
breves

Intertransversarii
medialis
lumborum

Intertransversarii
laterales
lumborum

Interspinalis
lumborum

Transversus
abdominis

Thoracolumbar
fascia, deep layer

Multifidus

Quadratus
lumborum

Fig. 4.8 Muscles of the thoracic and lumbar spines.

Spinous
process

T1–T12
vertebrae

Costal
facets

Articular
processes

Intervertebral
foramina

L1–L5
vertebrae

Intervertebral
disk

Sacral
promontory

Fig. 4.9 Joints of the thoracic and lumbar spines.

Thoracic and Lumbar: Exam for Somatic Dysfunction

This exam is performed with the patient sitting. Patients are asked to forward and backward bend the trunk in order to identify the sagittal plane component. If a patient is unable to sit or make the appropriate movements, the exam can be performed with the patient prone. Adjustments may be made to test sagittal plane PROM, such as asking the patient to rise up onto the elbows to backward bend. When examining the thoracic and lumbar spines, recall anatomic landmarks to aid in identifying vertebral levels (**Fig. 4.10**).

> **WATCH** ▷ ▶ ▷
> ─────────────────────
> ▶ *Video 4.4 Exam for Thoracic and Lumbar Somatic Dysfunction, T1–L5*

Positioning and Preparation

▶ Patient: the positions shift based on the exam being performed.

▶ Physician: the positions shift based on the exam being performed.

Observational Assessment

• Visually inspect the trunk for symmetry, including acromion processes, scapular positions, iliac crest heights, thoracic cage, and pelvis position as described in the standing postural screening exam and scoliosis screen.

• Visually inspect the skin of the trunk. Note any rashes, asymmetrical hair patterns, or muscular asymmetry.

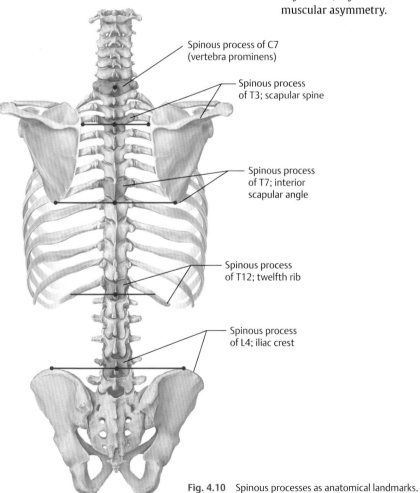

Spinous process of C7 (vertebra prominens)

Spinous process of T3; scapular spine

Spinous process of T7; interior scapular angle

Spinous process of T12; twelfth rib

Spinous process of L4; iliac crest

Fig. 4.10 Spinous processes as anatomical landmarks.

Regional AROM Testing

- Ask the patient to move the torso in planes of motion: right/left rotation, right/left side bending, flexion, extension. Observe motion.
  - Determine if motions are full and symmetrical, or limited.

Palpation: TTC, Tenderness, and Position Assessment

Temperature

- Place the dorsal surface of your hands about 1 cm posterior to the surface of the skin of the upper back. Use your right hand to assess the patient's right side and left hand to assess the patient's left side.
- Slowly move your hands inferiorly along the back.
  - ✓ Identify regions with temperature differentials (warmth/coolness).

Skin Provocation Test

- Contact both sides of the paraspinal musculature with the pads of the second, third, and fourth fingers, about 1 to 2 cm lateral to the spinous process of T1.
- Layer palpate to the superficial fascial layer.
- Briskly rub the fingers down the spine two to three times.
  - ✓ Observe both sides for changes.
    - If there are no changes, the test is negative.
    - If there are changes, identify if it is acute, the side, and the vertebral level.
      - ▫ Acute changes: prolonged erythema.
      - ▫ Chronic changes: some erythema followed by blanching.
- Superficial fascia/musculature: "skin drag".
  - Ask the patient to identify areas that are tender when palpated.
  - Contact the paraspinal musculature about 1 or 2 cm lateral to the spinous process of T1 with the pads of the second, third, and fourth fingers. Use your right hand to contact the patient's right musculature and your left hand to contact the left.
  - Layer palpate to the superficial fascia layer.
  - Slowly glide fingers inferiorly down to the L5.
  - ✓ Identify regions where gliding is restricted.

- Deep paraspinal musculature and transverse processes.
  - Return your fingers to the tissue contact used in the skin drag test.
  - Gently press into the musculature with the fingertips noting the textural qualities and tone of the skin, superficial fascia, muscle, and deep fascia. Also note if a transverse process is prominent.
    - Move your fingers inferiorly, one vertebral level at a time, and palpate all musculature and transverse processes down to L5.
    - A vertebral prominence indicates a posterior transverse process of a rotated vertebra.
  - ✓ Identify areas of TTC and tenderness.

Optional: Thoracic/Lumbar Musculature Somatic Dysfunction Diagnosis

- Somatic dysfunction is named by the spinal level, muscle group, or specific muscles and identified TTCs.
  - Example: right/left/bilateral paraspinal musculature hypertonicity.

Vertebral (Segmental) PROM Testing

- Contact the transverse processes of T1 with the pads of the thumbs. Use your right thumb to contact the patient's right transverse process and left thumb to contact the left.
- Layer palpate to the transverse processes.
- Rotation motion testing: perform on all vertebrae or only those with identified asymmetries and/or associated TTCs.
  - Apply an anteriorly directed force with the pad of one thumb to rotate the vertebra. Use your right thumb to rotate the vertebra to the left and left thumb to rotate the vertebra to the right.
  - ✓ Determine if all motions are full and symmetrical, or limited in one direction. If limited, the sagittal plane component must be identified.
- Sagittal plane motion testing.
  - The patient should flex or extend only enough that the vertebra being tested flexes or extends slightly.

- Flexion.
    - T1–T5 vertebrae: ask the patient to flex the neck (or look downward toward the floor).
    - T6–L5 vertebrae: ask the patient to flex the spine (curve forward).
    - Ask the patient to hold this position.
    - Repeat rotational motion testing.
- Extension.
    - T1–T5 vertebrae: ask the patient to extend the neck (look upward).
    - T6–L5 vertebrae: ask the patient to extend the spine (backward bend/push out belly).
    - Ask the patient to hold this position.
    - Repeat rotational motion testing.
- ✓ Determine if the rotation motion improves when also flexed or extended or neither. If range of motion does not change with flexion or extension, the sagittal plane component is neutral. If range of motion improves with flexion the vertebra is flexed. If range of motion improves with extension, the vertebra is extended.
- If right and left rotation are both limited, assess for bilateral flexion/extension somatic dysfunction. Do this by palpating the spinous process in relationship to the one above and below the affected vertebra. Then ask the patient to bend forward and backward. Note if the vertebra moves into one position easier than the other.

T1–L5 Vertebra Somatic Dysfunction Diagnosis

- SD is named by the positions and directions of motion of the inferior articular facets of one vertebra as they are oriented and move upon the superior vertical facets of the vertebra below. There are two types, the first type is in the sagittal plane only, the other occurs in three planes, so is called triplanar.
    - Sagittal Plane: T1–L5: flexion/extension.
    - Triplanar: there are three components: sagittal plane, side bending, and rotation. Side bending and rotation are coupled motions, but the coupling depends on the sagittal plane component.

- Recall the principles of spinal motion/Fryette principles.
    - If rotational motion testing did not change in flexion or extension, the vertebra has type I (neutral) biomechanics, with side bending and rotation to opposite sides, in neutral. Typically, these dysfunctions occur in groups of adjacent vertebrae.
        - T1–L5: NS_XR_Y.
    - If rotational motion testing rotation improves with flexion or extension, the vertebra has type II (non-neutral) biomechanics, with side bending and rotation to the same side. Identify the sagittal plane component by motion ease. Typically, these dysfunctions occur in one vertebra.
        - T1–L5: $F/E\ S_XR_X$.

Costal/Rib Somatic Dysfunction

All ribs move with thoracoabdominal respiration, but because rib shapes and articulations vary, there are multiple types of rib somatic dysfunctions (**Fig. 4.11**, **Fig. 4.12**, and **Fig. 4.13**). These various types are divided into two broad categories of somatic dysfunction: respiratory and structural. Respiratory rib somatic dysfunctions are physiological and correlate to respiratory phase range of motion. Structural somatic dysfunctions are nonphysiological and are best correlated to very slight slippages of the rib at any articulation as well as compressions of the ribs that are more flexible. Finally, respiratory and structural rib somatic dysfunction may also be secondary to sympathetic nervous system activity. Therefore, rib somatic dysfunctions should be correlated with the patient's presentation, and patients should be examined for associated visceral disease.

TART Criteria: Costal/Rib Somatic Dysfunction

T = TTC: iliocostalis, scalenes, pectoralis major/minor and/or intercostal musculature

A = Asymmetrical position: costal angles, shaft, costal margins, and intercostal spaces in relation to normal rib positions

R = Restriction of AROM (breathing) and PM

T = Tenderness: iliocostalis, scalenes, pectoralis major/minor and/or intercostal musculature, rib periosteum

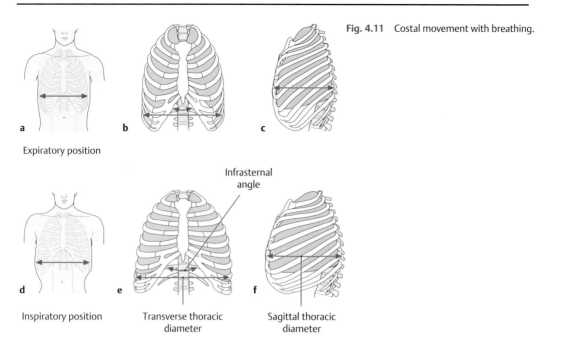

Fig. 4.11 Costal movement with breathing.

a | b | c

Expiratory position

Infrasternal angle

d | e | f

Inspiratory position

Transverse thoracic diameter

Sagittal thoracic diameter

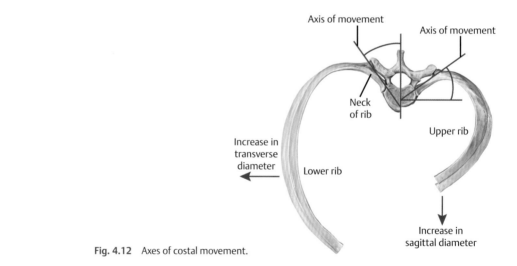

Axis of movement

Axis of movement

Neck of rib

Upper rib

Increase in transverse diameter

Lower rib

Increase in sagittal diameter

Fig. 4.12 Axes of costal movement.

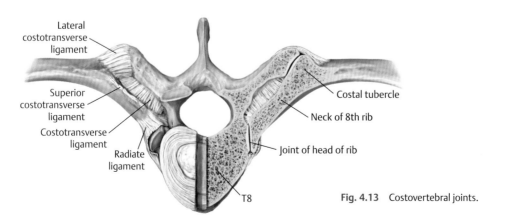

Lateral costotransverse ligament

Superior costotransverse ligament

Costotransverse ligament

Radiate ligament

Costal tubercle

Neck of 8th rib

Joint of head of rib

T8

Fig. 4.13 Costovertebral joints.

Exam for Rib Somatic Dysfunction

This exam is separated into two sections. The first is an exam for the first rib. The second examines ribs 2–12. Both include assessments for structural and respiratory somatic dysfunctions.

Positioning and Preparation

▶ Patient: the positions shift based on the regions examined and include supine, prone, and seated positions.

▶ Physician: the positions shift based on the regions examined such that the physician can easily and safely contact the ribs.

Observational Assessment

- Visually inspect the costal cage for position and acromion process levelness as described in the Standing Postural Screening Exam, including a scoliosis screen.
- Visually inspect the costal cage for sternal asymmetries, including pectus excavatum or carinatum, and the skin for lesions.
- Observe thoracic respiration for excursion and rate as described in the Respiratory Circulatory Screening Exam.

First Rib: Exam for Somatic Dysfunction

Both ribs are assessed at the same time in this exam.

> **WATCH** ▷ ▶ ▷
>
> ▶ *Video 4.5 Exam for Rib 1 Somatic Dysfunction*

Tissue Contact

Contact the head of the first rib with the tips of the second and/or third fingers. Which hand is used to contact which side of the patient depends on the patient/physician positioning. Tissue contact does not change for the remainder of the exam.

Palpation: TTC, Tenderness Assessment

- Ask the patient to identify areas that are tender when palpated.
- Contact the skin superior to the head of the first rib.
- Gently press inferiorly into the musculature with the fingertips, noting the textural qualities and tone of the skin, superficial fascia, muscle, and deep fascia.
  - ✓ Identify areas of TTC and tenderness.

Palpation: Position Assessment

- Layer palpate to contact the heads of both the first ribs and assess the first ribs for levelness in the horizontal plane.
- ✓ Determine if one rib is superior or inferior compared to the other rib.

AROM Testing: Respiratory Motion

- Layer palpate to contact the heads of both the first ribs.
- Ask the patient to take a few deep breaths. Follow rib motion with the tissue contacts.
  - ✓ Determine if rib motion is full or limited with each respiratory phase: inhalation/exhalation, or limited in both inhalation/exhalation.
  - – If limited, determine which phase of respiration is more full; this somatic dysfunction is respiratory.
  - – If limited in both phases of respiration; this somatic dysfunction is likely structural.

PM Testing

Note: This test is intended to determine the compliance, or spring, of the first rib at the costovertebral articulation, not to assess directional range of motion.

- Layer palpate to contact the heads of both the first ribs.
- Apply a gentle, inferiorly directed springing force along the plane of the articular facet on one rib at a time.
  - ✓ Determine if each rib has good compliance/spring or has poor compliance/spring.

First Rib Somatic Dysfunction Diagnosis

- Structural somatic dysfunction: somatic dysfunction is named for the position of the rib in relationship to the costovertebral articulation.
  - – Right/left superior/inferior first rib.
- Respiratory somatic dysfunction: somatic dysfunction is named for the breath cycle that is unrestricted.
  - – Right/left first rib inhalation/exhalation somatic dysfunction.

Ribs 2–12 and Ribs 2–10, Structural: Exam for Somatic Dysfunctions

Rib excursion is easiest to palpate on the anterior and lateral surfaces where rib motion is maximal; however, this exam may be performed entirely on the posterior costal cage.

> **WATCH** ▷ ▶ ▷
>
> ▶ *Video 4.6 Exam for Ribs 2–12 Somatic Dysfunction*

Palpation: TTC, Tenderness Assessment

- Ask the patient to identify areas that are tender when palpated.
- Contact the right and left posterior iliocostalis and intercostal musculature with the finger pads of both hands. Use as many finger pads as desired.
  - – The anterior musculature is usually not initially examined for modesty reasons in this sensitive area. However, the intercostals and pectoralis major/minor musculature can be assessed, especially if a patient complains of anterior chest wall pain.
- Gently press into the musculature with the fingertips, noting the textural qualities and tone of the skin, superficial fascia, muscle, deep fascia, and bone.
- Move the fingers inferiorly and palpate all musculature down to rib 12.
  - ✓ Identify areas of TTC and tenderness.

Palpation: Positional Asymmetry Assessment

- The posterior rib angles, anterior shafts, and lateral margins of the ribs can all be assessed for positional symmetry. Begin with the posterior assessment and use the anterior/lateral assessment for confirmation. This can be performed on both right and left sides simultaneously.
- Posterior rib angle assessment.
- Contact the posterior rib angle of the second rib with the tips of the fingers.
- Examine the rib angle for prominence (speed bump–shaped) or flatness (divot-shaped).
- Contact rib 3 and repeat assessment on all ribs down to rib 10.
  - ✓ Identify positional asymmetries.
  - – A prominent rib angle may indicate a posterior somatic dysfunction, and a flattened rib angle may indicate an anterior somatic dysfunction.
- Anterior/lateral assessment.
  - – Be sure to explain this exam to the patient before performing it because the anterior costal cage is a sensitive area. Adjust tissue contact as necessary, moving laterally as necessary to best palpate each rib.
- Contact the anterior shaft of the second rib near the midclavicular line or chondral junction with the tips of the fingers.
- Examine the rib shaft for prominence or flatness.

- Contact rib 3, moving laterally as necessary, and repeat assessment on all ribs down to rib 10.
  - ✓ Determine if ribs 2–10 are positioned anteriorly or posteriorly, correlating findings.
- Optional: intercostal space assessment
  - The superior/inferior space between adjacent ribs can be assessed. Palpate the posterior, anterior, and/or lateral intercostal spaces for size—those that are decreased/narrowed or increased/widened compared to those that are normal. Correlate with AROM testing findings.
    - Example: the anterior intercostal space between left ribs 2 and 3 is widened but narrowed between ribs 1 and 2. This indicates that the left rib 2 may have inhalation somatic dysfunction (pump handle mechanics). Correlate with AROM testing.

AROM Testing: Respiratory Motion

Although ribs 2–10 all exhibit some component of pump and bucket handle motions, ribs 2–5/6 are assessed anteriorly to best palpate pump handle motion and ribs 5/6–10 are assessed laterally to best palpate bucket handle motion. Ribs 11–12 are assessed posteriorly. In all cases, assess for the range of motion by following rib motion with hand contacts.

Tissue Contact: Ribs 2–5/6, Exam for Pump Handle Motion

- Contact the anterior shafts of ribs 2–5 or 6 near the costochondral junctions along the midclavicular line with the pads of each finger and/or thumb.
  - Use the hypothenar sides of the hands and fifth digit to assess motion of the upper ribs if breast tissue does not permit palpation of the rib shafts with the finger pads.

Tissue Contact: Ribs 5/6–10, Exam for Bucket Handle Motion

- Contact the lateral shafts of the ribs with the fingers and thumbs. Follow the contour of the ribs with the fingers.

Tissue Contact: Ribs 11–12, Exam for Caliper Motion

- Contact the shafts of the ribs with the fingers and/or thumbs. Follow the contour of the ribs with the fingers.

Assessment of Rib Respiratory Motion

- Ask the patient to take a few slow and deep breaths.
  - ✓ Determine if rib motion is full with each respiratory phase. If limited, determine which phase of respiration is more full because this will be the named respiratory somatic dysfunction.
    - If a rib exhibits restriction in both phases of respiration, this somatic dysfunction is likely structural.

Ribs 2–12 Respiratory Somatic Dysfunction Diagnosis

- Somatic dysfunction is named by the breath cycle that is unrestricted.
  - Right/left rib number inhalation/exhalation rib.
  - Right/left rib number inhalation/exhalation somatic dysfunction.
- Note: Respiratory rib somatic dysfunction is also described by the restricted phase of respiration.
  - Example: left ribs 2–6 restricted in inhalation.

PM testing

- Contact the posterior angle and the anterior shaft of each rib with identified asymmetry and/or AROM restriction with the pads of the second and third fingers. Use one hand to contact the posterior angle and the other to contact the anterior shaft.
  - Alternatively, contact only the posterior angle.
- Apply a gentle, springing motion directed first anteriorly, then posteriorly, along the plane of the articular facet.
  - ✓ Determine if the motion is symmetrical or limited in one direction. Correlate findings with identified positional asymmetry.

Ribs 2–10 Structural Somatic Dysfunction Diagnosis

- Somatic dysfunction is named by the position and direction of motion ease of the rib in relationship to the costovertebral articulation.
  - Right/left anterior/posterior rib number.

Pelvis

Somatic dysfunction in the pelvis refers to the innominate articulation with the sacrum and/or with the other innominate at the pubic symphysis (**Fig. 4.14**, **Fig. 4.15**, **Fig. 4.16**, **Fig. 4.17**, and **Fig. 4.18**). Pelvic somatic dysfunctions often occur with lower extremity, sacral, and lumbar somatic dysfunctions owing to muscular and ligamentous attachments, as well as gravitational influences and fascial support in gait and posture. So, in cases of innominate somatic dysfunction, those adjacent regions should also be examined for somatic dysfunction.

TART Criteria: Pelvis

T = TTC: pelvic floor musculature/fascia, piriformis, gluteus musculature

A = Asymmetrical position: anterior superior iliac spine, posterior superior iliac spine, pubic symphysis

R = Restriction of AROM and PM: standing flexion test and sacroiliac joint compression test

T = Tenderness: pelvic musculature, sacroiliac joint, pubic symphysis

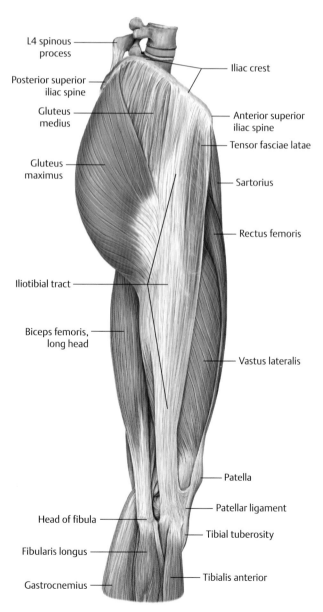

Fig. 4.14 Pelvic musculature, lateral view.

Fig. 4.15   Pelvic musculature, posterior view.

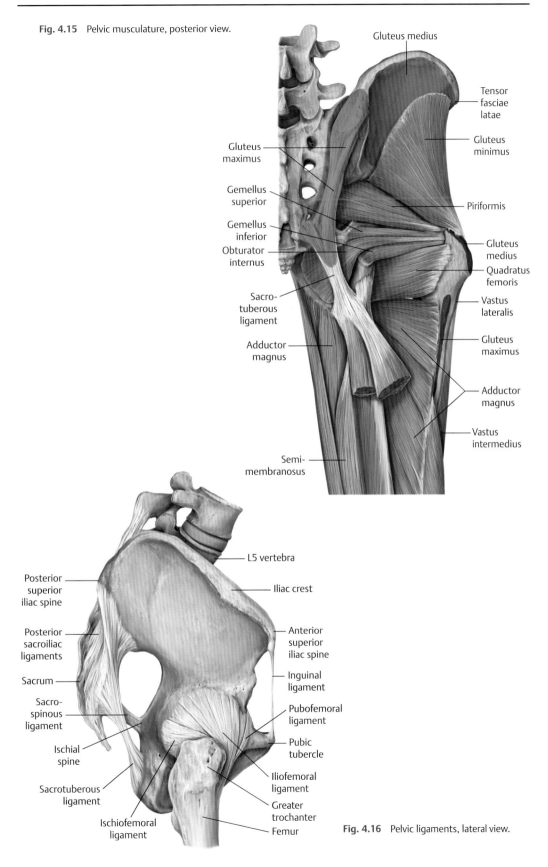

Gluteus medius

Tensor fasciae latae

Gluteus minimus

Gluteus maximus

Piriformis

Gemellus superior

Gemellus inferior

Obturator internus

Gluteus medius

Quadratus femoris

Vastus lateralis

Sacro-tuberous ligament

Gluteus maximus

Adductor magnus

Adductor magnus

Vastus intermedius

Semi-membranosus

L5 vertebra

Iliac crest

Posterior superior iliac spine

Posterior sacroiliac ligaments

Anterior superior iliac spine

Sacrum

Inguinal ligament

Sacro-spinous ligament

Pubofemoral ligament

Ischial spine

Pubic tubercle

Sacrotuberous ligament

Iliofemoral ligament

Ischiofemoral ligament

Greater trochanter

Femur

Fig. 4.16   Pelvic ligaments, lateral view.

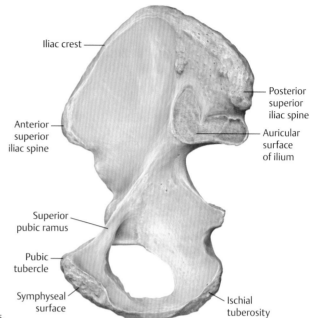

Fig. 4.17 Medial innominate articular surfaces.

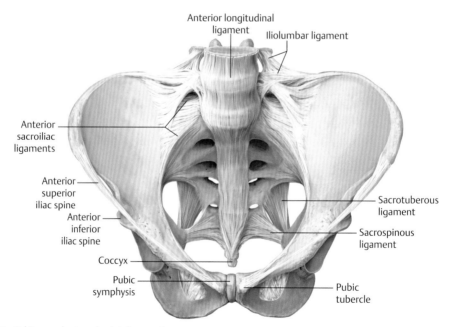

Fig. 4.18 Pubic symphysis and pelvic ligaments.

Screening Exams: Lateralization Tests

Because the right and left innominates are compared with each other to determine landmark positional asymmetry, it is prudent to first identify which innominate has somatic dysfunction and which does not. To do this, screening exams or lateralization tests are performed first.

Standing Flexion Test

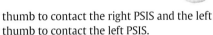

Key Elements

- End goal: to identify the side of innominate somatic dysfunction with active motion testing.
- Positive test: the innominate that rotates further anteriorly than the other has somatic dysfunction.
    - All subsequent landmark assessments are named for this innominate.

> **WATCH ▷ ▶ ▷**
>
> ▶ *Video 4.7 Standing Flexion Test*

Positioning and Preparation

▶ Patient: standing, with feet spaced apart.
▶ Physician: standing behind the patient approximately an arm's length away.

Tissue Contact

- Contact the most inferior surface, or underslope, of both posterior superior iliac spines (PSISs) with the thumbs. Use the right thumb to contact the right PSIS and the left thumb to contact the left PSIS.
    - Abduct thumbs and orient them so the long axes of the thumbs are horizontal.

Movements, Barriers, and Forces

Use both hands to do the following:

- Layer palpate to the PSISs.
- Ask the patient to very slowly bend forward as far as possible.
    - If the patient moves too quickly, have the patient return to an upright position and repeat the test.
- While the patient is bending forward, maintain contact with the PSISs, and follow them as they rotate anteriorly.
- Carefully and continuously observe and palpate the last few degrees of innominate rotation, comparing sides for differences.
    - ✓ The innominate that rotates anteriorly the farthest (or moves last) is the one with somatic dysfunction.
        - If both innominates stop moving at the same time, or it is difficult to determine, either pelvic somatic dysfunction is not present or both innominates have somatic dysfunction. In this case, correlate findings with the Sacroiliac Joint Compression Test.

Sacroiliac Joint Compression Test

This test is also called the anterior superior iliac spine (ASIS) compression test because the ASISs are compressed to assess compliance or spring of the sacroiliac joint. This test is nonspecific in that it does not distinguish innominate from sacral somatic dysfunction. However, it is useful to perform as a second test, especially in cases where the standing or seated flexion test yields ambiguous results.

Key Elements

- End goal: to assess passive motion at the sacroiliac joint to identify pelvic and sacral somatic dysfunction.
- Positive test: compression through the ASIS yields poor compliance/spring, indicating pelvic or sacral somatic dysfunction on that side.
  - Pelvic somatic dysfunction: correlate findings with the standing flexion test.
  - Sacral somatic dysfunction: correlate findings with the seated flexion test.
  - It is possible that both sacroiliac joints have poor spring. Consider performing an articulatory technique on the sacrum or an indirect technique to both sacroiliac joints in order to improve motion, and then perform the sacroiliac joint compression test again.

Positioning and Preparation

▶ Patient: supine.
▶ Physician: standing on one side of the table at the level of the patient's upper thighs, facing the patient's head, with the dominant eye closer to the patient.

Tissue Contact

- Performing hands: contact both ASISs with the palms of the hands.

Movements, Barriers, and Forces

- With the palms of both hands, layer palpate to the ASISs.
- With the palms of both hands, apply gentle and equal posteriorly directed forces to stabilize the pelvis on the table.
- With one hand, apply additional posteriorly directed force along the plane of the sacroiliac joint articulation in a springing fashion toward the sacroiliac joint on the same side.
- Repeat step 3 with the other hand, apply additional posteriorly directed force in a springing fashion toward the sacroiliac joint on the same side.
  - ✓ Determine if spring/compliance is good on both sides or if one sacroiliac joint exhibits poor spring. The side with poor spring is the positive side.

Innominate Bone and Pubic Symphysis: Exam for Somatic Dysfunction

> **WATCH ▷ ▶ ▷**
>
> ▶ *Video 4.8 Exam for Innominate Bone and Pubic Symphysis Somatic Dysfunction*

Positioning and Preparation

▶ Patient: shifting from standing to supine to prone based on the exam.

▶ Physician: standing on one side of the patient.

Observational Assessment

- Observe the pelvis for symmetry, the iliac crests and greater trochanters for levelness, as described in the Standing Postural Exam.

Palpation: TTC, Tenderness Assessment

- Tissue texture changes and tenderness are not globally assessed because the pelvis is a sensitive area. Instead, palpate specific musculature, such as the piriformis or gluteus muscles if clinically indicated, being sure to inform the patient of the exam you wish to perform.

Palpation: Position Assessment: Anterior Innominate and Pubic Bone Landmarks

- Patient positioning: supine.
- Physician positioning: standing at the foot of the table.
- Align the pelvis: because the patient may not be lying straight on the treatment table, the pelvis should be repositioned for landmark position assessment.
  - Ask the patient to bend the knees, lift the hips (pelvis) off the table a few inches, then return the pelvis back down onto the table.
  - Ask the patient to allow you to straighten the legs.
  - Grasp the ankles and slowly straighten the patient's legs into neutral position. Avoid tugging or pulling.
    - If desired, examine for a leg length discrepancy by assessing the medial malleoli for levelness.

Innominate Bone

- Physician positioning: move to one side of the table at the level of the patient's pelvis, facing the patient's head. Lean in medially as necessary to assess landmarks.
- Contact each ASIS with one thumb. Abduct the thumbs and line them horizontally along the long axis of the thumb.
  - Determine if the ASISs are horizontally level or if one is superior or inferior compared to the other.
    - Identify the ASIS on the side of the positive lateralization tests.
- Optional: identify the distance between the ASIS and the umbilicus by observation or by using the hands or a ruler.
  - Determine if the ASISs are equidistant from the umbilicus. Identify the ASIS on the side of the lateralization tests as inflared or outflared.
  - Note that this exam is not in the video.

Pubic Bone

- Inform patient that you will be examining the pubic bones and explain the steps of the exam.
- Contact the anterior aspect of each pubic ramus just lateral to the pubic symphysis with the tips of the second fingers. Use your right hand to contact the patient's left side and left hand to contact the patient's right side.
  - To find the pubic symphysis, it is common to first palpate the patient's umbilicus with the palm of the hand, and carefully move the heel of the hand inferiorly until contact with the pubic bone is made. Then replace the heel of the hand with your fingertips.
  - ✓ Determine if the pubic rami are level in a coronal plane or if one is anterior or posterior.
  - Identify the pubic ramus on the side of the positive lateralization tests.
- Shift your fingers to contact the superior aspect of each pubic ramus.
  - ✓ Determine if the pubic rami are horizontally level, or if one is superior or inferior compared to the other.
  - Identify the pubic ramus on the side of the positive lateralization tests.

Palpation: Position Assessment: Posterior Innominate Landmarks

- Patient positioning: prone.
- Physician positioning: standing on one side of the patient at the level of the patient's pelvis.
- Align the pelvis by bending the patient's knees to end range of motion to slightly stretch the quadriceps. Then return the legs slowly back to the table.
  - Contact each PSIS with one thumb. Abduct thumbs and orient them so the long axes of the thumbs are horizontal.
  - ✓ Determine if the PSISs are horizontally level, or if one is superior or inferior compared to the other.
  - Identify the PSIS on the side of the positive lateralization tests.

Innominate Somatic Dysfunction Diagnosis

- Somatic dysfunction is named for the position of the innominate in relationship to the sacrum at the sacroiliac joint.
  - Right/left superior/inferior innominate shear, anterior/posterior innominate rotation, innominate inflare/outflare.
  - Synonyms include anteriorly rotated right innominate, left inflared innominate.

Pubic Symphysis Somatic Dysfunction

- Somatic dysfunction is named by the position of the side of the dysfunctional pubic bone.
  - Right/left superior/inferior pubic shear.

Sacrum

Somatic dysfunction of the sacrum can occur at any of the sacral articulations: the lumbosacral joint, or at one or both of the sacroiliac joints (**Fig. 4.19**, **Fig. 4.20**, and **Fig. 4.21**). Although there are numerous types of sacral somatic dysfunctions, this exam primarily focuses on those dysfunctions related

to gross body movements, such as gait or a fall on the sacrum. Sacral somatic dysfunctions related to thoracoabdominal breathing and inherent cranial motion are assessed in a different manner. Refer to chapter 9 for more details on sacral somatic dysfunction related to inherent cranial motion and this chapter for details about sacral somatic dysfunction related to thoracoabdominal breathing.

TART Criteria: Sacrum

T = TTC: pelvic musculature

A = Asymmetrical position: sacral base/sacral sulcus, inferior lateral angle (ILA)

R = Restriction of AROM and PM: sacroiliac joint: seated flexion test, lumbosacral joint: spring test and backward bending test

T = Tenderness: pelvic musculature, sacrum, sacroiliac joint

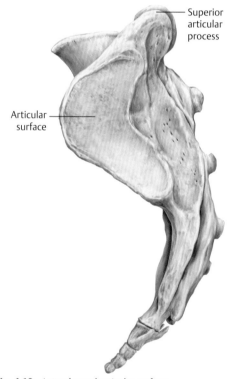

Fig. 4.19 Lateral sacral articular surface.

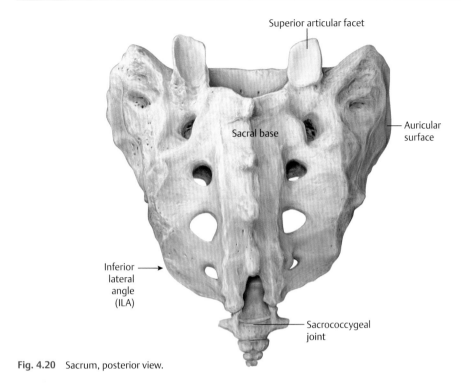

Superior articular facet

Sacral base

Auricular surface

Inferior lateral angle (ILA)

Sacrococcygeal joint

Fig. 4.20   Sacrum, posterior view.

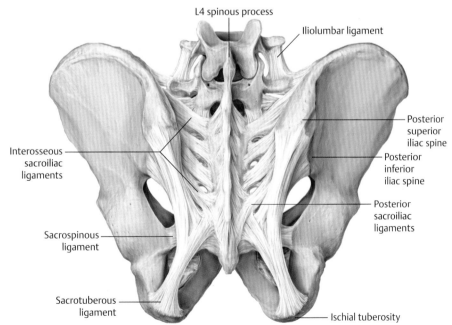

L4 spinous process

Iliolumbar ligament

Interosseous sacroiliac ligaments

Posterior superior iliac spine

Posterior inferior iliac spine

Posterior sacroiliac ligaments

Sacrospinous ligament

Sacrotuberous ligament

Ischial tuberosity

Fig. 4.21   Pelvic ligaments posterior view.

Seated Flexion Test

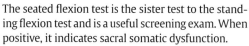

The seated flexion test is the sister test to the standing flexion test and is a useful screening exam. When positive, it indicates sacral somatic dysfunction.

When using the Muscle Energy Model, the side of the positive seated flexion test is correlated to make a somatic dysfunction diagnosis only after the physician has determined if the sacrum has a torsion or a shear.

Using a Muscle Energy Model, when a sacral shear is identified, the side of the positive seated flexion test is the side of the sacral shear. When a sacral torsion is identified, the side of the positive seated flexion test is opposite that of the oblique axis that the sacrum is rotated around.

Key Elements

- End goal: to determine if the sacrum has somatic dysfunction.
- Positive test: when one innominate moves more than the other, sacral somatic dysfunction is likely present.

WATCH ▷ ▶ ▷

▶ *Video 4.9 Seated Flexion Test*

Positioning and Preparation

▶ Patient: sitting, with feet touching the floor and widely spaced apart.

▶ Physician: sitting or standing behind the patient approximately an arm's length away.

Tissue Contact

- Performing hands: contact the most inferior surface, or underslope, of both PSISs with the thumbs. Use the right thumb to contact the right PSIS and the left thumb to contact the left PSIS.
  - Abduct thumbs and orient them so the long axes of the thumbs are horizontal.

Movements, Barriers, and Forces

Use both hands to do the following:

- Layer palpate to the PSISs.
- Ask the patient to very slowly bend forward as far as possible.
  - If the patient moves too quickly, have the patient return to upright position and repeat the test.
- While the patient is bending forward, maintain contact with the PSISs and follow them as they rotate anteriorly.
  - Continuously observe and palpate innominate movement.
- ✓ Carefully observe and palpate the last few degrees of PSIS rotation, comparing sides, for differences in range of motion.
  - If both innominates stop moving at the same time, there is no sacral somatic dysfunction.
  - If one innominate moves farther (or moves last), the test is positive and named for this side.
  - If a positive side is challenging to identify, and/or general motion restrictions are appreciated and sacral somatic dysfunction is possibly related to the patient's condition, continue examining the sacrum. The patient may have a sacral somatic dysfunction that is not a torsion or shear.

AM: Lumbosacral Backward Bending/Sphinx Test

This test identifies sacral motion at the lumbosacral junction, specifically to determine if the sacrum does or doesn't move anteriorly when the lumbar spine is extended. Both sides of the base (or sulci) and both ILAs are assessed for changes in position from neutral. The results of this test are described qualitatively.

WATCH ▷ ▶ ▷

▶ *Video 4.10 Lumbosacral Backward Bending/Sphinx Test*

Key Elements

- End goal: to observe any positional changes in the sacrum when the sacrum is in a flexed position while the lumbar spine is extended.
- Improved landmark symmetry: indicates that the sacrum is positioned (or has moved) anteriorly.
  - Somatic dysfunctions possible: forward torsion, sacral base anterior, superior sacral shear.
- Unchanged landmark symmetry: indicates that the sacrum is positioned (or has moved) posteriorly.
  - Somatic dysfunctions possible: backward torsion, sacral base posterior, inferior sacral shear.

Positioning and Preparation

- ▶ Patient: prone.
- ▶ Physician: standing on the side of the table at the level of the patient's sacrum, facing the patient.

Tissue Contact

- With both hands, contact the sacral base with the second fingers and the ILAs with the thumbs. Contact the right sacral base and ILA with one hand and the left sacral base and ILA with the other hand. Note the positions of the landmarks.

Movements, Barriers, and Forces

- This extends (backward bends) the lumbar spine and flexes the sacrum(sacral base moves anterior). Effectively, the patient looks like a sphinx, hence the name of the test.
- ✓ Determine if the positions of the sacral base and ILAs shift such that symmetry improves with backward bending or if the asymmetrical findings remain unchanged.

PM: Lumbosacral Spring Test

The lumbosacral joint is sprung upon to infer permitted anterior motion of the sacrum at its articulation with the lumbar spine. The terms *positive* and *negative* are somewhat of a misnomer; be sure to clearly distinguish the nuances.

Key Elements

- End goal: to determine if sacral motion at the lumbosacral joint is intact or restricted by "springing" upon the lower lumbar spine.
- Negative test: intact PM, or "good" spring; the lumbosacral junction yields slightly and quickly returns to neutral position.
  - Dysfunctions possible: forward torsion, sacral base anterior, superior sacral shear, unilateral/bilateral flexion.
- Positive test: limited PM, or "poor" spring; motion is stiff or very slight.
  - Dysfunctions possible: backward torsion, sacral base posterior, inferior sacral shear, unilateral or bilateral sacral extension.

WATCH ▷ ▶ ▷

▶ *Video 4.11 Lumbosacral Spring Test*

Positioning and Preparation

- ▶ Patient: prone.
- ▶ Physician: standing on the side of the table at the level of the patient's sacrum, facing the patient.

Tissue Contact

- Performing hand: use the hand that is nearer the head. Contact the spinous processes of the low lumbar spine with the heel of the hand such that the thenar edge of the heel is on L5 and the remainder of the heel of the hand is on the superior vertebra(e).
- Place your other hand on top of this one.

Movements, Barriers, and Forces

- With both hands, apply a gentle anteriorly directed, springing force.
- ✓ Determine if the lumbosacral junction has intact PROM or "good" spring, indicating a negative test. Or, if the lumbosacral junction has limited PROM or "poor" spring, indicating a positive test. Synthesize this information with the rest of the exam findings.

Sacrum: Exam for Somatic Dysfunction

> **WATCH** ▷ ▶ ▷
>
> ▶ *Video 4.12 Exam for Sacral Somatic Dysfunction*

Positioning and Preparation

▶ Patient: standing for observational assessment, prone for all others.

▶ Physician: standing on one side of the patient at the level of the patient's pelvis.

Observational Assessment

- Visually inspect the pelvis for symmetry, the iliac crests and greater trochanters for levelness as described in the standing postural exam.

Align the Pelvis

Because the patient may not be lying straight on the treatment table, the patient is asked to level the pelvis as follows:

- Bend the patient's knees to slightly stretch the quadriceps. Allow the legs to slowly fall back to the table.
- Move to one side of the table at the level of the patient's pelvis, facing the patient's head. Lean medially as necessary.

Palpation: Position Assessment

- Contact the right and left sides of the sacral base with the thumbs or index fingers.
- ✓ Determine if the sacral base is level in a coronal plane or if one side is anterior compared to the other.
- Alternative assessment: contact the right and left sacral sulci (space between the midline sacral base and the PSISs). Determine if the sacral sulci are symmetrically deep, or if one is deeper than the other.
  - Contact the posterior aspect of the right and left inferior lateral angles (ILAs) of the sacrum with the thumbs or fingers.

- ✓ Determine if the ILAs are level in a coronal plane or if one ILA is posterior compared to the other.
- Contact the most inferior aspect, or underslope, of the ILAs with the thumbs. Abduct the thumbs and align them horizontally.
- ✓ Determine if the ILAs are horizontally level. If not, identify the ILA that is inferior. Of note, ILAs tend to be both posterior/inferior or superior/anterior, owing to the shape of the sacrum and the sacroiliac articulation.

Optional: PROM Testing: Sacral Torsions

- If a sacral torsion is suspected, determine the axis and direction of rotation by motion testing the sacrum around each oblique axis.
- Contact the sacral base on one side of the sacrum, and on the opposite side, contact the sacrum near the ILA.
- Rotate the sacrum anteriorly by applying anterior pressure in a springing fashion on the right sacral base to create left rotation around a left oblique axis.
- Rotate the sacrum posteriorly in a springing fashion on the left side of the sacrum at the ILA to create right rotation around a left oblique axis.
  - ✓ Determine if the sacrum rotates anteriorly or posteriorly or has poor compliance.
- Switch hands and rotate the sacrum around the other oblique axis.
  - ✓ Determine if the sacrum rotates anteriorly or posteriorly or has poor compliance.
    - The axis about which rotation is most limited is the named axis of the sacral torsion. The direction of the easiest motion is the direction of the sacral rotation.

Somatic Dysfunction Diagnosis: Sacral Torsions

- Somatic dysfunction is named for the position of the sacrum in relationship to the lumbar articulation.
  - Forward torsions: right rotation about a right oblique axis, left rotation about a left oblique axis (R on R, L on L).

– Backward torsions: right rotation about a left oblique axis, left rotation about a right oblique axis (R on L, L on R).

Somatic Dysfunction Diagnosis: Sacral Shears

- Somatic dysfunction is named for the position of the sacrum in relationship to one or both the sacroiliac joints. Muscle energy model terminology is in parentheses.
  - Superior sacral shear (unilateral sacral flexion).
  - Inferior sacral shear (unilateral sacral extension).
  - Anterior sacral base (bilateral sacral flexion).
  - Posterior sacral base (bilateral sacral extension).

Sacral Rotation around a Vertical Axis

- Somatic dysfunction is named by the direction the sacrum is rotated around a vertical axis in relationship to L5.
  - Rotated right/left on a vertical axis.

Upper Extremities

Upper extremity somatic dysfunctions should be carefully distinguished from more significant injuries, such as moderate to severe ligamentous or muscular tears, fractures, dislocations, and radiculopathy. Perform a thorough physical examination that includes orthopedic exams, which may be integrated into the exam for somatic dysfunction at any point. In cases of specific joint complaints, examine the joints that are proximal and distal to the one the patient identifies as problematic because most extremity musculature crosses two joints. In cases of joint replacements or rheumatoid or osteoarthritis, perform the exam within the joint's permitted range of motion.

This section describes exams for locations in which somatic dysfunction is common, and those for which techniques are available in this manual. These include the clavicle (sternoclavicular and acromioclavicular joints), shoulder (glenohumeral joint), forearm (radioulnar joint and interosseous membrane), and wrist (radiocarpal and ulnocarpal joints).

TART Criteria: Upper Extremity

T = TTC: joints, upper extremity musculature, interosseous membrane

A = Asymmetrical position: clavicles, humerus, carpal bones

R = Restriction of AROM and PROM: clavicle, shoulder (humerus), forearm (radius), wrist

T = Tenderness: upper extremity musculature, tissues surrounding joints

Clavicle: Exam for Somatic Dysfunction

The clavicle is one bone, but the sternal and acromial ends are shaped differently so each articulation has slightly different predominant motions. Thus it is easier to examine each end independently for somatic dysfunctions. The two clavicles are functionally joined by an interclavicular ligament that spans the manubrium of the sternum, so it is recommended that both clavicles be examined for somatic dysfunction, regardless of the patient's complaint (**Fig. 4.22** and **Fig. 4.23**).

> **WATCH ▷ ▶ ▷**
>
> ▶ *Video 4.13 Exam for Clavicle Somatic Dysfunction*

Exam for Sternoclavicular Joint Somatic Dysfunction

Positioning and Preparation

- ▶ Patient: standing, supine, or sitting.
- ▶ Physician: shifting position based on the exam being performed.

Observation

- Observe the sternal ends of the clavicle and acromion processes for levelness in the horizontal plane as described in the standing postural exam.

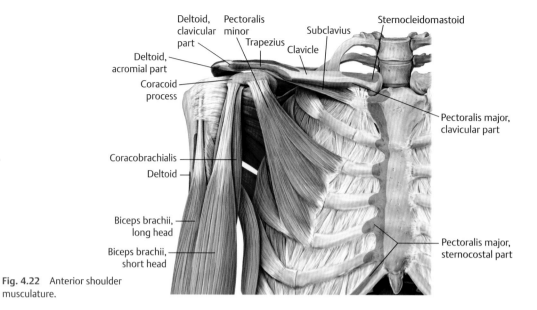

Fig. 4.22 Anterior shoulder musculature.

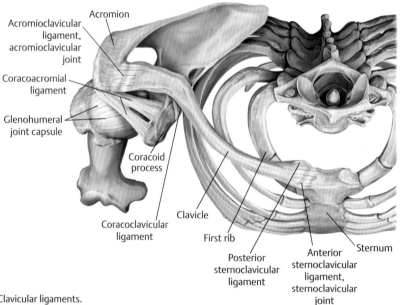

Fig. 4.23 Clavicular ligaments.

Palpation: TTC and Tenderness

- Contact the superior aspects of both sternoclavicular joints and palpate the joint by moving the fingers around the joint region.
- ✓ Identify areas of TTC and tenderness.

AROM Testing

- Contact the superior aspects of both sternoclavicular joints with the pads of the second and third fingers.
- Ask the patient to shrug both shoulders. This moves the sternal end of the clavicle inferiorly.
- ✓ Determine if the motions are full and symmetrical or restricted.

- Ask the patient to move the shoulders backward (posteriorly) and forward (anteriorly).
  - As the patient moves the shoulders backward, the sternal ends of the clavicles move anteriorly. As the patient moves the shoulders forward, the sternal ends of the clavicles move posteriorly.
  ✓ Determine if the motions are full and symmetrical or restricted.

PM Testing

- With the fingertips, contact the superior margin of both sternal ends of the clavicles near the articulation.
- Apply a gentle, inferiorly directed springing force along the plane of each sternoclavicular articulation, one at a time, to assess for compliance/spring.
- Repeat testing, applying force in a posterior direction.
  ✓ Determine if one or both sternoclavicular joints have good or poor compliance/spring in both directions. Correlate with positional asymmetry and AROM findings.

Sternoclavicular Joint Somatic Dysfunction

- Somatic dysfunction is named for the position and motion ease of the sternal end of the clavicle in relationship to the manubrium.
- Right/left/bilateral sternoclavicular joint: superior/inferior, anterior/posterior.

Acromioclavicular Joint: Exam for Somatic Dysfunction

The humerus is used as a long lever to move the acromioclavicular joint into internal and external rotation.

Positioning and Preparation

▶ Patient: supine, sitting, or standing.
▶ Physician: shifting position based on the exam being performed.

Observational Assessment

- Visually inspect the acromion processes for levelness in the horizontal plane as described in the standing postural exam.

Palpation: TTC and Tenderness

- Contact the superior aspects of both acromioclavicular joints and palpate the joint by moving the fingers around the joint region.
  ✓ Identify areas of TTC and tenderness.

AROM Testing

- Ask the patient to abduct the arms to 90 degrees and bend the elbows to 90 degrees.
- Ask the patient to then rotate the arms and hands superiorly and then inferiorly, and return to starting position.
  ✓ Determine if the motions are full and symmetrical or restricted.

PROM Testing

- Ask the patient to abduct the arms to 90 degrees and bend the elbows to 90 degrees.
- Contact the anterior acromioclavicular joint with the fingertips of one hand.
- With the other hand, grasp the patient's arm or forearm in order to move the acromioclavicular joint.
- Move the patient's arm into internal and external rotation.
  ✓ Determine if one or both acromioclavicular joints have intact or limited PROM.

Acromioclavicular Joint Somatic Dysfunction

- Somatic dysfunction is named for the position and motion ease of the acromioclavicular joint.
  - Right/left/bilateral acromioclavicular joint: internally/externally rotated.

Shoulder Somatic Dysfunction

The scapulothoracic articulation may also be assessed for somatic dysfunction but is not presented in this manual.

Glenohumeral Joint: Exam for Somatic Dysfunction

This exam is focused on range of motion testing of the glenohumeral joint. The joint is challenging to palpate because of its deep location (**Fig. 4.24** and **Fig. 4.25**).

> **WATCH ▷ ▶ ▷**
>
> ▶ *Video 4.14 Exam for Glenohumeral Joint Somatic Dysfunction*

Positioning and Preparation

▶ Patient: sitting or standing.
▶ Physician: shifting positions based on the exam being performed.

Observational Assessment

• Visually inspect the acromion process heights, scapular angles, and inferior lateral angles of the scapula as described in the standing postural exam.
• Also note the roundedness of the shoulders, which may indicate that the humerus is internally rotated.

Palpation: TTC and Tenderness Assessment

• Palpate the biceps tendons, pectoralis major/minor, deltoids, trapezius, and rotator cuff muscles.
✓ Identify areas of tissue texture changes and tenderness.

Palpation: Positional Asymmetry Assessment

• Palpate the contour of the anterior shoulder.
✓ Identify if one or both shoulders are rounded and correlate with observational assessment.

AROM Testing

• Ask the patient to slowly abduct both arms and touch the backs of the hands overhead, then return to neutral.
✓ Determine if one or both glenohumeral joints have intact and symmetrical motions or if they are restricted.
• If desired, perform the Apley scratch test to assess for abduction/external rotation and adduction/internal rotation motion.

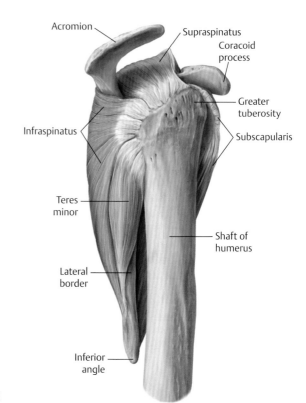

Fig. 4.24 Rotator cuff.

PROM Testing

- Move the patient's shoulder into flexion, extension, abduction, adduction, internal and external rotation.
    - ✓ Determine if one or both glenohumeral joints have intact and symmetrical motions or if motions are restricted.

Glenohumeral Joint Somatic Dysfunction

- Somatic dysfunction is named for the position and motion ease of the humeral head in relationship to the glenoid fossa.
    - Right/left/bilateral glenohumeral joint: flexed, extended, abducted, adducted, internally/externally rotated.

Radioulnar Joint and Interosseous Membrane

Somatic dysfunctions of the radioulnar joint and interosseous membrane are functionally linked, although the structures and specific somatic dysfunctions are distinct. Radial head and interosseous membrane somatic dysfunctions commonly found in cases of lateral epicondylitis, carpal tunnel syndrome, and after falls onto an outstretched hand (**Fig. 4.26** and **Fig. 4.27**).

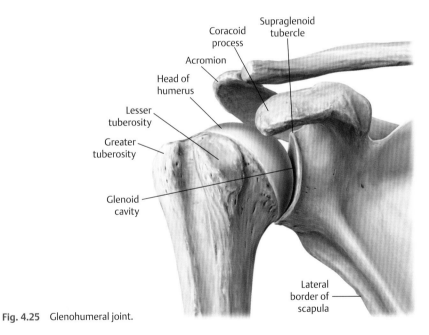

Fig. 4.25   Glenohumeral joint.

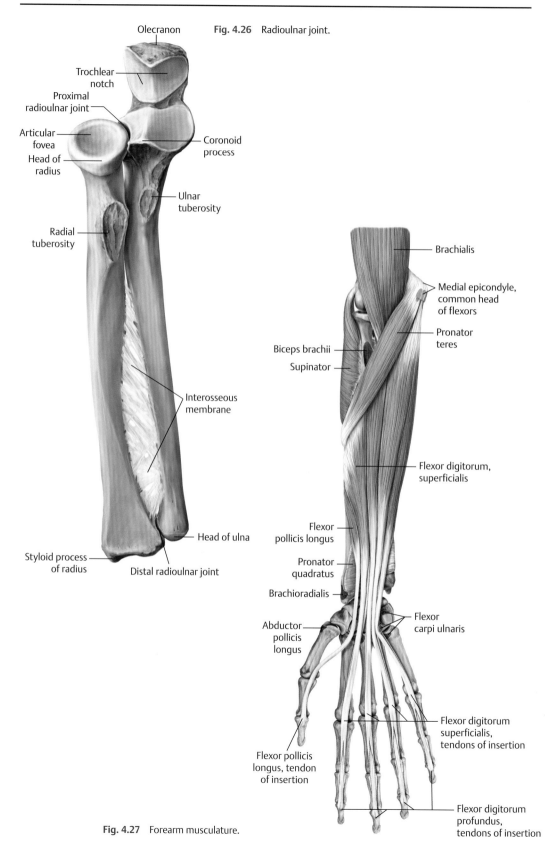

Olecranon

Fig. 4.26   Radioulnar joint.

Trochlear notch

Proximal radioulnar joint

Articular fovea

Head of radius

Coronoid process

Ulnar tuberosity

Radial tuberosity

Interosseous membrane

Head of ulna

Styloid process of radius

Distal radioulnar joint

Brachialis

Medial epicondyle, common head of flexors

Biceps brachii

Pronator teres

Supinator

Flexor digitorum, superficialis

Flexor pollicis longus

Pronator quadratus

Brachioradialis

Flexor carpi ulnaris

Abductor pollicis longus

Flexor digitorum superficialis, tendons of insertion

Flexor pollicis longus, tendon of insertion

Flexor digitorum profundus, tendons of insertion

Fig. 4.27   Forearm musculature.

Radioulnar Joint: Exam for Somatic Dysfunction

> **WATCH ▷ ▶ ▷**
>
> ▶ *Video 4.15 Exam for Radioulnar Somatic Dysfunction*

Positioning and Preparation

▶ Patient: supine or sitting.
▶ Physician: shifting positions based on the exam being performed.

Observational Assessment

- Visually inspect the forearms for muscular symmetry, hypertrophy, and atrophy.

Palpation: TTC and Tenderness Assessment

- Ask the patient to identify areas that are tender when palpated.
- Contact the proximal forearm with the pads of the second, third, and fourth fingers of one or both hands.
- Layer palpate to the muscle layer.
- Gently press into the musculature with the fingertips noting the textural qualities and tone of the skin, superficial fascia, muscle, and deep fascia. The deep fascia is the interosseous membrane.
- ✓ Identify areas of TTC and tenderness.

Upper Extremity Musculature/ Interosseous Membrane: Somatic Dysfunction Diagnosis

- Somatic dysfunction is named for the location of identified tissue texture changes, which can globally be termed restriction.
  - Musculature: right/left/bilateral, muscle group (wrist flexors/extensors)/specific muscle: restriction/hypertonicity.
  - Upper extremity interosseous membrane: right/left/bilateral interosseous membrane restriction.

AROM Testing

- Ask the patient to bend the elbows to 90 degrees and turn the forearms so that the thumbs are superior and the palms are facing one another. This is the neutral position.
- Ask the patient to supinate both forearms, then return to neutral.
- Ask the patient to pronate both forearms, then return to neutral.
- ✓ Determine if one or both radioulnar joints have intact and symmetrical motions or if they are restricted.

PROM Testing

- Grasp the patient's wrist as if shaking hands. Flex the elbow to 90 degrees.
- This should orient the patient's forearm in neutral position (described in AROM testing).
- Contact the radial head anteriorly, posteriorly, and laterally with the fingers of the other hand to monitor it for anterior movement with supination and posterior movement with pronation.
- Move the patient's forearm into supination and pronation.
- ✓ Determine if one or both radioulnar joints have intact and symmetrical motions or if they are restricted.

Radioulnar Joint Somatic Dysfunction

- Somatic dysfunction is named by the position and motion ease of the radial head in relationship to the ulna. Note that there are two different, but synonymous, ways to name this dysfunction. During forearm pronation, the radial head moves posteriorly while when supinated, the radial head moves anteriorly.
  - Right/left/bilateral forearm/radioulnar joint: supinated or pronated.
  - Right/left/bilateral radial head: anterior or posterior.

Wrist Somatic Dysfunction

The carpal bones do not have any direct muscular attachments. Instead, motions are guided and limited by ligaments and the forearm musculature that spans the radiocarpal and radioulnar joints (**Fig. 4.28** and **Fig. 4.29**). This exam specifically focuses on the radiocarpal articulations of the wrist joint and the individual carpal bones of that joint. The distal row of carpal bones can also be assessed in a similar fashion as the proximal ones.

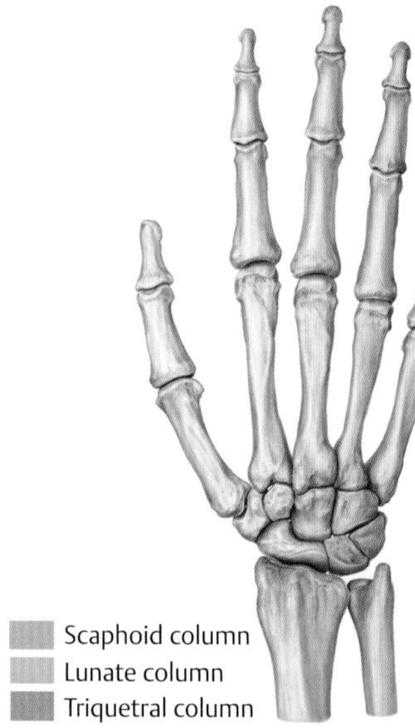

■ Scaphoid column
■ Lunate column
■ Triquetral column

Fig. 4.28 Carpal bones, right hand.

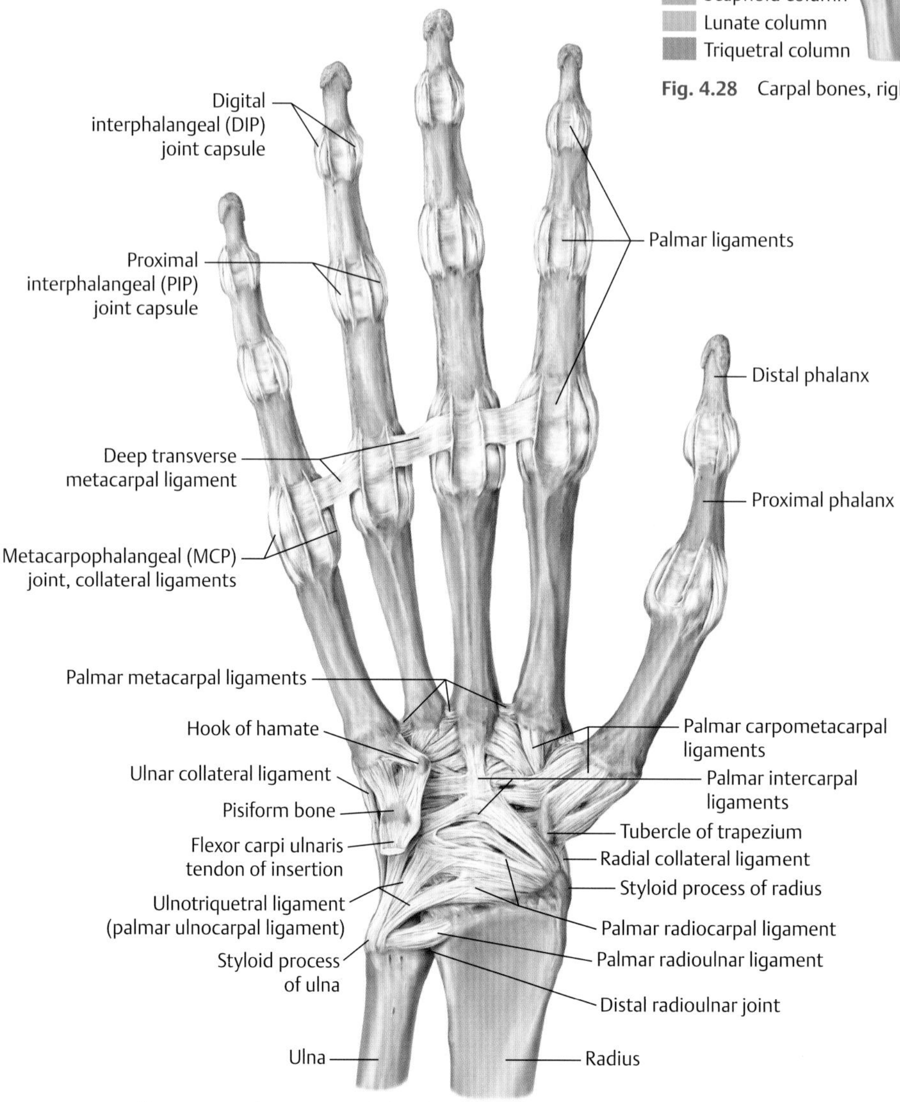

Digital interphalangeal (DIP) joint capsule

Proximal interphalangeal (PIP) joint capsule

Palmar ligaments

Distal phalanx

Deep transverse metacarpal ligament

Proximal phalanx

Metacarpophalangeal (MCP) joint, collateral ligaments

Palmar metacarpal ligaments

Hook of hamate

Ulnar collateral ligament

Pisiform bone

Flexor carpi ulnaris tendon of insertion

Ulnotriquetral ligament (palmar ulnocarpal ligament)

Styloid process of ulna

Ulna

Palmar carpometacarpal ligaments

Palmar intercarpal ligaments

Tubercle of trapezium

Radial collateral ligament

Styloid process of radius

Palmar radiocarpal ligament

Palmar radioulnar ligament

Distal radioulnar joint

Radius

Fig. 4.29 Hand ligaments, palmar view, right hand.

Wrist: Exam for Somatic Dysfunction

WATCH ▷ ▶ ▷

▶ *Video 4.16 Exam for Carpal Somatic Dysfunction*

Positioning and Preparation

▶ Patient: supine or sitting.

▶ Physician: shifting positions based on the exam being performed.

Observational Assessment

- Visually inspect the carrying angles or alignment/deviation and the wrist for bony or cystic prominences.

Palpation: TTC and Tenderness and Positional Asymmetry Assessment

- Ask the patient to identify areas that are tender when palpated.
- Contact the proximal row of carpal bones with the thumbs or finger pads.
- Gently press into the fascia (flexor retinaculum), noting the textural qualities and bony prominences.
- ✓ Determine if any of the bones are more prominent on the dorsal or volar surface.

AROM Testing

- Ask the patient to bend the elbows to 90 degrees, keeping the hands straight with the palms facing upward (supinated) or downward (pronated). Either one is acceptable. This is the neutral position.
- Ask the patient to move the wrist in flexion, extension, abduction (radial deviation), and adduction (ulnar deviation).
- ✓ Determine if the motions are full and symmetrical.

PROM Testing

- Move the patient's wrist into flexion, extension, abduction (radial deviation), and adduction (ulnar deviation). Perform on one wrist at a time.

✓ Determine if the motions are full and symmetrical.

Radiocarpal Joint and Carpal Bone Somatic Dysfunction

- Somatic dysfunction is named by the position and motion ease of the proximal carpal bones in relationship to the radius. Each wrist can have somatic dysfunction in more than one direction. Also, each bone can have dysfunction.
  - Right/left wrist flexion/extension, abduction/adduction somatic dysfunction.
  - Right/left scaphoid/lunate/triquetrum: internally/externally rotated, flexed/extended.

Lower Extremities

Lower extremity somatic dysfunctions should be carefully distinguished from more significant injuries, such as moderate to severe ligamentous or muscular tears, fractures, dislocations, and radiculopathy. Perform a thorough physical examination that includes orthopedic exams, which may be integrated into the exam for somatic dysfunction at any point. In cases of specific joint complaints, examine the joints that are proximal and distal to the one the patient identifies as problematic because most extremity musculature crosses two joints. In cases of joint replacements, rheumatoid or osteoarthritis, perform the exam within the joint's permitted range of motion.

This section describes exams for locations in which somatic dysfunction is common, and those for which techniques are available in this manual. These include the hip (femoroacetabular joint), knee (tibiofemoral joint), leg (proximal tibiofibular joint and interosseous membrane), ankle (talocrural joint), and foot (cuboid and navicular bones).

TART Criteria: Lower Extremity

T = TTC: lower extremity musculature, interosseous membrane

A = Asymmetrical position: any bone or joint of the lower extremity: fibular head, talus, cuboid, navicular

R = Restriction of AROM and PROM: femoroacetabular joint, tibiofemoral joint, tibiofibular joint, tibiotalar joint

T = Tenderness: any lower extremity muscle or joint

Hip Somatic Dysfunction

Hip somatic dysfunction often accompanies other lower extremity or innominate somatic dysfunctions. Beyond the joint itself, keep in mind the musculature that influences hip motion, especially the piriformis, which can be a cause of low back, gluteal, and leg pain (**Fig. 4.30**).

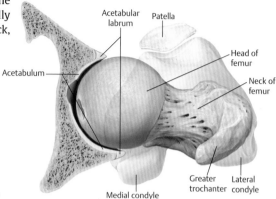

Fig. 4.30 Hip joint, superior view.

Femoroacetabular Joint: Exam for Somatic Dysfunction

> **WATCH ▷ ▶ ▷**
>
> ▶ *Video 4.17 Exam for Femoroacetabular Joint Somatic Dysfunction*

Positioning and Preparation

▶ Patient: supine or prone.
▶ Physician: shifting positions depending on the exam being performed.

Observational Assessment

• Visually inspect the heights of the iliac crests, greater trochanters, lateral condyles of the femurs, and tibia/femur angulation, as described in the standing postural exam.

Palpation: Positional Asymmetry

• Positional asymmetry of the femoral head is challenging to palpate so it is omitted in this exam.

AROM Testing

• Ask the patient to move the lower extremities, one at a time in the following directions: flexion, extension, abduction, adduction, internal rotation, external rotation.

✓ Determine if the motions are full and symmetrical or restricted.

Palpation: TTC and Tenderness Assessment

• Ask the patient to identify areas that are tender when palpated.
• Contact the inguinal ligament with the pads of one or two fingers.
• Layer palpate to the inguinal ligament.
✓ Identify lymphadenopathy, masses, fullness, passive congestion, tension, and textures of the inguinal ligament.
• The posterior pelvic musculature may also be examined for TTCs and tenderness. Examine one muscle at a time in this sensitive area, being sure to describe the exam to the patient.

PROM Testing

• Move each hip through its ranges of motion: flexion, abduction, adduction, internal rotation, external rotation, extension.
• Move around the table as needed to perform each motion. Extension is usually assessed with the patient prone, or the Thomas test can be performed.
✓ Determine if the motions are full and symmetrical or restricted.

Femoroacetabular Joint Somatic Dysfunction

- Somatic dysfunction is named by the motion ease of the femur in relationship to the acetabulum.
  - Right/left femoracetabular joint (hip): flexion/extension, abduction/adduction, internal/external rotation.
- Alternatively, somatic dysfunction can be named by individual muscles or groups of musculature that are hypertonic and thus impair PROM of the hip as "restricted."
  - Example: right/left/bilateral hamstrings/ quadriceps/adductor/abductor restriction.

Knee Somatic Dysfunction

The knee joint, because of its relatively large but securely guarded articulations, is prone to somatic dysfunctions in directions other than flexion and extension. Flexion somatic dysfunction, however, is often present after knee arthroplasty. Although postsurgical dysfunction can be challenging or impossible to completely correct with OMT, OMT can improve joint motion and aid in normalizing muscle and fascial tensions (**Fig. 4.31** and **Fig. 4.32**).

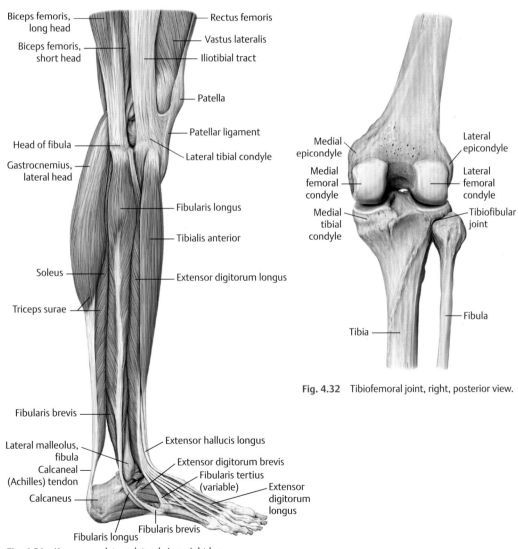

Fig. 4.32   Tibiofemoral joint, right, posterior view.

Fig. 4.31   Knee musculature, lateral view, right leg.

Tibiofemoral Joint: Exam for Somatic Dysfunction

> **WATCH** ▷ ▶ ▷
>
> ▶ *Video 4.18 Exam for Tibiofemoral Joint Somatic Dysfunction*

Positioning and Preparation

▶ Patient: supine.

▶ Physician: shifting positions depending on the exam being performed.

Observational Assessment

- Visually inspect the lower extremities for genu varum, valgum, ankle angulation, and feet arches as described in the standing postural examination. Additionally, assess for genu recurvatum and muscular hypertrophy/atrophy.

AROM Testing

- Ask the patient to move each leg, one at a time, in flexion and extension.
- ✓ Determine if the motions are full and symmetrical or restricted.

Palpation: TTC and Tenderness Assessment

- Ask the patient to identify areas that are tender when palpated.
- Contact the medial and lateral aspects of the knee with the palms of the hands and allow the fingers to wrap posteriorly.
- Layer palpate to the musculature with all tissue contacts.

- Gently press into the tissues, noting the textural qualities and tone of the skin, superficial fascia, muscle, and deep fascia.
- Shift the hands and palpate the medial and lateral joint lines. Gently press into the deeper fascial layer.
- ✓ Identify areas of TTCs and tenderness.

Palpation: Positional Asymmetry

- Optional: assessment of the tibial plateau in relationship to the femur can be added. Note that this is a nonspecific exam, but it may be helpful to correlate with PROM testing of internal/external rotation.

PROM Testing

- Contact the distal femur with one hand and the proximal tibia with the other so as to firmly grasp the joint.
- Layer palpate to the bony layer.
- Use both hands to move the tibiofemoral joint through its ranges of motion: internal rotation, external rotation, anterior glide, posterior glide, medial glide (valgus), lateral glide (varus).
- ✓ Determine if the motions are full and symmetrical or restricted.

Tibiofemoral Joint Somatic Dysfunction

- Somatic dysfunction is named for the position and motion ease of the tibia in relationship to the femur.
  - Right/left tibiofemoral joint: flexion/extension, internal/external rotation, anterior/posterior, varus/valgus.

Fibula Somatic Dysfunction

The fibula has two articulations (**Fig. 4.33**). However, the proximal and distal tibiofibular joints have reciprocal motions, so typically only the proximal joint is assessed because it is easier and has a greater range of motion. The indirect technique for the fibula corrects somatic dysfunction in both joints and the interosseous membrane.

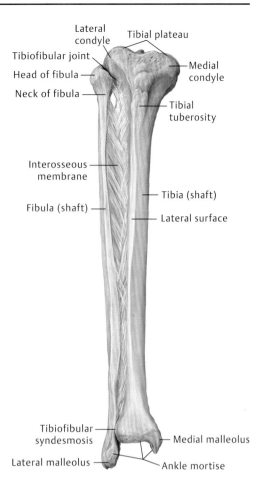

Fig. 4.33   Fibula and tibia, anterior view.

Proximal Tibiofibular Joint and Interosseous Membrane: Exam for Somatic Dysfunction

> **WATCH ▷▷▷**
>
> ▶ *Video 4.19 Exam for Proximal Tibiofibular Joint and Interosseous Membrane Somatic Dysfunction*

Positioning and Preparation

▶ Patient: supine or sitting.
▶ Physician: shifting positions based on the exam being performed.

Observational Assessment

• Visually inspect the lower extremities for genu varum, valgum, ankle angulation, and feet arches as described in the standing postural examination. Additionally, assess for genu recurvatum and muscular hypertrophy/atrophy.

Palpation: TTC and Tenderness Assessment

• Ask the patient to identify areas that are tender when palpated.
• Contact the proximal interosseous membrane. Layer palpate to the deep fascial layer (interosseous membrane).

- Press into the membrane with the fingertips. Proceed distally along the length of the leg.
- ✓ Identify areas of tissue texture changes and tenderness.

Lower Extremity Interosseous Membrane Somatic Dysfunction Diagnosis

- Somatic dysfunction is named for the location and identified tissue texture changes, which can globally be termed restriction.
  - Musculature: right/left/bilateral, muscle group/specific muscle: restriction/hypertonicity.
  - Lower extremity interosseous membrane: right/left/bilateral interosseous membrane restriction.

AROM Testing

The proximal fibula glides with ankle movement, but the direction of the glide may change depending on whether or not the knee is flexed or extended. To avoid confusion (or remembering which is which), test both with the knees flexed and extended.

- Contact the proximal fibular head so as to grasp the anterior and posterior aspects.
- Ask the patient to invert and evert the ankle.
- ✓ Determine if one or both proximal tibiofibular joints have intact and symmetrical motions or are restricted.

PROM Testing

- Contact the proximal fibular head with one hand so as to grasp the anterior and posterior aspects. Grasp one aspect with the thumb and one with the fingers.
- Apply anterior and slightly laterally directed force on the posterior aspect to move the fibular head anteriorly.
- Apply posterior and slightly medially directed force on the anterior aspect to move the fibular head posteriorly.
- ✓ Determine if one or both proximal tibiofibular joints have intact and symmetrical motions or are restricted.

Tibiofibular Joint Somatic Dysfunction

- Somatic dysfunction is named for the position and motion ease of the fibular head in relationship to the tibia.
  - Right/left/bilateral proximal tibiofibular joint/fibular head: anterior/posterior.

Ankle Somatic Dysfunction

The talocrural joint is only one of three joints at the ankle; the others are the subtalar (talocalcaneal) and distal tibiofemoral joint (**Fig. 4.34**). The talus glides posteriorly with foot dorsiflexion and anteriorly with plantar flexion. The talocalcaneal joint may additionally be assessed for somatic dysfunction, especially in situations in which talocrural or proximal tibiofibular joint somatic dysfunction is not successfully corrected with OMT.

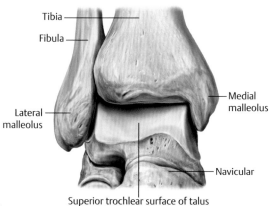

Fig. 4.34 Talocrural joint, anterior view.

Talocrural Joint: Exam for Somatic Dysfunction

> **WATCH ▷ ▷ ▷**
> ─────────────────
> ▶ *Video 4.20 Exam for Talocrural Joint*
> *Somatic Dysfunction*

Positioning and Preparation

▶ Patient: supine or sitting.

▶ Physician: facing the patient's feet.

Palpation: Asymmetry

- Contact the anterior talus near the articulation with the tibia with the thumb or fingers.
- Layer palpate to the bony layer.
- Move the thumb or finger along the contour of the talus and note the shape of the angle the tibia and talus make, as well as the prominence of the talus.
- ✓ Determine if the talus is prominent dorsally.

AROM Testing

- Ask the patient to dorsiflex and plantar flex the feet, either simultaneously or one at a time.
- ✓ Determine if the motions are full and symmetrical or restricted.

PROM Testing

- Perform testing on the ankles one at a time.
- Contact the patient's feet, either near the ankle or on the plantar surfaces, with one or both hands.
- Move the patient's feet, one at a time, into dorsiflexion and plantarflexion.
- ✓ Determine if the motions are full and symmetrical or restricted.

Talocrural Joint Somatic Dysfunction

- Somatic dysfunction is named for the position and motion ease of the talus in relationship to the tibia, either as ankle/talocrural joint motion or as the position of the talus.
  – Right/left/bilateral ankle/talocrural joint: dorsiflexion/plantarflexion.
  – Right/left/bilateral talus anterior/posterior.

Foot Somatic Dysfunction

This exam is limited to assessing the plantar fascia and cuboid and navicular bones for somatic dysfunction (**Fig. 4.35** and **Fig. 4.36**). This particular version forgoes AROM testing because the permitted motion between the tarsal bones is quite limited, owing to the dense fascial and ligamentous structures required for weight bearing. The cuneiforms can be assessed in a similar fashion as the cuboid and navicular, keeping in mind their relatively small sizes.

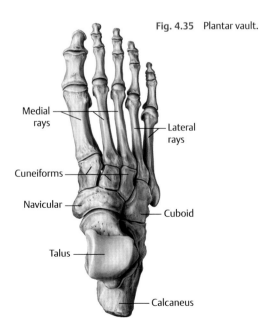

Fig. 4.35   Plantar vault.

Medial rays
Lateral rays
Cuneiforms
Navicular
Cuboid
Talus
Calcaneus

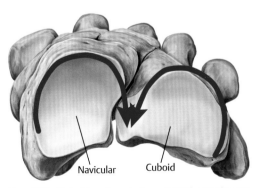

Navicular   Cuboid

Fig. 4.36 Cuboid and navicular proximal articular surfaces. Red arrows indicate direction of movement when the arch flattens.

Cuboid and Navicular: Exam for Somatic Dysfunction

WATCH ▷ ▶ ▷

▶ *Video 4.21 Exam for Cuboid and Navicular Bone Somatic Dysfunction*

Positioning and Preparation

▶ Patient: supine or sitting.

▶ Physician: shifting positions based on the exam being performed.

Observational Assessment

• Visually inspect the skin of the bottom of the foot.

Palpation: TTC, Tenderness and Asymmetry Assessment

• Ask the patient to identify areas that are tender when palpated.

• Contact the plantar surface of the foot.

• Layer palpate to the plantar fascia (deep fascial layer).

• Press into the plantar fascia with the finger tips, noting TTCs and prominences of the navicular and cuboid bones.

✓ Identify areas of TTC and tenderness and bony prominence.

PROM Testing

• Perform on both the navicular and the cuboid bones.

• Contact the bone so as to grasp it. Layer palpate to the tarsal bones.

• Move the bone into eversion and inversion.

✓ Determine if the motions are full and symmetrical.

Cuboid and Navicular Bone Somatic Dysfunction

• Somatic dysfunction is named for the position of the tarsal bone in relationship to the long axis of the foot. Typically, the navicular rotates medially and the cuboid rotates laterally. Colloquially these dysfunctions are also called dropped because the foot arch also flattens, or drops. More than one tarsal bone can have somatic dysfunction in an extremity.

– Right/left/bilateral navicular: medially rotated/inverted.

– Right/left/bilateral cuboid: laterally rotated/everted.

Abdomen

Structures that are examined for somatic dysfunction in the abdomen include abdominal wall musculature and fascia, the thoracoabdominal diaphragm, and the visceral organs and their attachments (**Fig. 4.37**). Abdominal wall musculature and fascial somatic dysfunction diagnoses are found in chapter 6 (see Abdomen, Linea Alba). Visceral dysfunction is identified by fascial restrictions, mobility, or motility and is identified in chapter 14.

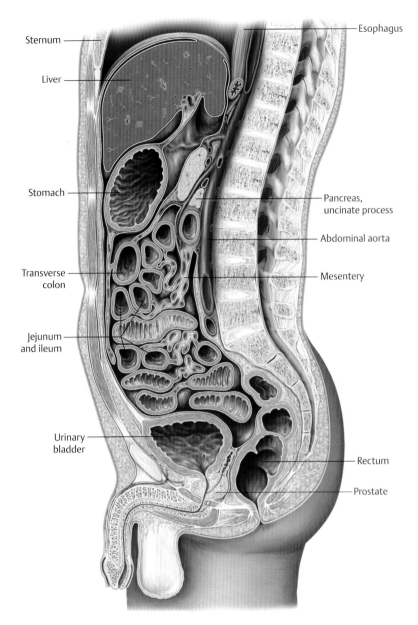

Esophagus

Sternum

Liver

Stomach

Pancreas,
uncinate process

Abdominal aorta

Transverse
colon

Mesentery

Jejunum
and ileum

Urinary
bladder

Rectum

Prostate

Fig. 4.37   Abdominal organs.

Thoracoabdominal Diaphragm: Exam for Somatic Dysfunction

The examination for thoracoabdominal diaphragm (TAD) somatic dysfunction is very similar to the exam for respiratory rib somatic dysfunction. It is included here because the TAD is often considered as an abdominal region for documentation purposes but may be categorized in the costal or thoracic region (**Fig. 4.38**).

> **WATCH ▷ ▶ ▷**
>
> ▶ *Video 4.22 Exam for Thoracoabdominal Diaphragm Somatic Dysfunction*

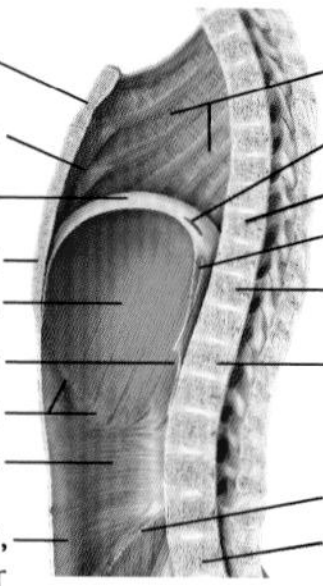

Labels: Manubrium, Transversus thoracis, Central tendon, Body of sternum, Diaphragm, costal part, Aortic hiatus, Costal arch, Transversus abdominis, Rectus sheath, posterior layer, Internal intercostals, Caval opening, T8 vertebral body, Esophageal hiatus, T10 vertebral body, T12 vertebral body, Iliac crest, L5 vertebral body

Fig. 4.38   Thoracoabdominal diaphragm, lateral view.

Positioning and Preparation

- ▶ Patient: supine with knees flexed and feet on the table for relaxation of the musculature of the abdominal wall.
- ▶ Physician: standing on one side of the table, leaning over to be near the midline of the patient.

Observational Assessment

- Visually inspect the costal cage and abdomen for respiratory rate, ratio of inhalation/exhalation, and type of breathing, as described in the respiratory circulatory exam.

Palpation: TTC, Tenderness, and Positional Assessment

- Contact the inferior margins of the costal cage with the thumbs and thenar eminences of both hands.
- Abduct thumbs and place the thumb tips on the inferior costal margins about a centimeter from the xiphoid process.
- Gently layer palpate and identify TTCs: skin → superficial fascia → bone → diaphragm musculature, and related fascias.
- ✓ Identify whether right and left sides are symmetrically shaped, positioned (whether one side is superior/inferior compared to the other, or twisted).

AROM: Respiratory Motion

- Ask the patient to take a few slow and deep breaths.
- ✓ Determine if diaphragmatic motion is full on both sides (right and left) with each respiratory phase (inhalation/exhalation). If limited, determine which phase of respiration is more full because this will be the named somatic dysfunction.

Thoracoabdominal Somatic Dysfunction Diagnosis

- Somatic dysfunction is named for the breath cycle that is unrestricted.
  - Right/left/bilateral thoracoabdominal: inhalation/exhalation.
  - Note: TAD somatic dysfunction can also described by the general term *restriction* to indicate and imply decreased motion, without specifying respiratory phase.
    - Example: left TAD restriction.

Chapter Summary

This chapter presents an ordered approach for the osteopathic manual diagnosis for somatic dysfunction. The repeating pattern of observation, examination for tissue texture changes, asymmetries, tenderness, and active and passive ranges of motion is used in each body region. After examination, the physician analyzes and synthesizes all gathered data to determine the naming, or diagnosis of, somatic dysfunction.

Clinical Cases and Review Questions

Q1. A 42-year-old man presents with back pain. Physical exam reveals tenderness, bogginess, warmth, and redness in the right lumbar paravertebral musculature region. Based on this information, you classify these findings as which type of somatic dysfunction?

　A. Acute.
　B. Chronic.
　C. Primary.
　D. Secondary.
　E. Type II.

Q2. A 52-year-old woman presents to the clinic for a routine exam and medication refills for chronic obstructive pulmonary disease. Examination is positive for a few bilateral expiratory wheezes. Which of the following will you also find during your structural exam, indicating the chronicity of her condition?

　A. Increased skin temperature.
　B. Localized muscle contraction.
　C. Moist skin.
　D. Soft, boggy musculature.
　E. Stiff articular motion.

Q3. A 13-year-old girl presents with left shoulder pain. What is the first step in performing a structural examination on this patient?

　A. Active range of motion testing.
　B. Observational assessment.
　C. Palpation for positional asymmetry.
　D. Palpation for tissue textural changes.
　E. Passive range of motion testing.

Q4. A 27-year-old woman presents with right jaw pain and popping for 4 weeks, since beginning orthodontic treatment for what she calls crooked teeth. Exam reveals that, upon jaw opening, her symphysis menti deviates to the right. There is also a palpable displacement of the right mandible, and an audible click is heard with jaw opening. The right temporomandibular joint is tender. Her temporomandibular joint somatic dysfunction diagnosis is

　A. Jaw displacement to the left with opening.
　B. Jaw displacement to the right with opening.
　C. Left temporomandibular joint restriction.
　D. Restricted jaw opening.
　E. Right medial ptyergoid muscle restriction.

Q5. A 63-year-old woman comes to your office with neck pain and difficulty turning her head when driving. Active range of motion testing reveals decreased left rotation. Passive range of motion testing, with the patient supine with the neck flexed, reveals that right rotation is limited to about 30 degrees, but left rotation is full. What joint is being examined?

　A. OA joint.
　B. AA joint.
　C. C2 facet joint.
　D. C3 facet joint.
　E. C4 facet joint.

Q6. A 32-year-old man presents with neck pain. Structural examination reveals decreased motion at the OA joint when translating it from left to right, while translation from right to left is not limited. Upon extension of the OA joint, the translator motion improves. The somatic dysfunction diagnosis is

　A. OA E $S_R R_L$.
　B. OA E $S_L R_R$.
　C. OA F $S_R R_L$.
　D. OA F $S_L R_R$.

Q7. A 51-year-old man presents with neck pain. On structural exam, you contact the vertebral arch and perform passive range of motion testing by translating the spine from right to left. The motion tested is

　A. Extension.
　B. Flexion.
　C. Left side bending.
　D. Right side bending.

Case 1

A 23-year-old woman presents with midthoracic pain after painting baseboards. She denies paresthesias. The pain is worse with bending forward and prolonged sitting.

Q8. After observational assessment, you contact the paraspinal musculature and layer palpate by pressing gently with your finger pads. You are

A. Determining tenderness by tissue qualities.

B. Identifying tissue textural changes.

C. Passive motion testing the vertebrae.

D. Performing a skin drag test.

E. Performing a skin provocation test.

Q9. Examination also reveals that at T7, the right transverse process is posterior compared to the left. Motion testing the right transverse process by pressing anteriorly reveals restriction. Which motion is being tested in this vertebra?

A. Left rotation.

B. Left side bending.

C. Right rotation.

D. Right side bending.

Q10. A 70-year-old man presents to your office complaining of low back pain. Palpation of L4 reveals that the transverse process of L4 is prominent on the right side. The spinous process of L5 is closer to the spinous process of L4 than L3 is. Motion testing reveals that L4 resists left rotation when also flexed. The somatic dysfunction diagnosis of L4 is

A. $E\ R_R S_R$.

B. $E\ R_R S_L$.

C. $F\ R_L S_L$.

D. $F\ R_R S_R$.

E. $N\ S_L R_R$.

Q11. A 35-year-old man presents with right upper shoulder pain. Examination reveals tissue texture changes around the head of the right first rib. Which of the following exams should be performed in order to make an accurate somatic dysfunction diagnosis of his first rib?

A. Active range of motion testing.

B. Palpation of the costomanubrial articulation.

C. Passive motion testing.

D. Tenderness assessment.

E. No further exam is necessary.

Q12. A 54-year-old woman presents to the clinic with right-sided rib pain. Structural examination reveals that the third rib on the right is more posterior compared to the others. Without further examination, which somatic dysfunction is most likely?

A. Posterior rib.

B. Anterior rib.

C. Superior rib.

D. Exhalation somatic dysfunction.

E. Inhalation somatic dysfunction.

Q13. A 23-year-old woman presents with right-sided chest wall pain. She says the pain is sharp and worse when she tries to take a deep breath. Examination reveals tissue texture changes in the pectoralis major muscle and upper iliocostalis musculature on the right. Active range of motion testing reveals that the anterior shafts of ribs 2–5 on the right have full anterior and superior motion during inhalation but movement is limited with exhalation. What is the somatic dysfunction diagnosis?

A. Anterior rib.

B. Exhalation somatic dysfunction.

C. Inhalation somatic dysfunction.

D. Posterior rib.

E. Superior rib.

Case 2

A 31-year-old woman presents with left hip pain after misstepping while hiking and landing hard on her left foot. Her foot doesn't hurt, but she awoke the next day with left hip pain. Structural exam is positive for a left standing flexion test, and the left anterior superior iliac spine and left posterior superior iliac spine are both superior.

Q14. Which of the following is correct about performing the standing flexion test?

A. Ask the patient to bend forward about 20 degrees.

B. Ask the patient to extend as far as she can while you observe pelvic motion.

C. Contact the iliac crests and follow their movement as the patient bends forward.

D. Evaluate for levelness of the posterior superior iliac spines while the patient is standing.

E. The underslope of the posterior superior iliac spines is contacted.

Q15. What is the somatic dysfunction diagnosis?
- A. Left anterior innominate rotation.
- B. Left inferior innominate shear.
- C. Left posterior innominate rotation.
- D. Left superior innominate shear.
- E. Right inferior innominate shear.

Q16. Which of the following pelvic somatic dysfunctions is considered to be nonphysiological?
- A. Innominate inflare.
- B. Innominate rotation.
- C. Pubic symphysis shear.

Case 3

A 22-year-old man presents with right-side buttocks pain after a fall while playing soccer where he landed on his bottom. The pain is sharp and limits his ability to walk and bend.

Q17. What examination or test should be performed in order to determine if the patient has a sacral somatic dysfunction?
- A. Backward bending test.
- B. Lumbosacral spring test.
- C. Sacral landmark assessment.
- D. Seated flexion test.
- E. Standing flexion test.

Q18. The patient is found to have a right anterior sacral base and a right posterior/inferior, inferior lateral angle of the sacrum. The seated flexion test is positive on the right. What is the somatic dysfunction diagnosis?
- A. Inferior sacral shear/unilateral extension.
- B. Right on right sacral torsion.
- C. Left on right sacral torsion.
- D. Superior sacral shear/unilateral flexion.

Q19. Which of the following exam findings is most consistent with a left on left sacral torsion?
- A. A negative seated flexion test.
- B. A posterior/inferior, inferior lateral angle of the sacrum on the right.
- C. An anterior sacral sulcus on the left.
- D. Decreased passive motion testing around the right oblique axis of the sacrum.
- E. Poor spring at the lumbosacral joint.

Q20. A 23-year-old man presents with right elbow pain. Structural exam reveals tenderness around the right radial head. What exam or test should also be performed to diagnose somatic dysfunction of the radial head?
- A. Assessment for textural changes in the interosseous membrane.
- B. Muscle strength testing of the wrist extensor muscles.
- C. Neurological testing of the upper extremities.
- D. Passive motion testing of the elbow.
- E. Passive range of motion testing of the forearm.

Q21. A 35-year-old man presents with right shoulder pain. Structural exam reveals that the right acromion process is inferior compared to the left and both active and passive range of motion are restricted in internal rotation at the acromioclavicular joint. What is the acromioclavicular joint somatic dysfunction diagnosis?
- A. Externally rotated.
- B. Inferior.
- C. Internally rotated.
- D. Superior.

Q22. A 23-year-old woman presents with right ankle pain. Examination reveals decreased active and passive range of motion of the ankle, with motion most limited in dorsiflexion. The somatic dysfunction diagnosis is
- A. Talocrural joint dorsiflexed.
- B. Talus anterior.
- C. Talus everted.
- D. Talus inverted.
- E. Talus posterior.

Q23. A 34-year-old woman has been training for the Boston marathon for 4 months, and about 1 week ago she began having pain in her left shin and ankle, which has been getting worse.
    Structural examination reveals tenderness in the interosseous membrane and fibular head. Further examination includes
- A. Active range of motion testing of the ankle in dorsi- and plantarflexion.
- B. Active range of motion testing of the knee.
- C. Passive motion testing of the fibula in anterior and posterior directions.
- D. Passive motion testing of the fibula in internal and external rotation.

Q24. A 47-year-old man presents with right-sided foot pain that is worse with prolonged standing. Examination reveals palpation of a bony prominence that is also tender in the lateral plantar surface of the foot. What somatic dysfunction is most likely?

A. Cuboid everted.
B. Navicular inverted.
C. Plantar fascia restriction.
D. Talus anterior.

Q25. A 12-year-old boy with a history of mild intermittent asthma presents with increasing shortness of breath after starting basketball practice. Physical examination is unremarkable at this time. Structural examination reveals that, with inhalation, his thoracoabdominal diaphragm has limited motion and his ratio of inhalation to exhalation is 1:1. What is this patient's diaphragm somatic dysfunction?

A. Exhalation.
B. Inhalation.

Answers to Review Questions

Q1. The correct answer is **A**.

Q2. The correct answer is **E**.

Q3. The correct answer is **B**.

Q4. The correct answer is **B**.

Q5. The correct answer is **B**.

Q6. The correct answer is **A**.

Q7. The correct answer is **D**.

Q8. The correct answer is **B**.

Q9. The correct answer is **A**.

Q10. The correct answer is **A**.

Q11. The correct answer is **C**.

Q12. The correct answer is **A**.

Q13. The correct answer is **C**.

Q14. The correct answer is **E**.

Q15. The correct answer is **D**.

Q16. The correct answer is **C**.

Q17. The correct answer is **D**.

Q18. The correct answer is **D**.

Q19. The correct answer is **D**.

Q20. The correct answer is **E**.

Q21. The correct answer is **A**.

Q22. The correct answer is **B**.

Q23. The correct answer is **C**.

Q24. The correct answer is **A**.

Q25. The correct answer is **A**.

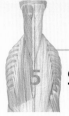

5 Soft Tissue Techniques

LEARNING OBJECTIVES

1. Explain the goals of performing soft tissue techniques.
2. Identify the clinical considerations, including indications, contraindications, and precautions for performing soft tissue techniques.
3. Compare and contrast the types of soft tissue techniques.
4. Identify the end goal for performing each soft tissue technique.
5. Visualize, verbalize, and identify the preparation, positioning, tissue contact, movements, barriers, and forces for each soft tissue technique.
6. Perform soft tissue techniques using appropriate: somatic dysfunction diagnosis, preparation and positioning, tissue contact, movements, barriers, and forces, retest for effectiveness, communication and safe tissue handling

Soft Tissue Techniques Introduction

Goals

Though simple in description and relatively simple to perform, there is power in including soft tissue (ST) techniques as a part of an osteopathic manipulative treatment (OMT) plan. These are foundational techniques and are used by novices and experts alike.[1] ST techniques in this chapter are used on hypertonic paraspinal musculature with an end goal of tissue relaxation and restoration of normal resting tone. ST techniques can be used as a primary treatment of somatic dysfunction, as a method to make a more specific bony somatic dysfunction diagnosis, or as a preparatory treatment for other techniques, such as high velocity, low amplitude

techniques. By restoring normal muscle tone, ST techniques can achieve the following:

- Improve local arterial, venous, and lymph circulation.
- Increase regional range of motion.
- Decrease muscular tenderness.

Background

The history of the use of ST techniques is not traceable to a particular individual in the osteopathic profession. There are numerous accounts, by early students of osteopathic medicine, recognizing the importance of treating soft tissues to correct underlying bony somatic dysfunctions.

Research

ST has been used as part of the protocol in many OMT basic science and clinical research studies. In particular, head/cervical inhibitory pressure, also called suboccipital inhibition, has been studied more extensively because OMT to the suboccipital region substantially affects vagal nerve function and muscle balance. A short research bibliography is presented at the end of this chapter.

Clinical Considerations

Some common clinical applications for using ST techniques are listed in Table 5.1. Always acquire adequate data in the form of an appropriate history, a thorough physical exam, and relevant diagnostic tests to exercise best clinical judgment before performing OMT.

Somatic Dysfunction Corrected

ST techniques in this chapter are performed on musculature with somatic dysfunction. Tissue texture abnormalities that are corrected with ST techniques include those related to muscle hypertonicity, such as tightness, ropiness, firmness, and bogginess. Because muscle somatic dysfunction is not a positional diagnosis, the term *somatic dysfunction* can be substituted as a generic term for specific tissue texture abnormalities.

Positioning and Preparation

▶ Patient: the patient must be comfortable and remain relaxed for the duration of the technique. ST techniques can be performed with the patient seated, supine, prone, or laterally recumbent.

▶ Physician: the physician must be comfortable and positioned to ensure safety, using the best ergonomic posture and movements possible.

Note: The videos include a narrated description of positioning only when not visually self-explanatory.

Tissue Contact

Finger and thumb pads, the heel of the hand, and thenar and hypothenar eminences may all be used to contact the skin over the affected musculature. Some techniques are performed with one hand and some with both hands.

It is customary to perform ST techniques in a general fashion along the entirety of a muscular region. Therefore techniques are written to begin at one end, such as the superiorly located musculature, and then continue inferiorly. The described directionality may be reversed.

Movements, Barriers, and Forces

ST is a direct technique and requires that patients remain in a relaxed, passive state. The end goal is to reduce tone in hypertonic musculature, and there are three methods to accomplish this: inhibitory pressure (inhibition), longitudinal stretching (longitudinal traction, linear stretching), and lateral stretching (kneading).

Physician movements begin with layer palpation. Slight pressure is applied perpendicularly into the affected musculature. Then, based on the method, movements and corrective forces are created in directions toward and into the restrictive barrier(s), or the hypertonic musculature. Movements and forces are then increased slowly to the point where the tissues first yield, or soften. After tissue softening is palpated, the physician can sustain, or hold, the forces for ~ 15 seconds or longer for further softening. Alternatively, the physician can perform short, repetitive movements into the restrictive barrier, holding forces for a few seconds. The physician should attempt to match the tension in the tissues with the force applied. Excessive forces can produce reflex muscle spasm or guard-

Table 5.1 Clinical considerations		
Indications	**Contraindications**	**Precautions**
Minor musculoskeletal injuries	Skin that is broken or infected	Modify or discontinue the
Mechanical neck and back pain	Fracture or suspected fracture	technique if it causes pain
Headache		
Muscle strains		
Muscle spasm		
Viscerosomatic, somatovisceral, and		
somatosomatic reflexes		

ing and should be avoided. Insufficient forces do not properly activate the tissues to initiate changes. Ergonomics and proper use of body weight, fulcrums, and levers should be employed to create a mechanical advantage and to minimize the energy required to create forces.

Table 5.2 compares and contrasts the movements, barriers, and forces used in the different methods.

Retest for Effectiveness

Changes in the tissues, such as softening, relaxation, loosening, and increased warmth, are signs that the technique has been effective and are col-

lectively referred to as a release. These changes indicate that the somatic dysfunction is resolving. When the tissues no longer exhibit the qualities of somatic dysfunction, the technique can be discontinued. Alternatively, if a complete release is not achieved the technique should be performed for about 2 minutes in each body or muscular region. The tissues are then retested to determine overall changes in somatic dysfunction. Two minutes is sufficient time to initiate tissue relaxation, but performing ST techniques for up to 5 minutes is not contraindicated. If tissue softening does not occur in about 2 minutes, rediagnosis of the patient's clinical condition and related somatic dysfunction is warranted.

Table 5.2 Soft tissue technique methods		
Method	**Movements, barriers, and forces**	**Force duration**
Inhibitory pressure	Apply pressure that is perpendicular, or into, the short axis of the muscle fibers	Sustained
Longitudinal stretching	Create a stretch that is parallel, or along, the long axis of the muscle fibers	Sustained or intermittent/repetitive
Lateral stretching	Create a stretch that is perpendicular, or 90 degrees away from, the long axis of the muscle fibers	Sustained or repetitive

Head/Cervical, Inhibitory Pressure

This technique is also known as suboccipital inhibition. It can bring immediate relief to patients with muscle tension headache. Since the vagus nerve lies deep to the suboccipital musculature, performing this technique can result in normalization of parasympathetic tone to structures innervated by the vagus nerve (**Fig. 5.1**).

Key Elements

- Somatic dysfunction corrected: right, left, or bilateral suboccipital musculature somatic dysfunction. Muscles included are the trapezius, semispinalis capitis, splenius capitis, rectus capitis posterior major and minor, obliquus capitis superior and inferior.
- End goal: to create sustained inhibitory forces directed perpendicularly into the fibers of the suboccipital musculature.

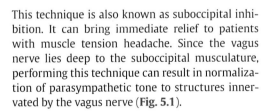

WATCH ▷▶▷

- ▶ *Video 5.1a Head/Cervical Inhibitory Pressure–Real Time*
- ▶ *Video 5.1b Head/Cervical Inhibitory Pressure–Narrated*

Example Somatic Dysfunction: Bilateral Suboccipital Musculature Hypertonicity

Position and Preparation

- ▶ Patient: supine.
- ▶ Physician: sitting at the head of the table facing the patient, with forearms contacting the edge of the table.

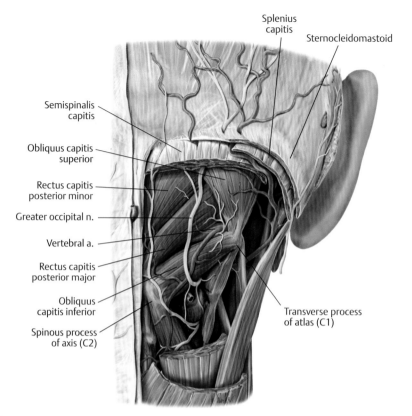

Fig. 5.1 Suboccipital musculature.

Tissue Contact

- The fingers of both hands create the corrective stretching forces.
- Performing hands: contact the patient's suboccipital musculature just inferior to the superior nuchal line with the pads of your second, third, and fourth fingers of both hands. Do not contact the temporal bones or occipitomastoid sutures. The patient's head will extend a bit, but avoid hyperextension and rotation.
    - Detailed suggestion: locate the external occipital protuberance with the fourth fingers of both hands. Then line up the second and fourth fingers horizontally so they fall along the superior nuchal line. Move all six contacting fingers inferiorly onto the bellies of the suboccipital musculature.

Movements, Barriers, and Forces

Use both hands to do the following:

- Layer palpate to the musculature.
- Apply anteriorly directed forces into the suboccipital musculature with the pads of contacting fingers. Use your forearms for leverage by leaning your body weight forward onto your arms.
- Continue increasing the anteriorly directed forces until a restrictive barrier is felt in all fingers. The patient's head may rise off the table and rest on your fingers.
- Hold forces and body positions until the tissues soften or for ~ 2 minutes.
- Release forces and return the patient's head to the neutral position.
- Retest the musculature for changes in tension.

Cervical, Longitudinal Stretching

This technique is useful in combination with other direct cervical techniques, such as high velocity, low amplitude and muscle energy techniques. Perform ST techniques first for preparation and identification of vertebral somatic dysfunction. Then consider performing ST techniques again after the direct technique prior to retesting for effectiveness (**Fig. 5.2**).

Key Elements

- Somatic dysfunction corrected: right, left, or bilateral somatic dysfunction of the cervical musculature from C2 to C7. Muscles included are the semispinalis capitis and cervicis, longissimus capitis, and splenius capitis and cervicis.
- End goal: to stretch the posterior cervical muscle fibers longitudinally.

WATCH ▷ ▶ ▷

- ▶ *Video 5.2a Cervical Longitudinal Stretching–Real Time*
- ▶ *Video 5.2b Cervical Longitudinal Stretching–Narrated*

Example Somatic Dysfunction: Bilateral Cervical Paraspinal Musculature Hypertonicity

Positioning and Preparation

▶ Patient: supine.
▶ Physician: sitting or standing at the head of the table, facing the patient.

Tissue Contact

- Both hands create the corrective arc-like stretching forces.
- Performing hands: contact the cervical musculature with the pads of the second through fourth fingers of both hands. Contact the right side of the patient's neck with your right fingers, and the left side of the patient's neck with your left fingers.

Movements, Barriers, and Forces

Use both hands to do the following:

- Layer palpate to the affected musculature.
- Apply anteriorly directed forces with all contacting fingers and hold this force.
- Add a traction force to stretch the muscle longitudinally by pulling the musculature from inferior to superior until a restrictive barrier is felt. The distance of the stretch should be approximately one to two vertebral levels.
- Hold the anterior and superior traction forces for 1 to 3 seconds, noting tissue changes.
- Release forces but not tissue contacts and allow tissues to return to neutral position.
- Repeat steps 2–5 in a rhythmic manner until the tissues soften and stretch with ease.
- Release forces and tissue contacts and move fingers superiorly. Repeat the technique on all affected musculature.
- Perform for ~ 2 minutes. Use more repetition on the areas of significant restriction.
- Retest the musculature for changes in tension.

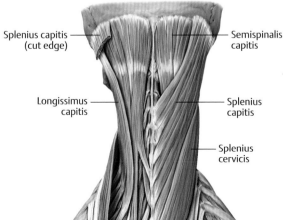

Splenius capitis (cut edge)
Semispinalis capitis
Longissimus capitis
Splenius capitis
Splenius cervicis

Fig. 5.2   Cervical paraspinal musculature.

Thoracic and Lumbar, Inhibitory Pressure

This technique is applicable beyond normalizing muscle tone. It is traditionally used to diminish sympathetic tone generated by a viscerosomatic or somatovisceral reflex via affecting the posterior and cutaneous dorsal rami nerves (**Fig. 5.3**). This technique also works well for bedridden and hospitalized patients.

Key Elements

- Somatic dysfunction corrected: right, left, or bilateral somatic dysfunction of musculature in the thoracic and/or lumbar region. Muscles included are the iliocostalis, longissimus, spinalis, and multifidus.
- End goal: to loosen musculature by creating sustained inhibitory forces perpendicularly directed into the muscle fibers of the paraspinal musculature.

WATCH ▷ ▶ ▷

▶ *Video 5.3 Thoracic and Lumbar Inhibitory Pressure–Narrated*

Example Somatic Dysfunction: Left Upper Thoracic Paraspinal Musculature Hypertonicity

---

Positioning and Preparation

▶ Patient: supine.

▶ Physician: sitting at the side of the table on the side of and near the region with somatic dysfunction.

Tissue Contact

- Both hands create the corrective inhibitory forces.
- Performing hands: contact the affected paraspinal musculature with the pads of all fingers, resting your forearms on the table. You may ask the patient to roll away from you to make contact.
  - Detailed suggestion: because the hand placement cannot be well visualized, first locate the spinous processes with your finger pads. Then retract your hands toward yourself, past the medial edge of the paraspinal musculature, until you are beneath the muscle bellies.

Movements, Barriers, and Forces

Use both hands to do the following:

- Layer palpate to the musculature.
- Apply anteriorly directed forces into the paraspinal musculature with the pads of all fingers. Use your forearms for leverage by keeping your wrists relatively stiff and leaning your body weight forward onto your arms.
- Continue increasing the anteriorly directed forces until a restrictive barrier is felt in all fingers.
- Hold forces and body positions until the tissues soften, or for ~ 2 minutes.
- Release forces and tissue contacts.
- Move hands and body inferiorly and repeat the technique, steps 2–5, on all affected musculature.
- Retest the musculature for changes in tension.

Fig. 5.3 Thoracic musculature and nerves.

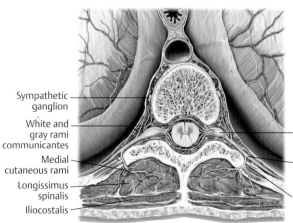

Sympathetic ganglion
White and gray rami communicantes
Medial cutaneous rami
Longissimus spinalis
Iliocostalis
Spinal ganglion
Anterior (ventral) ramus
Posterior (dorsal) ramus

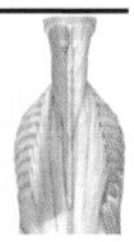

Thoracic and Lumbar, Longitudinal Stretching

This technique is useful in conjunction with thoracic and lumbar lateral stretching. Do not use too much anterior force or limit the patient's ability to breathe (**Fig. 5.4**).

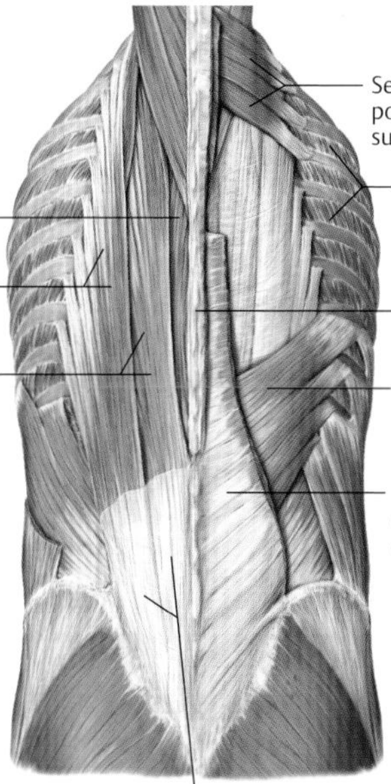

Key Elements

- Somatic dysfunction corrected: right, left or bilateral somatic dysfunction of musculature in the thoracic and/or lumbar region. Muscles included are the iliocostalis, longissimus, and spinalis.
- End goal: to longitudinally stretch the thoracic and lumbar paraspinal musculature on one side.

WATCH ▷▶▷

- ▶ *Video 5.4a Thoracic and Lumbar Longitudinal Stretching—Real-Time*
- ▶ *Video 5.4b Thoracic and Lumbar Longitudinal Stretching—Narrated*

Example Somatic Dysfunction: Right Upper Thoracic Paraspinal Musculature Hypertonicity

---

Fig. 5.4 labels: Serratus posterior superior; External intercostal muscles; Spinalis; Iliocostalis; Longissimus; Trapezius (cut); Serratus posterior inferior; Latissimus dorsi (cut) aponeurosis; Thoracolumbar fascia, superficial layer

Fig. 5.4 Posterior thoracic musculature.

Positioning and Preparation

- ▶ Patient: prone with the head resting in the head rest or turned to one side.
- ▶ Physician: standing beside the table on the side of the somatic dysfunction.

Tissue Contact

- Both hands create the corrective stretching forces.
- Performing hands: contact the bellies of the affected musculature with the heel of each hand. Place hands side by side so that the fingers of one hand point superiorly and the fingers of the other hand point inferiorly.

Movements, Barriers, and Forces

Use both hands to do the following:

- Layer palpate to the affected musculature.
- Apply an anteriorly directed force into the musculature until resistance is felt. Hold this force. This is best done by keeping the arms relatively stiff and leaning your body weight into the arms.
- Simultaneously apply traction forces with both hands along the longitudinal axis of the musculature.
  - Create a superior traction force using the hand with the fingers pointing superiorly. An inferior traction force is created by the other hand. The distance of the stretch is approximately one to two vertebral levels. Avoid twisting motions.
- Hold all forces for 1 to 3 seconds, noting tissue changes.
- Release forces but not tissue contacts and allow tissues to return to neutral position.
- Repeat steps 2–5 in a rhythmic manner once or twice more until the tissues soften and stretch with ease.
- Move hands and body inferiorly and repeat the technique on all affected musculature.
- Perform for ~ 2 minutes. Use more repetition on the areas of significant restriction.
- Retest the musculature for changes in tension.

Thoracic and Lumbar, Lateral Stretching

This technique is useful diagnostically because bilateral thoracic and lumbar regions can be quickly assessed for somatic dysfunction (**Fig. 5.5**).

Key Elements

- Somatic dysfunction corrected: right, left, or bilateral somatic dysfunction of musculature of the thoracic and/or lumbar region. Muscles included are the iliocostalis, longissimus, and spinalis.
- End goal: to laterally stretch the deep thoracic and lumbar paraspinal musculature.

WATCH ▷ ▶ ▷

▶ *Video 5.5a Thoracic and Lumbar Lateral Stretching—Real Time*

▶ *Video 5.5b Thoracic and Lumbar Lateral Stretching—Narrated*

Example Somatic Dysfunction: Right Upper Thoracic Paraspinal Musculature Hypertonicity

Positioning and Preparation

▶ Patient: prone, with head resting in the head rest or turned to one side.

▶ Physician: standing at one side of the table, at the level of the upper/midthoracic region, on the side opposite the somatic dysfunction.

Tissue Contact

- The heels of both hands create the stretching forces.
- Performing hands: contact the medial edge of the upper thoracic musculature, on the side opposite that on which you are standing, with the heels of both hands. Place hands side by side with fingers pointing laterally, or away from you.

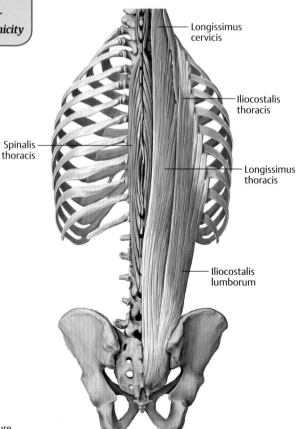

Longissimus cervicis

Iliocostalis thoracis

Spinalis thoracis

Longissimus thoracis

Iliocostalis lumborum

Fig. 5.5 Thoracic and lumbar paraspinal musculature.

- Detailed suggestion: locate the spinous processes with your fingertips. Move your fingertips away from you, laterally, until you feel a dip in the tissue contour. Continue moving fingertips laterally until the tissue contour raises. This is the medial edge of the paraspinal musculature.

Movements, Barriers, and Forces

Use both hands to do the following:

- Layer palpate to the affected musculature.
- Apply anteriorly directed forces into the musculature until resistance is felt. Hold these forces. Keep your arms relatively stiff and lean your body weight to create the forces.
- Add lateral traction to stretch the muscle until a restrictive barrier is felt.
- Hold the anterior and lateral forces for 1 to 3 seconds, noting tissue changes.
- Release forces but not tissue contacts and allow tissues to return to neutral position.

- Repeat steps 2–5 in a rhythmic manner once or twice more until the tissues soften and stretch with ease.
- Move your hands and body inferiorly and repeat the technique on all affected musculature.
- Perform for ~ 2 minutes on each side. Use more repetition on the areas of significant restriction.
- Retest the musculature for changes in tension.

Alternate Positioning: Lateral Recumbent

With patient laterally recumbent, stand in front of the patient. Contact the musculature on the side not in contact with the table. Create anterior, then laterally directed forces as described in the technique. Brace the patient to prevent excessive forward rotation by contacting the patient's hips and shoulders with your forearms. As you produce anteriorly directed forces, tractioning toward yourself, the patient will roll a bit forward, but you can brace the shoulders and hips with your forearms.

Upper Thoracic/Scapula, Lateral and Longitudinal Stretching

This technique affects both paraspinal and periscapular musculature simultaneously (**Fig. 5.6**). Perform this early on as part of a complete osteopathic manipulative approach for the treatment of any shoulder, upper thoracic, or upper rib condition.

Key Elements

- Somatic dysfunction corrected: right, left, or bilateral somatic dysfunction in the upper thoracic and/or medial periscapular region. Muscles included are the latissimus dorsi, levator scapulae, rhomboid major and minor, iliocostalis, longissimus, and spinalis.
- End goal: to longitudinally stretch the periscapular musculature and laterally stretch the spinal musculature.

WATCH ▷ ▶ ▷

▶ *Video 5.6a Upper Thoracic/Scapular Longitudinal and Lateral Stretching—Real-Time*

▶ *Video 5.6b Upper Thoracic/Scapular Longitudinal and Lateral Stretching—Narrated*

Example Somatic Dysfunction: Left Upper Thoracic/Scapular Musculature Hypertonicity

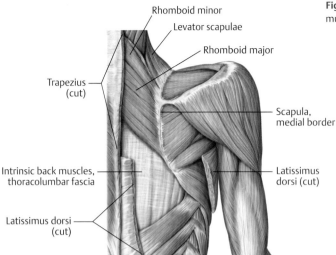

Rhomboid minor

Levator scapulae

Rhomboid major

Trapezius
(cut)

Scapula,
medial border

Intrinsic back muscles,
thoracolumbar fascia

Latissimus
dorsi (cut)

Latissimus dorsi
(cut)

Fig. 5.6 Upper thoracic and periscapular musculature.

Positioning and Preparation

▶ Patient: lying laterally recumbent on the side of the nondysfunctional shoulder with bent knees and with the head and neck in a neutral position, resting on a pillow or the arm, whichever is more comfortable for the patient.

▶ Physician: standing facing the front of the patient at the level of the patient's shoulders.

Tissue Contact

• Both hands create the corrective stretching forces and move the scapula for access to the deeper paraspinal musculature.

• Performing hands: tissue contact is best made sequentially, as follows:

– With the hand that is closer to the patient's head, contact the superior and lateral edge of the scapula with the side of your thumb and thenar eminence. Then contact the medial periscapular and spinal musculature with your finger pads.

– Drape the patient's arm over your arm as it contacts the scapula.

– With your free hand, contact the inferior and lateral edge of the scapula with the side of your thumb and thenar eminence. Then contact the medial periscapular and spinal musculature with your finger pads. Hands and fingers may overlap.

Movements, Barriers, and Forces

• With your finger pads that are contacting the more inferior musculature, layer palpate to the affected musculature.

• With both thumbs, gently push the scapula medially to release tension in the periscapular musculature.

• Apply anteriorly directed forces with your finger pads into the inferior periscapular musculature until resistance is felt. Hold these forces.

• Apply lateral traction forces directed at an angle toward the humeral head until a restrictive barrier is felt. Allow the scapula to move.

• Hold the forces for 1 to 3 seconds, noting tissue changes.

• Release forces but not tissue contacts and allow the scapula and tissues to return to neutral position.

• Repeat steps 2–6 in a rhythmic manner until the tissues soften and stretch with ease.

• Without releasing tissue contacts, layer palpate to the more superiorly located musculature and repeat the technique (steps 2–6) on all affected musculature.

• Perform for ~ 2 minutes. Use more repetition on the areas of significant restriction.

• Retest the musculature for changes in tension.

Lumbar, Lateral Stretching with the Hip as a Lever

This technique is very similar to thoracic and lumbar lateral stretching. The addition of pelvic rotation by using the patient's hip as a lever, improves tissue contact of the lumbar musculature by providing a counterforce (**Fig. 5.7**).

Key Elements

- Somatic dysfunction corrected: right, left, or bilateral somatic dysfunction of the lumbar musculature. Muscles included are the latissimus dorsi, iliocostalis, longissimus, quadratus lumborum, and multifidus.
- End goal: to laterally stretch the lumbar musculature using hip rotation as a counterforce.

WATCH ▷▶▷

- ▶ *Video 5.7a Lumbar Lateral Stretching With Hip as a Lever—Real Time*
- ▶ *Video 5.7b Lumbar Lateral Stretching With Hip as a Lever—Narrated*

Example Somatic Dysfunction: Right Lumbar Paraspinal Musculature Hypertonicity

Positioning and Preparation

- ▶ Patient: prone with head resting in the head rest or turned to one side, whichever is more comfortable for the patient.
- ▶ Physician: standing at one side of the table, at the level of the lumbar region on the side opposite the dysfunctional musculature.

Tissue Contact

- One hand creates the corrective stretching forces. The other hand assists by lifting the hip to create a counterforce for the performing hand.
- Performing hand: use the hand that is nearer the patient's head. Contact the medial edge of the paraspinal musculature with the heel of your hand at the level of the thoracolumbar junction on the side opposite to that on which you are standing.
- Assisting hand: with your other hand, contact the anterior superior iliac spine (ASIS) on the side opposite to that on which you are standing with your second, third, and/or fourth fingers. Gently grasp the ASIS and avoid digging into the tissues.

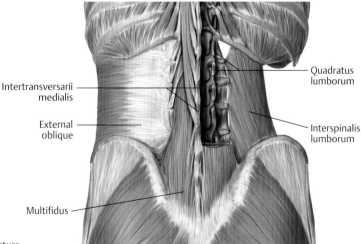

Fig. 5.7   Posterior lumbar musculature.

– If the patient is sensitive or ticklish, have the patient cover her ASIS with her hand. Place your fingers on top of the patient's and ask the patient to slowly remove her hand while your fingers replace hers to contact the ASIS.

Movements, Barriers, and Forces

- With the assisting hand, lift the ASIS in a posterior direction so it is off the table, until a slight stretch is felt with the performing hand. Do this by leaning forward, hold your arm relatively stiff, then lean backward using your body weight to lift the ASIS.
- With the performing hand, apply an anteriorly directed force into the musculature until resistance is felt. Hold this force.
- Add a laterally directed traction force to stretch the muscle away from the midline until a restrictive barrier is felt. Concurrently, with the assisting hand, guide the ASIS anteriorly as it rolls back onto the table due to your performing hand forces.
- With the performing hand, continue creating the anterior and lateral forces until the ASIS almost returns to the table. This should be a total of 3 to 5 seconds in duration.
- With the performing hand, release forces but not tissue contact and allow the tissues to return to neutral position.
- Repeat steps 1–5 in a rhythmic manner once or twice more until the tissues soften and stretch with ease.
- Move your performing hand inferiorly and repeat the technique (steps 1–7) on all affected musculature.
- Perform for ~ 2 minutes on each side. Use more repetition on the areas of significant restriction.
- Retest the musculature for changes in tension.

Chapter Summary

Soft tissue technique is a direct method of osteopathic manipulation that is ideal for beginners. It can be performed either as a primary treatment or in preparation for other techniques. This chapter presented relevant background information and addressed the specific soft tissue modalities of inhibitory pressure, lateral stretching, and longitudinal stretching. The most commonly performed techniques for treatment of spinal musculature were described. Included in each technique was an end goal, a description of the types of somatic dysfunction that can be treated, and a reminder to retest.

Clinical Cases and Review Questions

Case 1

A 44-year-old man presents with diffuse neck soreness and stiffness for 4 weeks, since moving and starting a new job. He is having difficulty turning his head to the right and feels like there are muscle knots in the back of his neck. He denies paresthesias, arm and hand weakness, and constitutional symptoms. His has no significant past medical history. Physical exam reveals decreased range of motion in right cervical rotation, right side bending, and extension. Neurological and orthopedic exams are negative.

Q1. After obtaining permission from the patient, you start performing cervical longitudinal stretching
   A. As a diagnostic process for identification of segmental vertebral somatic dysfunction.
   B. As a method of getting him to relax so you can counsel him about his stressors.
   C. To resolve his neck soreness and stiffness.
   D. To decrease sympathetic tone to alleviate some of his discomfort.
   E. To normalize parasympathetic tone to improve blood flow.

Q2. While performing cervical longitudinal stretching, you
   A. Apply repetitive superior traction forces into the bilateral cervical paraspinal musculature.
   B. Create and hold sustained inhibitory forces in the musculature that is just inferior to the superior nuchal line.
   C. Extend the head and neck to shorten the cervical musculature.
   D. Position the neck in right rotation, right side bending, and extension.
   E. Stretch the neck musculature by first rotating to the left and then side bending to the left.

Case 2

A 25-year-old woman has had back pain for 3 weeks. It began while she was working in her garden. She has pain on the right side that is worse with movement, especially going from sitting to standing, and when she lies supine. Her past medical history is remarkable for one uncomplicated spontaneous vaginal delivery 2 years ago. She takes no prescribed medications, but has taken ibuprofen at night with some relief. Once she falls asleep, she is able to stay asleep. She denies radiation, tingling, weakness, and loss of bowel or bladder control. The exam reveals tightness in the right paraspinal musculature from T10 to L3.

Q3. You start performing a lateral stretching technique by
   A. Using the pads of your fingers to contact the spinous processes of T10.
   B. Placing your elbow on her paraspinal musculature, starting at T10.
   C. Contacting the affected musculature with your thenar eminence and thumb.
   D. Lifting the ASIS superiorly and rotating it.
   E. Sitting at the side of the table.

Q4. You consider performing lateral traction to address her somatic dysfunction. Which of the following would be a contraindication to performing this technique?
   A. Pain that radiates to her groin.
   B. Paleness on the skin after performing a red reflex test.
   C. Suspected vertebral fracture.
   D. Suspected viscerosomatic reflex due to constipation.
   E. Tenderness of the lumbar muscles.

Answers to Review Questions

Q1. The correct answer is **A**. ST techniques can be used in this case as a diagnostic procedure because no somatic dysfunction diagnosis has been made yet.

B is incorrect. ST techniques may help him relax, but not for the purposes of using counseling as the primary treatment.

C is incorrect. ST techniques will not resolve his neck soreness necessarily because we do not know if he has somatic dysfunction beyond muscular.

D is incorrect. The sympathetic nervous system is usually affected with OMT directed at the chain ganglia in the thoracic/lumbar spine.

E is incorrect. This patient has no signs or symptoms related to abnormal parasympathetic nervous system function.

Q2. **A** is correct.

B is incorrect. This is a step of the head/cervical inhibitory pressure technique.

C–E are incorrect because they are not steps of ST techniques.

Q3. The correct answer is **C**. None of the other answer choices describe the tissue contact for this technique.

A is incorrect. This is the contact for thoracic and lumbar inhibition technique.

B is incorrect. This is not a contact for any ST technique.

D is incorrect. This is the contact for lumbar lateral stretching with the hip as a lever technique.

E is incorrect. This is the preparation and positioning for the thoracic and lumbar inhibition technique.

Q4. The correct answer is **C**.

Answers **A, B, D,** and **E** are not contraindications to performing any ST technique.

References

1. Johnson SM, Kurtz ME. Osteopathic manipulative treatment techniques preferred by contemporary osteopathic physicians. J Am Osteopath Assoc 2003;103(5):219–224

Research Bibliography

Antolinos-Campillo PJ, Oliva-Pascual-Vaca A, Rodríguez-Blanco C, Heredia-Rizo AM, Espí-López GV, Ricard F. Short-term changes in median nerve neural tension after a suboccipital muscle inhibition technique in subjects with cervical whiplash: a randomised controlled trial. Physiotherapy 2014;100(3):249–255

Aparicio ÉQ, Quirante LB, Blanco CR, Sendín FA. Immediate effects of the suboccipital muscle inhibition technique in subjects with short hamstring syndrome. J Manipulative Physiol Ther 2009;32(4):262–269

Heredia Rizo AM, Pascual-Vaca ÁO, Cabello MA, Blanco CR, Pozo FP, Carrasco AL. Immediate effects of the suboccipital muscle inhibition technique in craniocervical posture and greater occipital nerve mechanosensitivity in subjects with a history of orthodontia use: a randomized trial. J Manipulative Physiol Ther 2012;35(6):446–453

López E, Victoria G, Pascual-Vaca AO. Atlanto-occipital joint manipulation and suboccipital inhibition technique in the osteopathic treatment of patients with tension-type headache. Eur J Osteopathy Clin Related Res 2012;7(1):10–21

Oliveira-Campelo NM, Rubens-Rebelatto J, Martí N-Vellejo FJ, Alburquerque-Sendi NF, Fernández-de-Las-Peñas C. The immediate effects of atlanto-occipital joint manipulation and suboccipital muscle inhibition technique on active mouth opening and pressure pain sensitivity over latent myofascial trigger points in the masticatory muscles. J Orthop Sports Phys Ther 2010;40(5):310–317

6 Myofascial Release Techniques

LEARNING OBJECTIVES

1. Explain the goals of performing myofascial release techniques.
2. Identify the clinical considerations, including indications, contraindications, and precautions for performing myofascial release techniques.
3. Compare and contrast the indirect and direct methods of performing myofascial release techniques.
4. Outline the general movements, barriers, and forces used when performing myofascial release techniques.
5. Visualize, verbalize, and identify the preparation, positioning, tissue contact, movements, barriers, and forces for each myofascial release technique.
6. Perform the techniques using appropriate somatic dysfunction diagnosis, preparation, positioning, tissue contact, movements, barriers, forces, retest for effectiveness, communication, and safe tissue handling.

Myofascial Release Techniques Introduction

Fascia encircles and permeates every joint, bone, muscle, and organ throughout the body. When fascia is impaired, normal body processes and movement are affected. Myofascial release (MFR) techniques correct fascial somatic dysfunction, positively influencing a variety of disease processes from musculoskeletal to visceral. MFR is perhaps the gentlest of all osteopathic techniques for both the physician and the patient, and can be performed in the context of a wide variety of patient clinical conditions. The end goal of MFR techniques is to normalize abnormal fascial tensions through positioning fascia and use of mild forces. By restoring normal fascial tone, MFR techniques restore the following fascial properties:

- Viscoelasticity.
- Creep.
- Relaxation.
- Hysteresis.

MFR techniques also improve the following fascial functions:

- Biostructural support.
- Delivery of reparative fibroblasts.
- Biochemical signaling.

MFR techniques can be used as a primary treatment for somatic dysfunction, as a diagnostic aid, or as a preparatory treatment for other osteopathic manipulative techniques, such as high velocity, low amplitude.

Background

The history of the use of MFR in osteopathic medicine is traceable to its founder, Dr. Still. He wrote extensively about the fascia and its importance in the maintenance of health.

> I know of no part of the body that equals the fascia as a hunting-ground. . . . By its actions we live and by its failure we die.[1]

There are numerous variations to the foundational MFR techniques presented here, and all are effective. Those attributed to osteopathic physicians include integrated neuromuscular release, ligamentous articular strain, and the fascial distortion model. Two basic types of MFR techniques have been selected for this manual: single and multiple direction.

Research

MFR has been used as part of the protocol in many osteopathic manipulative treatment basic science and clinical research studies. An International Fascia Research Congress has met regularly since 2007 to discuss fascia research and clinical applications. A brief research bibliography is provided at the end of this chapter.

Clinical Considerations

Some common clinical points to consider for using MFR techniques are listed in Table 6.1. Always acquire adequate data in the form of an appropriate history, a thorough physical exam, and relevant diagnostic tests to exercise best clinical judgment before performing osteopathic manipulative treatment.

Table 6.1 Clinical considerations		
Indications	**Contraindications**	**Precautions**
Nerve entrapment syndromes	Skin that is broken or infected	Avoid performing techniques on the abdomen soon after the patient has eaten.
Enthesopathies	Fracture or suspected fracture	
Plantar fasciitis	Joint dislocation	
Chronic pain conditions	Necrotizing fasciitis	Modify or discontinue the technique if it causes pain.
Infectious or inflammatory conditions	Implanted medical equipment/ devices (e.g., intravenous line, feeding tube, pacemaker)	
	Acute compartment syndrome	
	Acute abdominal emergency	

Somatic Dysfunction Corrected

MFR techniques correct somatic dysfunction in the fascia, which is identified on exam by tissue texture changes or passive range of motion restriction. Routinely, tissue texture changes and specific passive range of motion directions are identified immediately before MFR technique performance. For this reason, somatic dysfunction diagnosis instructions are included in each Movements, Barriers, and Forces section of the technique steps. Identification of fascial tightness is a sufficient somatic dysfunction diagnosis for single-direction MFR techniques. However, identification of directions of fascial range of passive motion is required for multiple direction techniques.

Positioning and Preparation

▶ Patient: the patient must be comfortable and remain relaxed for the duration of the technique. MFR can be performed with the patient seated, supine, prone, or laterally recumbent.

▶ Physician: the physician must be comfortable and positioned to ensure safety, using the best ergonomic posture and movements possible.

Note: The videos include a narrated description of positioning when it is not visually self-explanatory.

Tissue Contact

Tissue contact is usually made directly over the affected fascia. The entire palmar surface or the finger pads of one or both hands may be used. Typically, both hands contact the tissues and are performing hands.

Movements, Barriers, and Forces

Fascia responds to positioning that is either toward or away from restrictive barriers. This means that MFR can be performed in a direct or an indirect method for somatic dysfunction correction. The physician chooses which method to use based on clinical judgment and the patient's condition. When fascias are positioned with either method, the body's inherent homeostatic mechanisms are activated and the fascias return to functional or normal tension. Therefore, it is important to continuously monitor the fascia to appreciate the body's responses to the changes created in the fascia. Movements should proceed slowly to allow time for fascia to respond (fascial creep, elasticity) and to avoid creating a guarding reflex or reflex spasm of associated musculature.

When performing multiple-direction MFR techniques, the fascias should be moved into one plane at a time, holding the fascia at each position, essentially "stacking" the motions. For example, with thoracolumbar fascial somatic dysfunction of superior, left translation, and clockwise twist, the fascia should first be positioned in a superior direction and held. Then the fascia is positioned left and held. Finally, the fascia is positioned in a clockwise direction. Because motion in one plane affects motion in all other planes, the fascial motion at the last position will be less than at the first.

Table 6.2 summarizes direct and indirect methods of MFR techniques.

Optional Technique Enhancements

• Fascial unwinding: fascial unwinding is an additional way to continuously release fascial tissues and can be used with most MFR techniques. To perform fascial unwinding, after the first change in tissue tension occurs, reposition the fascias in all directions of tightness when using direct method or looseness when using indirect method. Continue repositioning fascias as subsequent releases are palpated until restrictive barriers are eliminated or no further tissue changes occur.

• Respiratory cooperation: respiratory cooperation can be employed in any MFR technique when the physician is holding the fascias in position and awaiting their release. Refer to chapter 2 for a full description.

Retest for Effectiveness

Changes in fascial tensions and increased warmth are signs that the technique has been effective and are collectively referred to as a release. This is the indication that the somatic dysfunction is resolving

Table 6.2 Direct and indirect methods of myofascial release techniques

	Direct method MFR	Indirect method MFR
Type of MFR	Single direction Multiple direction	Multiple direction only
Best use	Smaller fascial regions Areas with limited access Tendons	Larger sheets of fascia Three-dimensional regions of fascia Tubes of fascia
Movements, barriers	Single direction: forces are perpendicular to the fascial plane Multiple direction: movements are in the directions of the restrictive barriers	Multiple direction: movements are in the directions of the physiological barriers (opposite the restrictive barriers)
Forces	Forces match or just exceed the tension in the fascia	Forces create fascial loosening Forces are usually lighter than those used in the direct method
Palpatory feel	Stretching, tightness, fascial pulls	Softness, neutrality, lack of fascial pulls

or is resolved. When performing a direct method, fascial changes are usually loosening or softening. Changes with an indirect method include further fascial loosening and may include a sense of movement or slippage of the tissues because the restrictive barrier is no longer present and range of motion is increased. When changes associated with a release are palpated, forces should be released but not the tissue contacts. Alternatively, if a release is not palpated, the technique should be performed continuously for ~ 2 minutes, which is sufficient time to initiate fascial changes. Then the forces should be released but not the tissue contacts. In either case, the fascia should be retested for changes in somatic dysfunction. If resolution of somatic dysfunction does not occur in ~ 2 minutes, the tissue contacts should be rechecked to ascertain that the correct fascial layer is being addressed, and then the technique can be performed again. Adding one of the technique enhancements should be considered. After the second attempt, rediagnosis of the patient's clinical condition and related somatic dysfunction is warranted.

MFR Technique Summary Steps

- Layer palpate to the affected fascial layer.
- Identify fascial somatic dysfunction in a single plane or multiple planes.
  - If the fascial somatic dysfunction is in a single plane, use a direct method for positioning.
  - If the fascial somatic dysfunctions are in multiple planes, choose a direct or an indirect method for positioning.
- Move the fascia into the appropriate position(s) for the technique type and chosen method.
- Hold forces and position(s).
- Monitor fascia(s) until release or for ~ 2 minutes.
  - Optional: add fascial unwinding and/or respiratory cooperation.
- Release forces and return fascias to a neutral position.
- Retest the fascia for changes in somatic dysfunction.

Cervical, Submandibular Fascia

MFR Type: Single Direction, Direct Method

This technique is helpful for patients with dysphasia or vocal disorders. Although not specifically categorized as a lymphatic technique, this technique also releases fascial restrictions around the submental lymph nodes. Thus this technique is applicable as an adjunct treatment in cases of upper respiratory tract infections, sinusitis, or dental infections (**Fig. 6.1**).

Key Elements

- Somatic dysfunction corrected: submandibular fascia tightness. Fascias include the cervical investing, muscular, and/or visceral pretracheal fascias.
- End goal: to decrease tension in the submandibular fascias.

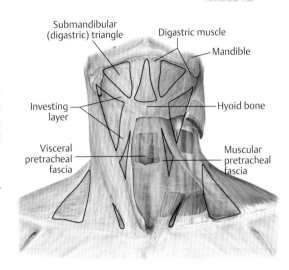

Fig. 6.1 Submandibular fascia.

WATCH ▷ ▶ ▷

▶ *Video 6.1 Cervical Submandibular Fascia—Narrated*

Example Somatic Dysfunction: Bilateral Submandibular Fascial Tightness

---

Note: Allow the patient to swallow during technique performance.

Positioning and Preparation

▶ Patient: supine.
▶ Physician: sitting at the head of the table.

Tissue Contact

- Both hands create the corrective stretching forces.
- Contact the submandibular fascia with the pads of the second fingers on either side of the inferior surface of the symphysis menti. Place the third and fourth fingers alongside the second fingers on the inferior surface of the symphysis menti. Slightly curl the fingers so they contact the posterior mandibular surface.

Movements, Barriers, and Forces

Use both hands to do the following:

- Layer palpate to the affected fascial layer: skin → superficial fascia → musculature → deep fascia.
- Apply gentle superiorly directed forces into the fascial layer and hold these forces.
  - Identify areas of tissue texture changes.
- Apply lateral and additional superiorly directed stretching forces until resistance is felt, maintaining contact with the mandible.
- Hold forces and positions.
- Monitor fascias until release or for ~ 2 minutes.
  - Optional: add fascial unwinding and/or respiratory cooperation.
- Release forces and return fascias to neutral position.
- Retest the submandibular fascia for changes in tension.
- Move fingers laterally if necessary and repeat the technique until all affected submandibular fascia has been addressed.

Upper Thoracic and Sternal Fascia

MFR Type: Multiple Direction, Direct or Indirect Method

This technique can be used to continue treatment of the anterior cervical fascias with the addition of a posterior contact. The posterior contact allows for treatment of a large three-dimensional body region and serves as an introduction to the use of two hands treating independently (**Fig. 6.2**). Be sure to first describe the hand contacts and steps of the technique to patients when working in this sensitive area.

Key Elements

- Somatic dysfunction corrected: upper thoracic vertebral and sternal fascia passive range of motion restrictions. Advance this technique by applying it to the deeper visceral endothoracic fascias.

- End goal: to release the posterior thoracic and anterior sternal fascias together as one functional unit.

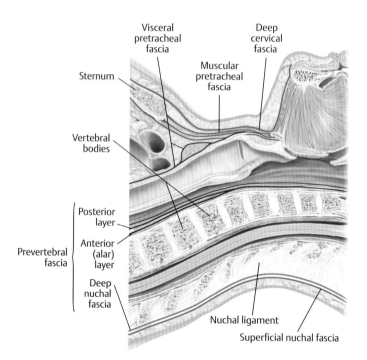

Fig. 6.2 Fascias of the upper thoracic and cervical regions.

WATCH ▷ ► ▷

► *Video 6.2 Upper Thoracic and Sternal Fascia—Narrated*

Example Somatic Dysfunction: Fascias are Extended, Rotated Left, and Twisted in a Clockwise Direction

Positioning and Preparation

► Patient: supine.

► Physician: sitting at the head of the table.

Tissue Contact

- Both hands position the fascias. Use one hand to contact the patient's posterior fascias, the other to contact the anterior fascias.
- Performing hand, posterior contact: contact the upper thoracic fascias with the palm and fingers of one hand.
  - Place the heel of the hand at the C7/T1 region, and make space between the second and third fingers for the spinous processes. Place the forearm on the edge of the table to be used as a fulcrum.
- Performing hand, anterior contact: contact the sternum with the palm on the sternal notch and the second and third fingers along the long axis of the sternum.
  - For female patients, adjust the hand contacts to avoid the breast tissue. Do this by contacting the sternum only with the middle finger (lift other fingers off of the patient), or use the ulnar side of the hand.

Movements, Barriers, and Forces

Use both hands to do the following:

- Layer palpate to the affected fascial layer: skin → superficial fascia → bone and musculature → endothoracic fascia → deep structural fascia.
- Test fascias for somatic dysfunction in three directions of motion.
  - Rotation: move the anterior fascias to the right and the posterior fascias to the left to test right rotation. Reverse motions to test left rotation.
  - Flexion/extension: move the anterior fascias inferiorly and the posterior fascias superiorly to test flexion. Reverse motions to test extension.
  - Twist: rotate the anterior fascias clockwise and the posterior fascias counterclockwise to test clockwise twist. Reverse motions to test counterclockwise twist. Clockwise motion is named for the motion of the anterior fascias, with the sternal notch at 12 o'clock.
- Move the fascia in all directions of motion ease (indirect method), or all directions of motion restriction (direct method). Move fascias in one direction at a time.
- Hold forces and positions.
- Monitor fascias until release or for ~ 2 minutes.
  - Optional: add fascial unwinding and/or respiratory cooperation.
- Release forces and return fascias to neutral position.
- Retest the thoracic and sternal fascias for changes in passive ranges of motion.

Thoracic, Thoracic Outlet

MFR Type: Multiple Direction, Direct or Indirect Method

MFR performed on the thoracic outlet releases fascial tensions around the terminal lymphatic ducts (**Fig. 6.3**). Therefore, this is often the first technique performed as part of a lymphatic treatment. Sometimes this technique is called the steering wheel technique, as hand movements mimic those of holding the steering wheel of a bus.

Key Elements

- Somatic dysfunction corrected: thoracic outlet fascia passive range of motion restrictions. Fascias include the prevertebral and pretracheal layers.
- End goal: to release fascial tensions in the right and left thoracic outlet regions.

WATCH ▷▶▷

- ▶ *Video 6.3 Thoracic, Thoracic Outlet— Narrated*

Example Somatic Dysfunction: Fascias are Rotated Right Flexed, and Translated to the Left

---

Positioning and Preparation

- ▶ Patient: seated so that the tops of the patient's shoulders can be contacted when the physician is standing.

- ▶ Physician: standing behind the patient, facing the patient's back.
- ▶ Alternate positioning: patient supine and physician sitting at the head of the table.

Tissue Contact

- Both hands position the fascias. Use your right hand to contact the patient's right thoracic outlet and your left hand to contact the patient's left side.
- Performing hands: contact as much fascia of the thoracic outlet as possible with the palms and fingers of both hands. Avoid leaving gaps between your hand contact and the patient's skin.
  - Contact the transverse or spinous processes of C7/T1 region with the thumbs.
  - Contact the lateral and anterior cervical fascias with the fingers, avoiding neurovascular structures.
  - Contact the fascia just above the clavicles with the fingertips of the second and third digits. The fourth and fifth digits may contact the clavicle or extend inferiorly near the first rib.
  - Contact the fascias around the trapezius with the remainder of the hand/palm.

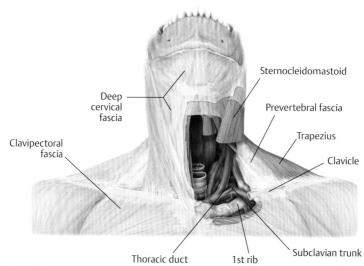

Fig. 6.3 Thoracic outlet.

Movements, Barriers, and Forces

Use both hands to do the following:

- Layer palpate to the affected fascial layer: skin → superficial fascia → musculature → deep fascia.
- Test fascias for somatic dysfunction in three directions of motion. The patient's shoulders may move slightly.
  - Rotation: turn fascias to the right (as if steering to the right) to test right rotation. Reverse directions to test left rotation.
  - Flexion/extension: move fascias inferiorly and thumbs superiorly to test flexion. Reverse directions to test extension.
  - Translation: move fascias to the right to test translation to the right. Reverse directions to test left translation.
- Move the fascia in all directions of motion ease (indirect method), or all directions of motion restriction (direct method).
- Hold forces and positions.
- Monitor fascias until release or for ~ 2 minutes.
  - Optional: add fascial unwinding and/or respiratory cooperation.
- Release forces and return fascias to neutral position.
- Retest the fascias of the thoracic outlet for changes in passive ranges of motion.

Abdomen, Thoracoabdominal Diaphragm

MFR Type: Single Direction, Direct Method

This technique has colloquially been called redoming or doming of the diaphragm, because a tightened diaphragm cannot ascend into its normal domed shape with exhalation. Perform in conjunction with an indirect technique for the 11th and 12th ribs to completely treat the thoracoabdominal diaphragm and related fascias (**Fig. 6.4**). This technique is written to be coordinated with the patient's breathing, and fascial unwinding is incorporated in the steps of this technique.

Key Elements

- Somatic dysfunction corrected: anterior thoracoabdominal diaphragm fascial tightness or range of motion restrictions.
- End goal: to release tension in the fascias of the anterior thoracoabdominal diaphragm and anterior abdominal wall.

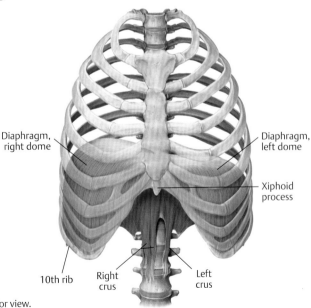

Fig. 6.4 Thoracoabdominal diaphragm, anterior view.

Positioning and Preparation

▶ Patient: supine with knees flexed and feet on the table for relaxation of the musculature of the abdominal wall.

▶ Physician: standing on one side of the table (for ease of contact, bend sideways at the waist toward the midline of the patient).

Tissue Contact

• Both thumbs and thenar eminences create the corrective stretching forces.
• Performing hands: contact the inferior margins of the costal cage with the thumbs and thenar eminences of both hands.
  – Detailed suggestion: abduct the thumbs and place the thumb tips on the inferior costal margins about a centimeter from the xiphoid process.

Movements, Barriers, and Forces

Coordinate movements with the patient's breath cycles. Use both hands to do the following:

• Ask the patient to breathe slowly and fully.
• During the patient's exhalation, layer palpate: skin → superficial fascia → abdominal musculature → diaphragm musculature and fascias.
  – Do this by extending the wrists so the thumbs and thenar eminences roll first inferiorly, then superiorly along the costal margins as the patient exhales. Maintain contact with the deeper tissues.
• On the patient's next inhalation, hold the forces and slightly limit diaphragmatic motion.
• During the patient's next exhalation, increase superiorly directed forces until tissue resistance is felt, matching forces with tissue tensions.
  – Note areas of somatic dysfunction.
• Continue alternating holding and increasing forces with the patient's breathing for three to four inhalation/exhalation cycles.
• Release forces.
• Retest the fascia for changes in tension and/or the thoracoabdominal diaphragm for improved motion.
• Move the thumbs laterally along the costal margin up to the level of the anterior axillary line and repeat the technique if somatic dysfunction is present in those fascias.

Abdomen, Thoracoabdominal Hemidiaphragm

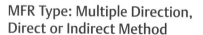

MFR Type: Multiple Direction, Direct or Indirect Method

This technique addresses both the anterior and the posterior thoracoabdominal diaphragm, one side at a time (**Fig. 6.5**). Therefore, it is an appropriate two-person technique.

Key Elements

• Somatic dysfunction corrected: thoracoabdominal diaphragm fascial passive range of motion restrictions.
• End goal: to release the fascias of the thoracoabdominal hemidiaphragm.

Positioning and Preparation

▶ Patient: supine with bent knees and feet resting on the table to relax the abdominal musculature.

▶ Physician: sitting at the side of the patient's dysfunctional hemidiaphragm at about the level of the hemidiaphragm, facing the patient.

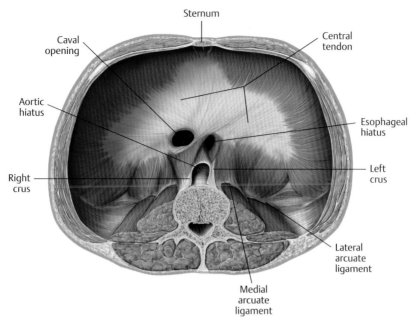

Fig. 6.5   Thoracoabdominal diaphragm, inferior view.

Tissue Contact

- Use one hand to contact the patient's posterior fascias, the other to contact the anterior fascias.
- Anterior performing hand contact: contact the anterior diaphragm fascias with the palm and second, third, and fourth fingers so that the heel of the hand is on the lateral costal margins and the fingers are near, but not contacting, the xiphoid process.
- Posterior performing hand contact: contact the posterior diaphragm fascias with the palm and second, third, and fourth fingers so that the heel of the hand is posterior to ribs 11 and 12 and the fingertips are near the costotransverse articulation.

Movements, Barriers, and Forces

Use both hands to do the following:

- Layer palpate to the affected fascial layer. The layers of the anterior and posterior regions will be different: skin → superficial fascia → muscle/bone → deeper fascia/musculature.
  - Test fascias for somatic dysfunction in three directions of motion.

- Rotation: move anterior fascias toward the right and posterior fascias to the left to test right rotation. Reverse directions to test left rotation.
- Flexion/extension: move anterior fascias inferiorly and posterior fascias superiorly to create flexion. Reverse directions to test extension.
- Side bending: move both anterior and posterior fascias into side bending away from the side you are contacting, so the fingers point at an angle inferiorly, toward the patient's opposite hip. Reverse directions to test side bending toward you (indicate right or left side bending).
- Move the fascia in all directions of motion ease (indirect method), or all directions of motion restriction (direct method). Position fascia in one direction at a time.
- Hold forces and positions.
- Monitor fascias until release or for ~ 2 minutes.
  - Optional: add fascial unwinding and/or respiratory cooperation.
- Release forces and return fascias to neutral position.
- Retest the diaphragmatic fascias for changes in passive ranges of motion.

Abdomen, Linea Alba

MFR Type: Single Direction, Direct Method

Beyond treating the abdominal wall fascia, this technique also improves the efficiency of breathing. When the anterior abdominal wall is unrestricted, the thoracoabdominal diaphragm can descend further, creating larger pressure differentials for more effective gas exchange and low pressure fluid flow. This technique can be extended inferiorly to the median umbilical ligament, located between the umbilicus and pelvic bone. Finally, this technique can be modified by directing forces more deeply and focused on the midline sympathetic ganglia: celiac, superior mesenteric, and inferior mesenteric (**Fig. 6.6**).

Note: Refer to chapters 4 and 14 for a complete list of contraindications and precautions.

Key Elements

- Somatic dysfunction corrected: linea alba tightness. Fascias include those that encapsulate the anterior abdominal wall musculature.
- End goal: to longitudinally stretch the linea alba and associated fascias.

> **WATCH ▷ ▶ ▷**
>
> ▶ **Video 6.6 Abdomen, Linea Alba—Narrated**
>
> **Example Somatic Dysfunction: Linea Alba Tightness**

Positioning and Preparation

▶ Patient: supine.

▶ Physician: standing at the side of the patient, at the level of the upper abdomen, facing the patient.

Tissue Contact

- Both hands create the corrective stretching forces.
- Performing hands: with the tips of the second, third, and fourth fingers of both hands, contact the fascias of the linea alba. The fingertips should be close together and the fingers bent.
  - Detailed suggestion: pronate forearms, and align the tips of the second, third, and fourth fingers so that the second fingertips of each hand are close together. Abduct the fingers enough so that the fifth digit

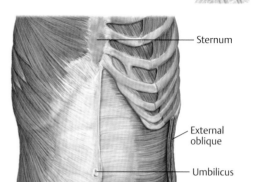

Fig. 6.6 Linea alba.

of the hand that is closer to the patient's head is about an inch from the xiphoid process and the fifth digit of the other hand is about an inch from the umbilicus.

Movements, Barriers, and Forces

Use both hands to do the following:

- Layer palpate to the affected fascial layer: skin → superficial fascia → linea alba.
- Apply posteriorly directed forces until resistance is felt. Hold these forces.
  - Note areas of somatic dysfunction.
- Add traction forces to longitudinally stretch the linea alba.
  - The hand that is nearer the patient's head moves superiorly and the other hand moves inferiorly.
  - If you easily and quickly feel the pulsation of the aorta, stop the technique and assess for an abdominal aortic aneurysm.
- Hold forces and positions.
- Monitor linea alba until release or for ~ 2 minutes.
  - Optional: add fascial unwinding and/or respiratory cooperation.
- Release forces and return fascias to neutral position.
- Retest the linea alba for changes in tension.

Thoracic/Lumbar, Thoracolumbar Fascia

MFR Type: Multiple Direction, Direct or Indirect Method

This technique is a prototype for treating planes of fascia (**Fig. 6.7**). Apply the principles and steps here to any other plane or sheet of fascia in the body, such as the lumbosacral or posterior cervical regions.

Key Elements

- Somatic dysfunction corrected: superficial or deep thoracolumbar fascial passive range of motion restrictions.
- End goal: to release the thoracolumbar fascia.

WATCH ▷ ▶ ▷

▶ *Video 6.7 Thoracic/Lumbar, Thoracolumbar Fascia—Narrated*

Example Somatic Dysfunction: Thoracolumbar Fascias are Left, Inferior and Clockwise Twist Positions

Positioning and Preparation

▶ Patient: prone with head resting in head rest or turned to one side, whichever is more comfortable.

▶ Physician: standing at one side of the table at the level of the pelvis, with body turned to face the head of the patient.

Tissue Contact

- Performing hands: with the entire palmar surface of both hands and fingers, contact the thoracolumbar fascia on both sides of the patient.

- Detailed suggestion: lean to the side at the waist to be closer to the midline of the patient's back. Extend wrists and place thumbs so that they are parallel to the spine and ~ 1 to 2 cm lateral to the spinous processes. The tip of the thumb should be about at the level of T10. Fingers can be close together or spread out for more extensive contact.

Movements, Barriers, and Forces

Use both hands to do the following:

- Layer palpate to the affected fascial layer: skin → superficial fascia → muscle → deep fascia.
- Test fascias for somatic dysfunction in three directions of motion.
  - Translation: move fascias to the right to test right translation, then to the left.
  - Superior/inferior: move fascias superiorly, then inferiorly.
  - Twist: twist fascias clockwise, then counterclockwise.
- Move the fascia in one direction at a time, into all positions of motion ease (indirect method), or motion restriction (direct method).
- Hold forces and positions.
- Monitor fascias until release or for ~ 2 minutes.
  - Optional: add fascial unwinding and/or respiratory cooperation.
- Release forces and return fascias to neutral position.
- Retest the thoracolumbar fascia for changes in passive ranges of motion.

Advance this technique by motion testing and positioning the fascias under each hand separately.

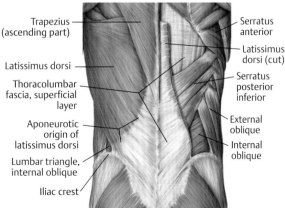

Fig. 6.7   Thoracolumbar fascia.

- Trapezius (ascending part)
- Latissimus dorsi
- Thoracolumbar fascia, superficial layer
- Aponeurotic origin of latissimus dorsi
- Lumbar triangle, internal oblique
- Iliac crest
- Serratus anterior
- Latissimus dorsi (cut)
- Serratus posterior inferior
- External oblique
- Internal oblique

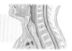

Pelvis, Pelvic Diaphragm Fascia

MFR Type: Single Direction, Direct Method

This technique can correct many innominate and sacral somatic dysfunctions and is helpful to perform before more specific articular techniques. It also can be used to improve lymphatic and venous circulation in the lower extremities. Be sure to briefly describe the steps to the patient prior to asking the patient to lie prone for osteopathic manipulative treatment in this sensitive area (**Fig. 6.8**).

Key Elements

- Somatic dysfunction corrected: pelvic floor fascial tightness. Fascias include those that encapsulate the levator ani musculature.
- End goal: to release the pelvic diaphragm musculature and related fascias.

WATCH ▷ ► ▷

► *Video 6.8 Pelvis, Pelvic Diaphragm Fascia—Narrated*

Example Somatic Dysfunction: Bilateral Pelvic Diaphragm Tightness

Positioning and Preparation

► Patient: prone.

► Physician: standing on one side of the patient near the patient's lower thighs.

Tissue Contact

- Both thumbs create the corrective stretching forces. Use your right thumb to contact the patient's right ischial tuberosity and left thumb to contact the patient's left ischial tuberosity.
- Performing thumbs: contact the medial border of the ischial tuberosities with the pads of the thumbs. Curl thumbs around the medial border of the ischial tuberosities and maintain contact with them at all times. Avoid contacting the patient with the fingers by keeping them extended.

Movements, Barriers, and Forces

Use both thumbs to do the following:

- Layer palpate to the affected fascial layer: skin → superficial fascia → musculature → deep fascia.
- Apply superiorly directed forces until resistance is felt. Hold these forces.
- Add laterally directed forces onto the ischial tuberosities until resistance is felt.
- Hold forces and positions.
- Monitor fascias until release or for ~ 2 minutes.
  - Optional: add fascial unwinding (in a superior direction only) or respiratory cooperation.
- Release forces and return fascias to neutral position.
- Retest the pelvic diaphragm musculature and related fascias for changes in tension.

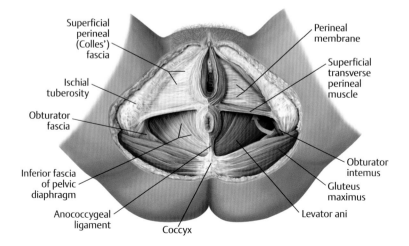

Fig. 6.8 Pelvic diaphragm.

Labels: Superficial perineal (Colles') fascia; Ischial tuberosity; Obturator fascia; Inferior fascia of pelvic diaphragm; Anococcygeal ligament; Coccyx; Perineal membrane; Superficial transverse perineal muscle; Obturator internus; Gluteus maximus; Levator ani

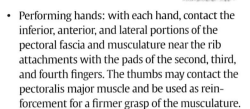

Upper Extremity, Pectoral Fascia

MFR Type: Single Direction, Direct Method

This technique can be used as part of a lymphatic treatment sequence. It releases tension in the upper ribs and anterior shoulders, thus improving thoracic cage motion, gas exchange, and lymph circulation. It can also be used to address the modern, forward-bent posture from prolonged sitting. Be sure to describe the tissue contact in this sensitive area (**Fig. 6.9**).

Key Elements

- Somatic dysfunction corrected: pectoral fascial tightness. Fascias include those that encapsulate the pectoralis major and minor muscles and portions of the anterior axillary region.
- End goal: to loosen the fascias of the anterior pectoral girdle, improving rib cage mechanics, lymphatic drainage of the arm, and internal rotation of the shoulder.

WATCH ▷ ▶ ▷

▶ **Video 6.9 Upper Extremity, Pectoral Fascia—Narrated**

Example Somatic Dysfunction: Bilateral Pectoral Fascia Tightness

---

Positioning and Preparation

▶ Patient: supine.
▶ Physician: standing at the head of the table.

Tissue Contact

- Both hands are used to create the corrective stretching forces.
- Use your right hand to contact the patient's right pectoral fascia and your left hand to contact the left side.

- Performing hands: with each hand, contact the inferior, anterior, and lateral portions of the pectoral fascia and musculature near the rib attachments with the pads of the second, third, and fourth fingers. The thumbs may contact the pectoralis major muscle and be used as reinforcement for a firmer grasp of the musculature.
  - Detailed suggestion: ask the patient to bend her elbows and place her hands on the upper abdomen. To avoid a tickle response, first locate and palpate the greater tubercle of the humerus and biceps tendon. Then slowly but firmly move inferiorly along the pectoralis major muscle until the inferior edge is palpated. Curl fingers underneath the musculature and move medially, close to the rib attachments.

Movements, Barriers, and Forces

Use the fingers of both hands to do the following:

- Layer palpate to the fascial layer: skin → superficial fascia → musculature → deep fascia.
- Apply gentle anteriorly directed forces to lift the musculature and related fascias anteriorly until resistance, or a restrictive barrier, is felt.
- Hold forces and position(s).
- Monitor fascia(s) until release or for ~ 2 minutes.
  - Optional: add fascial unwinding and/or respiratory cooperation.
- Release forces and return fascias to neutral position.
- Retest the pectoral fascia for changes in tension.

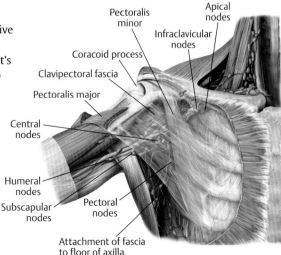

Fig. 6.9   Pectoral fascia.

119

Upper Extremity, Flexor Retinaculum

MFR Type: Single Direction, Direct Method

This technique is commonly performed on patients with carpal tunnel syndrome (**Fig. 6.10**).

Key Elements

- Somatic dysfunction corrected: flexor retinaculum fascial tightness.
- End goal: to laterally stretch the flexor retinaculum.

> **WATCH** ▷ ▶ ▷
>
> ▶ *Video 6.10 Upper Extremity, Flexor Retinaculum—Narrated*
>
> *Example Somatic Dysfunction: Right Flexor Retinaculum Tightness*

Positioning and Preparation

- ▶ Patient: sitting.
- ▶ Physician: standing or sitting, facing the patient.

Tissue Contact

- Both thumbs create the corrective stretching forces.
- Performing hands: contact the flexor surface of the patient's wrist, midline, over the creases, with the pads of both thumbs. Wrap remaining fingers around the contour of the patient's hand.

- Alternate contact: first interdigitate the space between your fourth and fifth fingers into the space between the patient's fourth and fifth fingers. Then interdigitate the space between your other fourth and fifth fingers into the space between the patient's thumb and index finger. Then contact the flexor surface of the patient's wrist as previously described.

Movements, Barriers, and Forces

Use both thumbs to do the following:

- Layer palpate to the fascial layer: skin → superficial fascia → flexor retinaculum.
- Apply gentle lateral traction forces with both thumbs to stretch the fascia apart from the midline to either side until resistance is felt. Adjust forces on each side so that the tension is equally distributed between your thumbs.
- Hold forces and positions.
  - Optional: extend the patient's wrist just until more tissue resistance is palpated.
- Monitor fascia(s) until release or for ~ 2 minutes.
  - Optional: add fascial unwinding and/or respiratory cooperation.
- Release forces and return fascias to neutral position.
- Retest the flexor retinaculum for changes in tension.

Fig. 6.10 Flexor retinaculum.

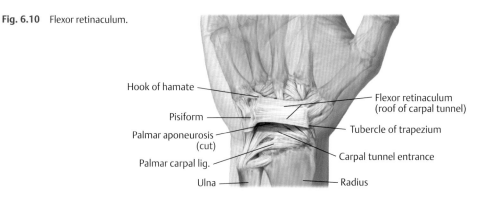

Hook of hamate

Pisiform

Palmar aponeurosis (cut)

Palmar carpal lig.

Ulna

Flexor retinaculum (roof of carpal tunnel)

Tubercle of trapezium

Carpal tunnel entrance

Radius

Lower Extremity, Popliteal Fossa

MFR Type: Single Direction, Direct Method

Perform this technique anytime you wish to improve lymph and venous drainage of the lower extremity. This is especially useful for cases of lower extremity edema, when passive congestion in the popliteal fossae is identified, or after minor injuries to the knee, ankle, or foot (**Fig. 6.11**).

Key Elements

- Somatic dysfunction corrected: popliteal fossa region fascial tightness, including the superficial and deep fascias that encapsulate the biceps femoris, semimembranosus, gastrocnemius tendons, and muscles.
- End goal: to release the fascias of the popliteal fossa.

> **WATCH ▷▶▷**
>
> ▶ *Video 6.11 Lower Extremity, Popliteal Fossa—Narrated*
>
> *Example Somatic Dysfunction: Bilateral Popliteal Fossa Fascial Restriction*

Positioning and Preparation

▶ Patient: supine, with legs extended.

▶ Physician: standing beside the leg with the popliteal fascial restriction, facing the head of the table.

Tissue Contact

- Both hands create the corrective stretching forces. Use one hand to contact the patient's medial popliteal fossa fascias and the other to contact the lateral fascias.
- Performing hands: contact the popliteal fossa with the pads of the second, third, and fourth fingers of both hands. Fingertips are ~ 1 to 2 cm apart from midline, avoiding the neurovascular structures. Thumbs and hypothenar eminence contact the lateral and medial one-third of the edges of the joint line. If an arterial pulse is felt, move the fingers laterally.
  - Detailed suggestion: The fingers contacting the lateral joint should be on the fascias surrounding the biceps femoris and lateral head of the gastrocnemius muscles. The

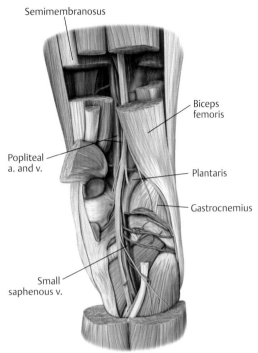

Fig. 6.11   Popliteal fossa.

fingers on the medial joint should be contacting the fascias surrounding the semimembranosus and medial head of the gastrocnemius muscles. Abduct elbows enough so that fingers are in a horizontal plane (versus wrist adduction only).

Movements, Barriers, and Forces

Use both hands to do the following:

- Lift the knee into slight flexion to loosen the posterior myofascial tissues. Hold this position.
- Layer palpate to the fascial layer: skin → superficial fascia → musculature → deep fascia.
- Apply gentle lateral traction forces to stretch the fascia from midline to either side until resistance is felt. Adjust forces on each side so that the tension is equally distributed between your fingers. Hold these forces.
- Monitor fascias until release or for ~ 2 minutes.
  - Optional: add fascial unwinding and/or respiratory cooperation.
- Release forces and return fascias to neutral position.
- Retest the fascias of the popliteal fossa for changes in tension.

Lower Extremity, Plantar Fascia

MFR Type: Single Direction, Direct Method

This technique is effective as part of a comprehensive treatment for plantar fasciitis. Often, though, this technique is a bit painful due to the richly innervated plantar aponeurosis and the amount of force needed to match the fascial tensions. Be sure to let the patient know this and slowly increase forces (**Fig. 6.12**).

Key Elements

- Somatic dysfunction corrected: plantar fascia tightness.
- End goal: to stretch the plantar aponeurosis laterally and distally.

WATCH ▷▶▷

- ▶ *Video 6.12 Lower Extremity, Plantar Fascia—Narrated*

Example Somatic Dysfunction: Left Plantar Fascia Tightness

Positioning and Preparation

- ▶ Patient: supine, with legs extended.
- ▶ Physician: sitting at the foot of the table.

Tissue Contact

- Both thumbs create the corrective stretching forces.
- Performing hands: contact the middle of the plantar fascia, near the calcaneal attachment, with the pads of both thumbs, with one crossed over the other. Fingers may wrap around the patient's foot, or not.

Movements, Barriers, and Forces

Use the pads of both thumbs to do the following:

- Layer palpate to the affected fascial layer: skin → superficial fascia → adipose → plantar aponeurosis.

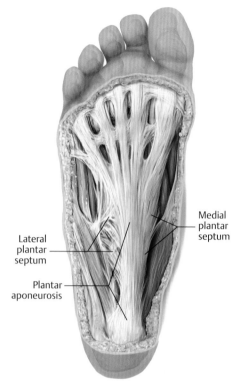

Fig. 6.12   Plantar fascia.

Labels: Medial plantar septum; Lateral plantar septum; Plantar aponeurosis

- Apply superiorly directed forces into the plantar fascia with both thumbs into the fascial layer. Hold forces.
  - Identify areas of somatic dysfunction.
- Slowly create forces that are lateral and at an angle directed toward the toes, until resistance is felt. This movement is only a few millimeters to a centimeter. Hold this force.
- Monitor plantar fascia until release or for ~ 2 minutes.
  - Optional: add fascial unwinding and/or respiratory cooperation.
- Release forces and return fascias to neutral position.
- Retest the plantar fascia for changes in tension.

The technique may be repeated along the length of the plantar fascia, up to the metatarsal bones.

Chapter Summary

Effective in both direct and indirect methods, MFR is a gentle, versatile technique suitable for most clinical conditions. MFR can be used as a primary treatment, a diagnostic technique, or in preparation for another technique. Several techniques can also be used as part of a lymphatic treatment sequence. This chapter presented many examples of direct and indirect MFR to allow for experience with fascia throughout the body. Included in each technique is a reminder that fascial unwinding and respiratory cooperation may be used to enhance fascial release.

Clinical Cases and Review Questions

Case 1

A 37-year-old woman presents with a 1-month history of midback pain. The exam is positive for multiple thoracic and lumbar vertebral positional asymmetries and soft tissue tightness, including findings of passive range of motion restrictions in the thoracolumbar fascia in superior, right, and counterclockwise directions.

Q1. What is the appropriate description for the thoracolumbar fascia positional somatic dysfunction diagnosis?
   A. Superior, right, and counterclockwise.
   B. Superior, left, and clockwise.
   C. Inferior, right, and clockwise.
   D. Inferior, left, and clockwise.
   E. Inferior, left, and counterclockwise.

Q2. When performing a multiple-direction MFR technique with direct method to correct this patient's somatic dysfunction, the fascias should be positioned in which directions?
   A. Superior, right, and counterclockwise.
   B. Superior, left, and clockwise.
   C. Inferior, right, and clockwise.
   D. Inferior, left, and clockwise.
   E. Inferior, left, and counterclockwise.

Q3. Which of the following structures is contacted when performing MFR: thoracic outlet?
   A. Pectoral fascia.
   B. Third rib, posterior angle.
   C. C4 spinous process.
   D. T1 transverse process.
   E. Longus colli muscles.

Case 2

A 25-year-old woman presents with abdominal pain and symptoms of acid reflux. The physical exam is positive for mild epigastric tenderness and increased tension in the linea alba.

Q4. You perform an MFR technique on the patient's somatic dysfunction. In which directions do you create the corrective forces?
   A. Anteriorly and medially.
   B. Superiorly with lateral compression.
   C. Posteriorly with superior/inferior traction.
   D. Inferiorly with medial compression.
   E. Posteriorly and laterally.

Q5. While performing a direct method MFR technique to correct her somatic dysfunction, which of the following findings warrants discontinuing the technique and pursuing a diagnostic workup instead?
   A. Mild tenderness.
   B. Radiating pain to the umbilicus.
   C. Restricted abdominal wall motion with breathing.
   D. A large pulsatile mass.
   E. Palpation of the aorta.

Answers to Review Questions

Q1. **D** is correct. The case gives the fascial movements that are restricted. Somatic dysfunction is named for the unrestricted, or freest, motion; therefore, inferior, left, and clockwise is the correct diagnosis.

Q2. **A** is correct. When treating with direct MFR, place the fascia in the restriction in all planes. In this case the restrictions are superior, right, and counterclockwise.

Q3. **D** is correct. The only answer choice that is a structure contacted during MFR to the thoracic outlet is the C7/T1. Other structures contacted include first rib, clavicle, sternocleidomastoid muscle, and trapezius muscle.

Q4. **C** is correct. This technique is performed by using the fingertips along the linea alba to create a posterior directed force with superior to inferior traction. This traction is added by approximating the wrists, which causes slight separation of the fingers. None of the other answer choices give the correct forces.

Q5. **D** is correct. This technique is contraindicated in a patient with a suspected or confirmed abdominal aortic aneurysm. Stop if you feel a large pulsatile mass during this technique. The other answer choices are not contraindications. The aortic pulse may be palpated, but without feeling a mass, it is normal.

References

1. Still AT. Philosophy and Mechanical Principles of Osteopathy. Kansas City, MO: Hudson-Kimberly; 1902:60

Research Bibliography

Barnes PL, Laboy F III, Noto-Bell L, Ferencz V, Nelson J, Kuchera ML. A comparative study of cervical hysteresis characteristics after various osteopathic manipulative treatment (OMT) modalities. J Bodyw Mov Ther 2013;17(1):89–94

Cao TV, Hicks MR, Zein-Hammoud M, Standley PR. Duration and magnitude of myofascial release in 3-dimensional bioengineered tendons: effects on wound healing. J Am Osteopath Assoc 2015;115(2):72–82

Castro-Sánchez AM, Matarán-Peñarrocha GA, Arroyo-Morales M, Saavedra-Hernández M, Fernández-Sola C, Moreno-Lorenzo C. Effects of myofascial release techniques on pain, physical function, and postural stability in patients with fibromyalgia: a randomized controlled trial. Clin Rehabil 2011;25(9):800–813

Chaudhry H, Schleip R, Ji Z, Bukiet B, Maney M, Findley T. Three-dimensional mathematical model for deformation of human fasciae in manual therapy. J Am Osteopath Assoc 2008;108(8):379–390

Danto JB. Review of integrated neuromusculoskeletal release and the novel application of a segmental anterior/posterior approach in the thoracic, lumbar, and sacral regions. J Am Osteopath Assoc 2003;103(12):583–596

Dodd JG, Good MM, Nguyen TL, Grigg AI, Batia LM, Standley PR. In vitro biophysical strain model for understanding mechanisms of osteopathic manipulative treatment. J Am Osteopath Assoc 2006;106(3):157–166

Kuchera ML. Applying osteopathic principles to formulate treatment for patients with chronic pain. J Am Osteopath Assoc 2007;107(10, Suppl 6):ES28–ES38

Meltzer KR, Cao TV, Schad JF, King H, Stoll ST, Standley PR. In vitro modeling of repetitive motion injury and myofascial release. J Bodyw Mov Ther 2010;14(2):162–171

O-Yurvati AH, Carnes MS, Clearfield MB, Stoll ST, McConathy WJ. Hemodynamic effects of osteopathic manipulative treatment immediately after coronary artery bypass graft surgery. J Am Osteopath Assoc 2005;105(10):475–481

Simmonds N, Miller P, Gemmell H. A theoretical framework for the role of fascia in manual therapy. J Bodyw Mov Ther 2012;16(1):83–93

7 Lymphatic Techniques

LEARNING OBJECTIVES

1. Explain the goals for performing lymphatic treatment and lymphatic techniques.
2. Identify the clinical considerations, including indications, contraindications, and precautions for performing lymphatic treatment and lymphatic techniques.
3. Compare and contrast the types of lymphatic techniques.
4. Outline the general movements, barriers, and forces required for performing lymphatic techniques.
5. Identify the end goal of each lymphatic technique.
6. Visualize, verbalize, and identify the preparation, positioning, tissue contact, movements, barriers, and forces for each lymphatic technique.
7. Perform lymphatic techniques using appropriate somatic dysfunction diagnosis, preparation, positioning, tissue contact, movements, barriers, forces, retest for effectiveness, communication, and safe tissue handling.

Lymphatic Techniques Introduction

The lymphatic system is important for the removal of larger extracellular particles, circulation of immune cells, and absorption and circulation of chyle. Somatic dysfunction in the structures that surround the lymphatic system (vessels, nodes, and ancillary organs) can limit circulation within this low pressure system. Somatic dysfunction of the body diaphragms and extremities can also restrict the effectiveness of these structures as lymphatic pumps. Thus somatic dysfunction leads to passive tissue congestion and impaired circulation of immune cells, which inhibits the natural healing process.

In general, osteopathic techniques that address the lymphatic system have the following effects:

- Increase the resorption of interstitial fluids and proteins.
- Restore tissue pH balance.
- Reduce fascial restrictions around lymphatic vessels for improved lymphatic fluid circulation.
- Improve the effectiveness of extrinsic (muscle contraction) and intrinsic lymphatic pumps (pressure differentials created during respiration).
- Maintain normal blood viscosity.

Often, it is beneficial to treat the lymphatic system as a unit with osteopathic manipulative treatment (OMT), whereby multiple techniques are sequentially performed and referred to as a lymphatic treatment. There is a recommended sequence for performing a lymphatic treatment with OMT.

Recommended Sequence of Lymphatic Treatment Steps

- Identify somatic dysfunction and perform OMT at the appropriate terminal drainage site(s): the thoracic duct or right lymphatic duct.
- Identify somatic dysfunction and perform OMT on any relevant sites of passive fluid congestion. Refer to chapter 3, Respiratory/Circulatory Model for identification of those sites.
- Identify somatic dysfunction and perform OMT at the thoracoabdominal and pelvic diaphragms.
- Identify somatic dysfunction and perform OMT on viscerosomatic and somatovisceral reflexes.
- Finally, promote lymph formation and circulation using lymphatic effleurage or pump techniques.

Remembering to "open the drain first" may help make the order easier to recall.

Background

What we meet with in all diseases is dead blood, stagnant lymph, and albumen in a semi-vital or dead and decomposing condition through the lymphatics and other parts of the body, brain, lungs, kidneys, liver and fascia. —Dr. Still[1]

Dr. Still discussed and wrote about the importance of unobstructed lymph circulation for resto-ration of health. He also described some lymphatic treatments, including the treatment of enlarged lymph nodes. Osteopathic medicine has continued this tradition, and to this day, there are no pharmaceuticals or surgical procedures that affect lymph circulation in a similar fashion to manual techniques.

Many early osteopathic physicians developed techniques for the lymphatic system. Fredrick Millard, DO, is notable for his work, *Applied Anatomy of the Lymphatics*,[2] which describes the lymphatic system and OMT approaches.

Research

The physiological effects of lymphatic techniques have been researched. One important study discovered that an osteopathic lymphatic pump circulated more lymph than was circulated during rest periods, but not as much as during active exercise.[3] A short research bibliography is provided at the end of this chapter.

Clinical Considerations

LYM techniques are appropriate to perform on patients who have impaired lymphatic circulation, including those with acute and chronic conditions, some of which are listed in Table 7.1. Always acquire adequate data in the form of an appropriate history, a thorough physical exam, and relevant diagnostic tests to exercise best clinical judgment before performing OMT.

Table 7.1 Clinical considerations

Indications	Contraindications	Precautions
Infections (especially when lymphadenopathy is present, although it is not a requirement) Inflammation Conditions that cause fluid congestion/edema	Unstable or life-threatening infections such as necrotizing fasciitis Anuresis Pharyngotympanic tube pump: blood in the middle ear or fluid/blood leakage from the ear Modified thoracic pump: moderate to severe obstructive lung diseases Mesentery pump: acute abdomen Pedal pump: deep vein thrombosis or leg injuries	Special precaution, cancer: Caution should be exercised in patients who have cancer. Treatment goals, expected outcomes, and precautions should be discussed with each patient.

Somatic Dysfunction Diagnosis Corrected

LYM techniques address a variety of somatic dysfunctions, including fascial somatic dysfunctions around lymphatic vessels and areas of passive fluid congestion. Lymphatic pump techniques are unique in that they can be performed empirically, or based on the patient's clinical condition, without a preceding tissue somatic dysfunction diagnosis.

Positioning and Preparation

▶ Patient: the patient must be comfortable and remain relaxed for the duration of the technique.
▶ Physician: the physician must be comfortable and positioned to ensure safety, using the best ergonomic posture and movements possible.

Note: The videos include a narrated description of positioning when not visually self-explanatory.

Movements, Barriers, and Forces

LYM techniques are direct techniques. There are two types presented in this manual: lymphatic pumps and effleurage. Both types use gentle forces because lymph circulates in thin-walled, low-pressure vasculature.

Extrinsic Lymphatic Pumps (Pharyngotympanic, Thoracic, Mesentery, Pedal)

Extrinsic lymphatic pumps are performed using oscillatory forces to help propel lymph through vessels with an end goal of promoting the uptake, or formation, of lymphatic fluid. Oscillatory forces should be sufficient to move the patient's tissues, span a short distance (usually ≤ 1 cm), and be performed at a rapid rate. Recommended rates for oscillations are listed for each technique. However, the exact rate should be adjusted for each patient, taking into account tissue resiliency and fluid dynamics to ensure that smooth oscillations are created. Pumps should be performed for 1 to 5 minutes, although the pedal pump can be continued for up to 10 minutes. Although only the mesentery pump is described in this manual, the spleen and liver can also be "pumped" in a similar fashion.

Effleurage (Anterior Cervical)

The end goal of effleurage is to manually move lymph inside the lymphatic vessel toward the terminal drainage site. Effleurage is performed over the skin of a body region where superficial lymph nodes and vessels are located. Gentle forces are essential because the lymphatic vessels treated are both superficial and thin. This manual describes only one effleurage technique; however, the movements, barriers, and forces can be used on any chain of lymph nodes, moving lymph toward the terminal drainage site.

Retest for Effectiveness

Tissue drainage resulting in a decreased amount of palpable extracellular fluid can occur immediately after lymphatic techniques but may take 24 hours or more for resolution. The rate of resolution depends on a variety of factors, including the effectiveness of the technique, the general health of the lymphatic system, and the removal or resolution of the causative agent or factors. Most LYM techniques do not require a retest for somatic dysfunction.

Pharyngotympanic Tube Pump

This technique is also known as the Galbreath technique and mandibular drainage technique. It is helpful for draining fluid out of the middle ear, which is commonly associated with conditions such as otitis media, allergies, upper respiratory viral illnesses, and eustachian tube dysfunction (**Fig. 7.1**). With a few minutes of demonstration and practice, parents can be shown how to perform this technique on their children at home, a few times daily, between office visits.

Key Elements

- Somatic dysfunction corrected: fluid in the middle ear. This technique can be performed empirically when fluid in the middle ear is identified.
- End goal: to rhythmically stretch the musculature and fascias around the pharyngotympanic tube, using the jaw as a lever. Moving the jaw opens the pharyngotympanic tube, and the rhythmic oscillations promote fluid and lymph drainage.

WATCH ▷ ▶ ▷

- ▶ *Video 7.1a Head, Pharyngotympanic Tube Pump—Real-Time*
- ▶ *Video 7.1b Head, Pharyngotympanic Tube Pump—Narrated*

Positioning and Preparation

- ▶ Patient: supine.
- ▶ Physician: sitting at the side of the table, near the patient's head and neck, on the side opposite that of the dysfunctional pharyngotympanic tube.

Tissue Contact

- One hand creates the corrective stretching forces. The other hand assists by stabilizing the head so it does not roll.
- Performing hand: use the hand that is nearer the patient's feet. Contact the posterior and superior aspect of the ramus of the mandible with the tips of the second and third fingers. Do this by reaching across and over the patient's chin. Curl the second and third fingertips around the posterior/superior ramus and allow the hand to contact and follow the contour of the mandible. Do not pinch the mandible with the fingers or thumb.
- Assisting hand: if needed, contact the forehead.

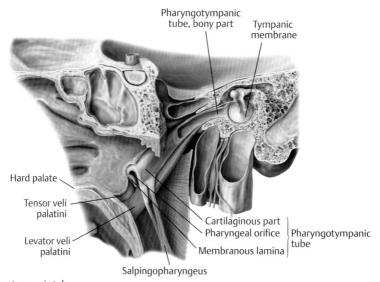

Fig. 7.1 Pharyngotympanic tube.

Movements, Barriers, and Forces

Precaution: movements and forces should be short and very gentle in patients who have temporomandibular joint dysfunction.

- Ask the patient to slightly open the mouth, relax it, and keep it relaxed.
- With the fingertips on the mandible, layer palpate to the bone.
- Apply an inferiorly and medially directed force to very gently stretch the mandibular ligament and associated soft tissues and musculature. The distance of the stretch is a few millimeters. If the patient's head moves, gently stabilize it with the assisting hand.

- Hold these forces for 2 to 3 seconds.
- Release forces but not hand contacts and allow the mandible to recoil to neutral position.
- Continue creating and releasing forces in a rhythmic, pumping fashion. Oscillations should be at a rate of 20 to 30 per minute (one stretch every 2–3 seconds).
- Perform continuously for at least 30 seconds, up to 2 minutes.
- Release forces and hand contacts.
- Retest the fascias for changes in tension. If performed empirically, no retest is required.

Anterior Cervical Effleurage

This technique is useful as an adjunct treatment of viral or bacterial infections of the sinuses, nasal cavities, oropharynx, face, and mouth. This technique can be extrapolated and used over the sinuses, extremities, and areas of superficial edema found elsewhere in the body (**Fig. 7.2**).

Key Elements

- Somatic dysfunction corrected: superficial fascial and/or muscular tissue texture changes in the anterior cervical region or cervical lymphadenopathy due to a related clinical condition
- End goal: to mobilize lymphatic fluid toward the thoracic outlet

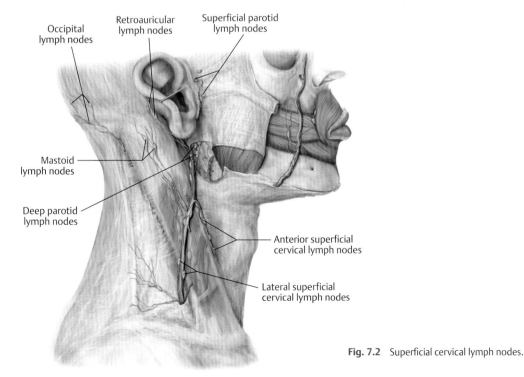

Occipital lymph nodes

Retroauricular lymph nodes

Superficial parotid lymph nodes

Mastoid lymph nodes

Deep parotid lymph nodes

Anterior superficial cervical lymph nodes

Lateral superficial cervical lymph nodes

Fig. 7.2   Superficial cervical lymph nodes.

Positioning and Preparation

▶ Patient: supine.

▶ Physician: sitting at the head of the table facing the patient.

Tissue Contact

This technique has two parts. The first part describes drainage of the lymphatics anterior to the sterno-cleidomastoid muscle. The second part describes drainage of the lymphatics posterior to the sterno-cleidomastoid muscle. Perform this technique on one side of the patient's neck at a time.

- One hand creates the gentle fluid mobilization forces. Use your right hand to contact the right sternocleidomastoid muscle and your left hand to contact the left sternocleidomastoid muscle.
- Part 1, anteriorly located lymphatics: contact the medial edge of one sternocleidomastoid muscle just inferior to the attachment at the mastoid process with the fingertips of one hand. Place the fingertips side by side along the length of the muscle.
- Part 2, posteriorly located lymphatics: contact the lateral edge of one sternocleidomastoid muscle just inferior to the attachment at the mastoid process with the fingertips of one hand. Place the fingertips side by side along the length of the muscle.

Movements, Barriers, and Forces

Use one hand to do the following:

- Layer palpate to the superficial fascial layer.
- Apply a very gentle posterior and lateral force with the fingers in a rhythmic, rolling fashion starting with the finger that is most superior and ending with the most inferior one. The movements are like tapping, or like softly playing a piano.
  - Visualize the lymphatic fluid as being gently guided inferiorly by your movements.
- Repeat rhythmic, rolling movements from superior to inferior two or three times.
- Release tissue contact and reposition the fingertips inferiorly on the musculature not yet addressed.
- Repeat the technique on the entire length of the sternocleidomastoid muscle.
- Change contact to that described as part 2, to address the posterior lymphatics.
- Repeat the technique (steps 1–5). However, the forces in step 2 are directed anterior-medially.
- Perform the technique on the other sternocleidomastoid muscle.
- Retest the fascias and/or tissues for changes in tension and passive congestion.

Thoracic Pump

This lymphatic pump was first described by C. Earl Miller, DO.[5] The version explained here is similar to the original technique (**Fig. 7.3**).

Key Elements

- Somatic dysfunction corrected: clinical conditions, such as infections and edema (this technique is performed empirically in such clinical conditions)
- End goal: to augment negative intrathoracic pressure to improve lymph circulation

Positioning and Preparation

▶ Patient: supine, with head turned comfortably to one side.

▶ Physician: standing at the head of the table facing the patient.

Note: Perform this technique only one time per OMT session.

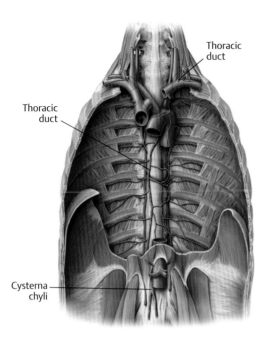

Fig. 7.3 Thoracic duct.

Tissue Contact

- Performing hands: contact the superior and lateral thoracic cage just below the clavicle, in the region of ribs 2–4, with the fingers and palms of both hands. Avoid sudden movements and digging your fingertips into the patient to avoid stimulating a nociceptor-mediated tickle response.
  - Detailed suggestion: abduct your thumbs, extend your fingers. Place fingers so they curl around the lateral edges of the upper ribs in the axillary region and thumbs and hypothenar eminences contact the anterior shafts of the upper ribs.

Movements, Barriers, and Forces

Note: The patient should breathe normally throughout the procedure.
  Use both hands to do the following:

- Use thumbs and thenar eminences to apply posteriorly directed forces on the ribs until they depress slightly, about 0.5 cm.
- Gently release forces for rib recoil.
- Immediately use the fingers to apply anteriorly directed forces until the ribs elevate.
- Continue creating posteriorly, then anteriorly directed forces (depression and elevation

of the ribs) in a rhythmic, pumping fashion. Oscillations should be at a rate of ~ 60 to 120 per minute (1–2 per second).
- Perform continuously for 1 to 5 minutes.
- Release forces and tissue contacts.
- Retest for effectiveness is not necessary.

Modified Thoracic Pump Technique: Optional Movements, Barriers, and Forces for the Thoracic Pump

The sudden-release maneuver produces an abrupt change in intrathoracic pressure. The idea is to temporarily limit expansion of the rib cage, then to suddenly permit full motion. This creates a negative intrathoracic pressure that is greater than normal, which draws air in. The negative intrathoracic pressure also draws more lymphatic fluid and venous blood back into central circulation. This technique is not to be performed on patients with moderate to severe obstructive lung disease.

Note: The patient can be asked to take four deep, slow breaths, or can breathe normally. Physician forces must be coordinated with the patient's breathing.

> **WATCH ▷ ▶ ▷**
>
> ▶ *Video 7.4 Modified Thoracic Pump—Real-Time*

Movements, Barriers, and Forces

Use both hands to do the following:

- As the patient starts the exhalation phase of respiration, apply two to three pumping motions (as described in steps 1–2 previously) throughout the duration of the patient's exhalation cycle.
- Hold the last posteriorly directed force just prior to the patient's next inhalation.
- Limit the anterior motion of the ribs on the patient's inhalation.
- Repeat steps 1–3 for the patient's next two inhalation–exhalation cycles.
- As the fourth inhalation begins, release forces by immediately and suddenly lifting both hands off the costal cage. The patient should take in a deep and full inhalation and may even make a gasping noise.
- Retest for effectiveness is not necessary.

Mesentery Pump

The intestinal lymphatics are contained within the mesenteries and are reached via the small intestines (**Fig. 7.4**). The mesentery pump is useful in constipation, irritable bowel syndrome, and viral infections.

Key Elements

- Somatic dysfunction corrected: circulation of the intestinal mesenteries (this technique is performed empirically in clinical conditions where improved lymph circulation of the intestinal mesenteries is desired)
- End goal: to promote lymph formation and circulation in the intestinal mesentery, using gentle, oscillatory forces

---

WATCH ▷ ▶ ▷

▶ *Video 7.5 Abdomen, Mesentery Pump—Narrated*

Positioning and Preparation

▶ Patient: supine.

▶ Physician: standing on the patient's right side.

Tissue Contact

- One hand creates the oscillatory, fluid mobilization forces.
- Performing hand: contact the midline of the patient's abdominal wall about an inch below the umbilicus, near the middle of the small intestines, with the heel of the hand.

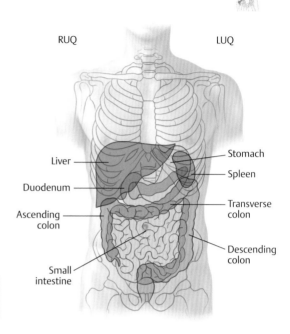

Fig. 7.4 Abdominal organs.

Movements, Barriers, and Forces

Use both hands to do the following:

- Layer palpate to the small intestines and mesenteries (skin, superficial fascia, adipose tissue, muscle, omentum/small intestines/mesentery).
- Hold these forces.
- Induce rhythmic, pumping, oscillatory forces directed superiorly toward the intestinal lymphatic trunk at a rate of ~ 20 to 30 per minute (one oscillation every 2–3 seconds).
- Perform continuously for ~ 2 minutes.
- Release forces and contacts.
- Retest for effectiveness is not necessary.

Pedal Pump

This technique is useful during systemic viral infections to support the patient's inherent healing mechanisms. Parents can be taught this technique, and children often think that the jiggling is playful (**Fig. 7.5**).

Key Elements

- Somatic dysfunction corrected: impaired lymphatic fluid circulation (this technique is performed empirically in clinical conditions that result in impaired lymphatic fluid circulation)
- End goal: to improve lymph circulation in the entire body

WATCH ▷ ▶ ▷

▶ *Video 7.6 Pedal Pump—Narrated*

Positioning and Preparation

▶ Patient: supine, preferably with shoes off.
▶ Physician: standing at the foot of the table, facing the patient's feet.

Tissue Contact

- Both hands create the oscillatory, fluid mobilization forces. Use your right hand to contact the patient's left foot, and your left hand to contact the right foot.
- Performing hands: contact the plantar surface of the foot with the palm of each hand at the level of the metatarsals. Use your right hand to contact the patient's left foot, and vice versa.

Movements, Barriers, and Forces

Use both hands to do the following:

- Simultaneously push both feet into dorsiflexion until resistance is met.
- Create a pumping force superiorly until the entire body moves. The nose should nod.
- As soon as the body moves, allow the foot to recoil back to neutral/upright position.
- Immediately on recoil, push the feet again superiorly.
- Continue creating and releasing forces in a rhythmic, pumping fashion. Oscillations should be at a rate of ~ 120 per minute (2–3 per second).
- Perform continuously for 1 to 5 minutes.
- Release forces and hand contacts.
- Retest for effectiveness is not necessary.

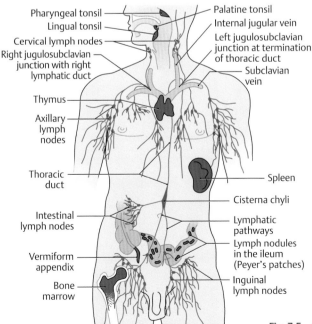

Fig. 7.5 Lymphatic system.

Chapter Summary

Lymphatic techniques are direct methods of osteopathic manipulation that promote the restoration of health in the body by improving lymphatic fluid circulation. They can be performed in a systematic fashion for treatment of systemic diseases. This chapter outlines specific lymphatic modalities, including multiple lymphatic pumps and effleurage, while emphasizing the utility, clinical relevance, and appropriate administration of lymphatic techniques.

Clinical Cases and Review Questions

Case 1

A 2-year-old boy presents with 2 days of ear tugging, fever, runny nose, and fussiness. The exam is positive for right-sided anterior cervical lymphadenopathy, a bulging ear drum, and bilateral tightness in the suboccipital musculature.

Q1. You perform a technique to most directly mobilize fluid and lymph drainage from his pharyngotympanic tube. Which of the following is true about this technique?

    A. Use an oscillatory activating force at a rate of 60 to 80 per minute.

    B. Hold sustained forces on the suboccipital musculature.

    C. Use gentle pressure to stretch the mandibular ligament.

    D. Allow the patient's head to turn from side to side to improve drainage.

    E. Contact the pharyngotympanic tube with your little finger.

Q2. You perform a technique to best directly address his cervical lymphadenopathy. Which label correctly identifies the structure in **Fig. 7.6** by location and name?

    A. Trapezius muscle.

    B. Posterior scalene muscle.

    C. Anterior scalene muscle.

    D. Sternothyroid muscle.

    E. Sternocleidomastoid muscle.

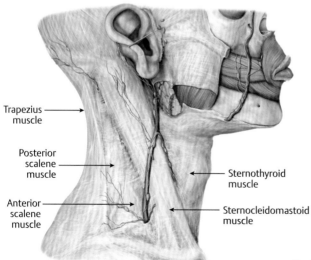

Fig. 7.6 Figure for Case 1, Q2.

Case 2

A 70-year-old man is hospitalized for bacterial pneumonia, secondary to influenza. His condition is stable, and he is continuing to receive intravenous antibiotics. Physical exam reveals coarse breath sounds in the right lower lung, decreased thoracoabdominal diaphragm motion with inhalation, seventh through tenth ribs with inhalation somatic dysfunction, thoracic outlet inlet fascial restriction bilaterally.

Q3. Your attending physician requests that you perform OMT to improve lymphatic flow. You begin with this technique:
   A. Thoracic outlet myofascial release.
   B. Thoracoabdominal diaphragm myofascial release.
   C. Ribs 7 through 10 muscle energy.
   D. Rib 5 muscle energy.
   E. Thoracic pump.

Q4. To perform a thoracic pump technique on this patient
   A. Be sure he does not have moderate to severe chronic obstructive lung disease.
   B. Create activating forces in the range of 5 to 10 per second.
   C. Direct forces posteriorly through the patient's upper rib cage.
   D. Instruct the patient to take four slow, deep breaths.
   E. Use the palm of your hand to contact the middle of his sternum.

Case 3

A 72-year-old woman is in the hospital for right lower leg cellulitis and is on IV antibiotics. There is erythema and moderate edema of the right leg from the middle thigh to the middle of the lower leg. Osteopathic exam reveals passive congestion in her right popliteal fossa and a compensated pattern on respiratory/circulatory exam.

Q5. What lymphatic technique would be most appropriate for this patient?
   A. Pharyngotympanic tube pump.
   B. Anterior cervical effleurage.
   C. Thoracic pump.
   D. Pedal pump.
   E. None, OMT is contraindicated in this patient.

Q6. What is the appropriate rate of oscillations when treating with a pedal pump technique?
   A. 30 per minute.
   B. 60 per minute.
   C. 90 per minute.
   D. 150 per minute.
   E. 200 per minute.

Answers to Review Questions

Q1. The correct answer is **C**.
   A is incorrect. The correct rate is 18 to 30 per minute, or one stretch every 2 to 3 seconds.
   B is incorrect. This is the description for suboccipital inhibition.
   D is incorrect. One should stabilize the head to prevent movement—see technique description.
   E is incorrect. This description is for a direct pharyngotympanic tube release that is not in this manual.

Q2. The correct answer is **E**. The others are incorrect. Refer to technique description for lymphatic techniques: Anterior Cervical Effleurage. The structures should be labeled correctly as follows:
   A. Trapezius muscle.
   B. Posterior scalene muscle.
   C. Anterior scalene muscle.
   D. Sternothyroid muscle.
   E. Sternocleidomastoid muscle.

Q3. The correct answer is **A**. It is best to release the thoracic outlet before starting lymphatic treatment. Answers **B–E** are regions other than the thoracic outlet.

Q4. The correct answer is **C**.
   A is incorrect. Severe chronic obstructive lung disease is a contraindication for modified thoracic pump only.
   B is incorrect. Five to 10 per second is too fast. The rate should be 1 to 2 per second.
   D is incorrect. This is for the modified thoracic pump.
   E is an incorrect contact.

Q5. The correct answer is **D**: pedal pump.

A. Pharyngotympanic tube pump is more appropriate for middle ear and upper respiratory symptoms.

B. Anterior cervical effleurage is more appropriate for upper respiratory symptoms.

C. Thoracic pump is more appropriate for respiratory symptoms.

E. No contraindications are apparent in this case.

Q6. The correct answer is **D**: 150 per minute.

A. Thirty per minute is much slower than the recommended 2 to 3 per second (120–180 per minute).

B. Sixty per minute is much slower than the recommended 2 to 3 per second (120–180 per minute).

C. Ninety per minute is slower than the recommended 2 to 3 per second (120–180 per minute).

E. Two hundred per minute is faster than the recommended 2 to 3 per second (120–180 per minute).

References

1. Still AT. Philosophy of Osteopathy. Academy of Applied Osteopathy; 1899
2. Millard D. Applied Anatomy of the Lymphatics. Health Research Books; 1964 It is open-access and can be found at http://www.archive.org/details/appliedanatomyof00milliala.
3. Knott EM, Tune JD, Stoll ST, Downey HF. Increased lymphatic flow in the thoracic duct during manipulative intervention. J Am Osteopath Assoc 2005;105(10):447–456
4. Chikly BJ. Manual techniques addressing the lymphatic system: Origins and development. J Am Osteopath Assoc 2005;105(10):457–464
5. Miller C. The lymphatic pump, its application to acute infections. J Am Osteopath Assoc 1926;25(Pt 1):443–445

Bibliography

Ehrlenbach, Heike. A preliminary investigation of the effect of the osteopathic lymphatic pump technique on salivary Immunoglobulin A levels in asymptomatic subjects: A single systems design pilot study. 2011

Falzon M. The effect of lymphatic pump techniques on the FEV and FVC measurements in people with asthma: a pilot study. Diss. Victoria University, 2003

Hodge LM. Osteopathic lymphatic pump techniques to enhance immunity and treat pneumonia. Int J Osteopath Med 2012;15(1):13–21

Hodge LM, Downey HF. Lymphatic pump treatment enhances the lymphatic and immune systems. Exp Biol Med (Maywood) 2011;236(10):1109–1115

Hodge LM, Creasy C, Carter K, Orlowski A, Schander A, King HH. Lymphatic pump treatment as an adjunct to antibiotics for pneumonia in a rat model. J Am Osteopath Assoc 2015;115(5):306–316

Huff JB, Schander A, Downey HF, Hodge LM. Lymphatic pump treatment augments lymphatic flux of lymphocytes in rats. Lymphat Res Biol 2010;8(4):183–187

Jackson KM, Steele TF, Dugan EP, Kukulka G, Blue W, Roberts A. Effect of lymphatic and splenic pump techniques on the antibody response to hepatitis B vaccine: a pilot study. J Am Osteopath Assoc 1998;98(3):155–160

Klucka G, Irwin J, Ferencz V, Myers N, Nelson J, Kuchera ML. Effects of abdominal shape on abdominal "slosh" during pedal pump osteopathic manipulative treatment. J Bodywork Movement Ther 2012;16(4):521

Mascarenhas SP, Pandit U, Yardi S. Effect of Thoracic Lymphatic Pump Technique on Pulmonary Function in COPD Patients. Indian Journal of Physiotherapy and Occupational Therapy-An International Journal 2013;7(4):235–240

Mckenzie S, Erin I, Jennifer B. P-204 Lymphatic Pump Technique Enhances Immunity in a DSS Colitis Model. Inflamm Bowel Dis 2014;20:S107

Noll DR. The short-term effect of a lymphatic pump protocol on blood cell counts in nursing home residents with limited mobility: a pilot study. J Am Osteopath Assoc 2013;113(7):520–528

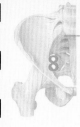

8 Indirect Techniques

LEARNING OBJECTIVES

1. Explain the goals of performing indirect techniques.
2. Identify the clinical considerations, including indications, contraindications, and precautions for performing indirect techniques.
3. Outline the general movements, barriers, and forces used to perform indirect techniques.
4. Identify the end goal for performing each indirect technique.
5. Visualize, verbalize, and identify the preparation, positioning, tissue contact, movements, barriers, and forces for each indirect technique.
6. Perform indirect techniques using appropriate somatic dysfunction diagnosis, preparation, positioning, tissue contact, movements, barriers, forces, retest for effectiveness, communication, and safe tissue handling.

Indirect Techniques Introduction

Indirect (IND) techniques are some of the oldest and gentlest osteopathic techniques. They are widely applicable for a range of patients and clinical conditions. IND techniques are especially useful in patient populations when direct method techniques are contraindicated, such as infants, children, and the elderly. When performed correctly, focused cognitive and palpatory attention is required to position, remain still, and monitor a joint for physiological changes. After practicing the basic IND techniques offered in this chapter, learners can apply the principles to correct somatic dysfunction in any joint in the body, including the cranial sutures. In general, IND techniques:

- Restore joint alignment.
- Normalize tension and tone of surrounding myofascial tissues, tendons, and ligaments.
- Improve local arterial, venous, and lymph circulation.
- Improve regional and joint active and passive range of motion.

Background

The IND techniques presented here represent one of three types of exaggeration techniques derived from the original techniques of Dr. Still. Through the years, IND techniques have been refined, modified, and probably even improved on. One popular derivative is balanced ligamentous tension (as developed by the A.T. Still Study Group in the New England region), in the style of William Garner Sutherland, DO. A second derivative of Dr. Sutherland's work is ligamentous articular strain (as developed by the Dallas Osteopathic Study Group). Another is functional technique. IND techniques in this manual follow the style described by Paul Kimberly, DO,[1] and are the most basic type, suited to a novice learner.

Research

IND techniques, including derivatives, are commonly used in research protocols, especially clinical trials involving pediatric patients. A research bibliography is not presented here because IND techniques themselves are rarely studied independently.

Clinical Considerations

Some common clinical things to consider when using IND techniques are listed in Table 8.1. Always acquire adequate data in the form of an appropriate patient history, a thorough physical exam, and relevant diagnostic tests in order to exercise best clinical judgment before performing osteopathic manipulative treatment (OMT).

Somatic Dysfunction Corrected

Somatic dysfunction diagnosis of a joint is required as IND techniques in this manual correct joint somatic dysfunction. The somatic dysfunction diagnosis can be made prior to the technique performance or after positional joint asymmetries and/or tissue texture changes are identified. In the latter case, as the joint is moved into the positions of ease, the somatic dysfunction diagnosis is made can be determined.

Positioning and Preparation

▶ Patient: the patient must be comfortable and remain relaxed for the duration of the technique. IND techniques can be performed with the patient sitting, supine, prone, or laterally recumbent.

▶ Physician: the physician must be comfortable and positioned to ensure safety, using the best ergonomic posture and movements possible. Levers and fulcrums are routinely employed.

Note: The videos include a narrated description of positioning when not visually self-explanatory.

Tissue Contact

Tissue contact is made with the finger pads, thenar or hypothenar eminences of one or both hands. Contact is relatively firm in order to move bones at a joint or joints.

- Performing contact: the performing hand is the contact that positions one bone of the joint, and it may also create the disengaging forces.
- Assisting contact: a second contact may be used to assist with positioning and/or create the disengaging force.

Movements, Barriers, and Forces

IND techniques are performed by positioning a joint in the position of ease, or the indirect position, as determined by the barrier concept. The end goal is to position and hold a joint in order for the patient's inherent, physiological, homeostatic mechanisms to restore joint alignment and normalize tensions of surrounding tissues. The bones of the joint are positioned into all directions of the greatest amount of physiologic motion, which are in the direction(s)

Table 8.1 Clinical considerations	
Indications	**Contraindications**
Minor musculoskeletal injuries such as sprains/strains	Fracture or suspected fracture
Mechanical back and neck pain	Joint dislocation
Tension and migraine headache	Joint infection
Newborns with minor birth trauma or in utero compression	Moderate–severe or full-thickness tendon, ligament, or meniscal tear
Enthesopathies	
Mild, stable joint effusions due to inflammation/degeneration	Moderate–severe bloody or infectious joint effusion
Peripheral nerve compression syndromes	
Postural Imbalances	

of the named somatic dysfunction diagnosis and opposite the restrictive barrier(s). The corrective forces are the patient's inherent homeostatic mechanisms. The motionless and virtually tensionless positioning creates the environment for joint nociceptors and proprioceptors to reset to physiological resting tone. Consider IND techniques as a method for creating ease or slack into the tightened tissues of a slightly misaligned joint. When the tissues sense ease, or release of tension, the nervous system is no longer facilitated and can reset to normal signaling, resulting in repositioning of the joint.

Disengagement

To achieve optimal positioning, the articular surfaces of a joint are first disengaged with a compression or traction force. Compression loosens surrounding soft tissues, and distraction creates space in the articulation. A variation of distraction is to shift one bone of a joint in one direction only, such as pushing anteriorly on a transverse process to glide the articular surfaces away from each other slightly. Both compression and distraction forces enable the positioning of one bone of the joint and should only be forceful enough to loosen the tissues. Avoid excessive compression or traction that can reflexively result in tissue contraction or guarding. Compressive and traction forces have both been identified in each technique as a "best practice." However, if one type of disengagement force does not produce correction of somatic dysfunction, the technique can be performed with the other disengagement force.

Positioning

After disengagement, one bone of the joint is moved in the direction of the somatic dysfunction until tissue tension is maximally decreased or the tissues feel relaxed. This is sometimes called the position of ease. Often, the position of maximal relaxation is palpated as a "floating" sensation, where the bone is freely suspended and tension is not palpable in any direction. Positioning recommendations are included in some techniques as a guide. Make minor adjustments as necessary to move the joint into a position that creates the least tissue tension.

Holding Positions

Once positioned, both the patient and the physician should remain still. This allows the body's nervous system to detect the new joint position and tissue tensions to reset nervous system activity to "nor-mal." Tissue responses include increased capillary blood flow, resulting in warmth and pulselike sensations of this fluid movement. Normal muscle tone is also restored, and these changes can be palpated as shifts in tissue tension. Subsequently, the joint articular surfaces realign, and this may be palpated as a slight shift in tissue position. Collectively, the moment when tissue tension and joint alignment is restored is called a subtle release. Tissue response should be monitored until the changes stop or release occurs. The physician should hold positions steady and wait for these changes to stop. The moment of release can be instantaneous. However, if a release is not palpated, hold forces and positions for about 2 minutes, the time it generally takes for a tissue response. Holding the position of ease gives the physician an opportunity to witness the phenomenon of the body's inherent healing forces at work.

Although it is preferred that the patient remain motionless, IND can be performed on infants and small children who may move. In this case, the physician should follow the patient's movement and maintain disengagement forces and joint positioning.

Retest for Effectiveness

Elimination of positional asymmetry and restoration of full passive range of motion are indicators that the joint somatic dysfunction has resolved. If a correction is not made after the first attempt, the technique can be repeated from the very beginning to the end once more. After that, it is appropriate to rediagnose the somatic dysfunction, consider another technique, or investigate other possible causes of the somatic dysfunction.

IND Technique Summary Steps

- Layer palpate to the bony layer with attention to the articular surfaces and surrounding joint soft tissues.
- Disengagement: apply compression or distraction. Hold forces.
- Positioning: move one bone in the direction of the somatic dysfunction, or the physiological barriers, opposite that of the restrictive barrier.
- Hold: remain still and hold all forces and positions until release occurs or for up to 2 minutes.
  - Optional: add respiratory cooperation.
- Release forces.
- Retest for changes in somatic dysfunction.

Cervical/Upper Thoracic, C2–T5

This technique is efficient because somatic dysfunction from C2 to T5 (**Fig. 8.1**) can be treated with a shift of hand contact, essentially working your way up or down the spine one vertebra at a time. This technique is especially useful for newborns, infants, and smaller children.

Key Elements

- Somatic dysfunction corrected:
  - C2–C7: N/F/E S_XR_X.
  - T1–T5: NS_XR_Y, FR_XS_X, ER_XS_X, bilateral E, bilateral F.
- End goal: to position a vertebra in order to restore facet joint alignment and resolve associated myofascial tensions.

WATCH ▷ ▶ ▷

▶ *Video 8.1 Cervical/Upper Thoracic, C2-T5—Narrated*

Example Somatic Dysfunction: C3 ER_LS_L

Positioning and Preparation

▶ Patient: supine.
▶ Physician: sitting at the head of the table.

Tissue Contact

- Both hands disengage and position the vertebra. Use your right hand to contact the right transverse process and your left hand to contact the left.

- Positioning hands: contact the vertebral arches (cervical vertebrae) or transverse processes (thoracic vertebrae) of the dysfunctional vertebra with the pads of the second and/or third fingers.

Movements, Barriers, and Forces

Use both hands to do the following:

- Layer palpate to the vertebra.
- Disengagement: apply anteriorly directed forces along the plane of the vertebral facets to disengage the vertebral articulations. Hold these forces.
- Positioning: move the vertebra into the position of the sagittal plane somatic dysfunction, if flexion or extension dysfunction is present.
  - Apply inferior traction forces if the vertebra is extended, superior traction forces if the vertebra is flexed.
- With the contact that is on the side opposite the rotation vertebrae, apply additional anteriorly directed force to rotate the vertebra further.
  - Side bending is not necessary because it occurs with rotation.
- Hold: remain still and hold all forces and positions until release occurs or for up to 2 minutes.
  - Optional: add respiratory cooperation.
- Release forces.
- Retest the vertebra for changes in position and/or passive range of motion.

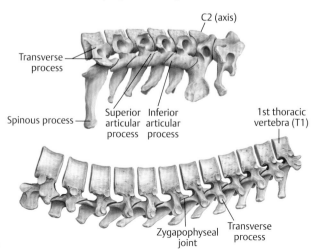

Fig. 8.1 Cervical and thoracic spines.

Costal, Ribs 2–10

Because this technique is performed in the seated position and universally applicable to any somatic dysfunction in ribs 2–10 (**Fig. 8.2**), it is useful in an emergency room or outpatient setting in cases of musculoskeletal chest wall pain. Be sure to describe the anterior hand contact to the patient prior to performing this technique, particularly when breast tissue can be encountered.

Key Elements

- Somatic dysfunction corrected: any somatic dysfunction in ribs 2–10.
- End goal: to position a rib in order to restore costotransverse and costovertebral joint alignment and resolve associated myofascial tensions.

> **WATCH** ▷ ▶ ▷
>
> ▶ *Video 8.2 Costal, Ribs 2-10—Narrated*
>
> *Example Somatic Dysfunction: Left Rib 2 Anterior*

Positioning and Preparation

▶ Patient: sitting.

▶ Physician: sitting beside the patient at the side of the dysfunctional rib and facing the same or the opposite direction as the patient.

- Alternate patient positioning: supine without using rotation of the torso.
- Alternate physician positioning: sitting beside the supine patient, on the side of the dysfunctional rib, facing the patient (this is especially useful for newborns and hospitalized patients).

Tissue Contact

- Both hands disengage and position a dysfunctional rib at the anterior (costosternal or costochondral) and posterior (costotransverse and/or costovertebral) articulations.

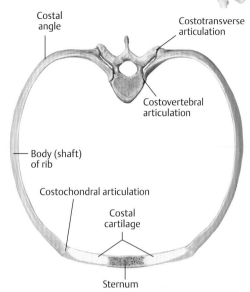

Fig. 8.2   Rib articulations.

- Anterior performing hand: contact the anterior shaft of the dysfunctional rib just lateral to the costochondral articulation with the pad(s) of the second and/or third finger(s). Allow the fingers to wrap around the contour of the rib, if possible, and contact the shaft of the rib at the midaxillary line with the thumb.
  - Note: if the underwire of a bra is significantly obstructing tissue contact, either request permission to move your hand underneath the underwire (remaining over the clothing), or ask the patient to shift or unhook the bra temporarily in order to perform the technique. If breast tissue is obstructing lateral rib contact, maintain anterior contact only.
- Posterior performing hand: contact the posterior angle of the dysfunctional rib near the costotransverse articulation with the pad(s) of the second and/or third finger(s). Allow the fingers to wrap around the contour of the rib so that this thumb is alongside the other thumb at the midaxillary line.

141

Movements, Barriers, and Forces

Use both hands to do the following:

- Layer palpate to the rib.
- Disengagement, part 1: with your anterior contact, apply posteriorly directed force to disengage the costochondral articulation. Hold this force.
- Disengagement, part 2: with your posterior contact, apply anteriorly directed force to disengage the costotransverse and costovertebral articulations. Hold this force.
- Positioning: move the rib in the directions of the somatic dysfunction (Table 8.2).

- Ask the patient to rotate the torso in one of the following directions, whichever creates maximal ease:
  - Rotation away from the side of the dysfunctional rib eases tension in the costotransverse articulation.
  - Rotation toward the side of the dysfunctional rib eases tension in the costovertebral articulation.
- Hold: remain still and hold all forces and positions until release occurs or for up to 2 minutes.
  - Optional: add respiratory cooperation.
- Release forces.
- Retest the rib for changes in position, active and/or passive range of motion.

Table 8.2 Indirect techniques: costal, ribs 2–10, positioning

Somatic dysfunction	Positioning
Inhalation somatic dysfunctions	Pump handle: move the anterior shaft superiorly and the posterior shaft inferiorly. Bucket handle: move the lateral rib margin superiorly.
Exhalation somatic dysfunctions	Pump handle: move the anterior shaft inferiorly and the posterior shaft superiorly. Bucket handle: move the lateral rib margin inferiorly.
Anterior rib somatic dysfunctions	Move the rib further anteriorly by creating more anteriorly directed force with your posterior hand.
Posterior rib somatic dysfunctions	Move the rib further posteriorly by creating more posteriorly directed force with your anterior hand.

Costal, Ribs 11–12

This technique is especially useful for treating stubborn somatic dysfunctions of the thoracoabdominal diaphragm as well as quadratus lumborum muscle strain, because these muscles attach to the lowest ribs (Fig. 8.3). It is also useful for treating the diaphragm when the anterior portion cannot be easily contacted, such as post–coronary artery bypass surgery or in pregnancy.

Key Elements

- Somatic dysfunction corrected: R/L rib 11 or 12 inhalation/exhalation.
- End goal: to position a rib in order to restore costovertebral joint alignment and improve rib motion, thoracoabdominal diaphragm movement, and function.

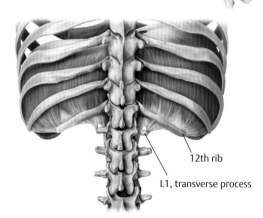

12th rib

L1, transverse process

Fig. 8.3 Ribs 11–12.

Positioning and Preparation

► Patient: supine.
► Physician: sitting on the side of the dysfunctional rib, facing the patient, with forearms resting on the table.

Tissue Contact

• Both hands disengage and position one dysfunctional rib at the costotransverse and costovertebral articulations.
• Performing hands: use the hand that is nearer the patient's head to contact the posterior shaft of the dysfunctional rib near the costotransverse articulation with the second and/or third finger pad. Place the remainder of your hand along the long axis of the rib, following the contour of the rib angle. Place your other hand beneath this hand. Adjust your body position to keep your wrists in neutral position with forearms resting on the table.
  – Detailed suggestion for finding the 12th rib: locate the posterior aspect of the iliac crest. Move your hand superiorly, pressing anteriorly, until a bony prominence is felt. This is the shaft of the 12th rib.

Movements, Barriers, and Forces

Use both hands to do the following:

• Layer palpate to the rib.
• Disengagement, part 1: apply an anteriorly directed force toward the costotransverse and costovertebral articulations with both hands.
• Disengagement, part 2: add lateral traction force for further disengagement.
• Positioning: with both hands, move the rib in the direction of the somatic dysfunction.
• Hold: remain still and hold all forces and positions until release occurs or for up to 2 minutes.
  – Optional: add respiratory cooperation.
• Release forces.
• Retest the rib for changes in position, active and/or passive range of motion.

Two-Person Technique

When both right and left 11th or 12th ribs have somatic dysfunction, two physicians can perform the technique simultaneously with one physician on each side of the patient. Keep tensions balanced between physicians so that one is not creating more anterior or lateral force than the other.

Pelvis, Innominate

If the patient has significant L5 lumbar paraspinal or iliopsoas muscular somatic dysfunction, consider treating those dysfunctions first to make positioning the innominate easier (**Fig. 8.4**).

Key Elements

• Somatic dysfunction corrected: innominate anterior/posterior rotation, superior/inferior shear, inflare/outflare.
• End goal: to position an innominate in order to restore sacroiliac joint position and resolve associated ligamentous tensions.

Positioning and Preparation

► Patient: supine.
► Physician: sitting beside the dysfunctional innominate.

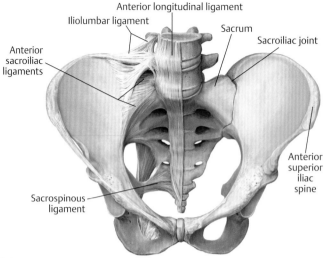

Fig. 8.4 Sacroiliac joint.

Tissue Contact

- The physician uses one hand to position the innominate and the other hand for disengagement.
- Positioning hand: contact the anterior superior iliac spine (ASIS) with the pads of the thumb, second, and third fingers so as to be able to grasp it. Alternatively, the ASIS can be contacted by the palm of the hand.
- Assisting hand: contact the lateral sacral margin near the sacroiliac joint with the pads of the second through fourth fingers.

Movements, Barriers, and Forces

Use the assisting hand as follows:

- Layer palpate to the sacrum.
- Disengagement: create an anteriorly directed force. Hold this force.

Use the positioning hand as follows:

- Positioning: move the ASIS in the direction of the innominate somatic dysfunction until the tissues ease (Table 8.3).
- Hold: remain still and hold all forces and positions until release occurs or for up to 2 minutes.
  - Optional: add respiratory cooperation.
- Release forces.
- Retest the innominate for changes in position and/or passive range of motion.

Table 8.3 Indirect techniques: pelvis, innominate positioning	
Somatic dysfunction diagnosis	**Positioning**
Innominate anterior rotation	Rotate the ASIS inferiorly
Innominate posterior rotation	Rotate the ASIS superiorly
Innominate superior shear	Shift or push the ASIS superiorly by creating force from the inferior aspect. Avoid rotation.
Innominate inferior shear	Shift or pull the ASIS inferiorly by creating force from the superior aspect. Avoid rotation.
Innominate inflare	Move the ASIS medially
Innominate outflare	Move the ASIS laterally

Abbreviation: ASIS, anterior superior iliac spine.

Sacrum

Because this technique can treat almost any somatic dysfunction of the sacrum, including dysfunctions related to cranial strain patterns, it can become an invaluable technique (**Fig. 8.5**). It is also appropriate to use this technique during two-person treatments when one person is treating the cranium. Be sure to explain the tissue contacts and steps of the technique to the patient prior to performing OMT in this sensitive area.

Key Elements

- Somatic dysfunction corrected: somatic dysfunction of the sacrum at the sacroiliac joints.
- End goal: to position the sacrum at both sacroiliac joints in order to restore both sacral movement and position, and to resolve associated ligamentous tensions.

WATCH ▷ ▶ ▷

▶ *Video 8.5 Sacrum—Narrated*

Example Somatic Dysfunction: Sacrum Rotated Left on a Left Oblique Axis

Positioning and Preparation

▶ Patient: supine, with knees bent and feet on the table.

▶ Physician: sitting at the side of the table at the level of the patient's pelvis, turned, facing the patient's head.

Tissue Contact

- One hand contacts the sacrum for positioning, and the other hand and forearm contact the ilia for disengagement.
- Performing hand: use the hand that is nearer the table. Contact the sacral base with the pads of the second through fourth fingers. Allow the palm of your hand to contact the rest of the sacrum with the inferior lateral angles of the sacrum near or on the palm of your hand. Do not put pressure directly on the sensitive coccyx.
  - Detailed suggestion: ask the patient to lift the hips off of the table slightly. Locate the posterior superior iliac spine (PSIS) nearer you and place the pad of your fourth digit medial to it. Ask the patient to return the hips onto the table and onto your hand.
- Assisting contact: with the finger pads of the second through fourth fingers, contact the anterior aspect of the ASIS on the side farther from you, and with your forearm contact the anterior aspect ASIS on the side nearer you.

Movements, Barriers, and Forces

- Disengagement: with the assisting contact, apply medially directed forces that bring the ASIS's closer together, effectively creating lateral traction forces of the innominates at the sacroiliac joints. Hold these forces.

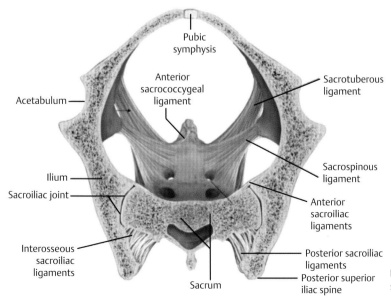

Fig. 8.5 Sacroiliac joints, superior view.

Pubic symphysis

Anterior sacrococcygeal ligament

Acetabulum

Sacrotuberous ligament

Sacrospinous ligament

Anterior sacroiliac ligaments

Ilium

Sacroiliac joint

Interosseous sacroiliac ligaments

Posterior sacroiliac ligaments

Posterior superior iliac spine

Sacrum

With your performing hand, layer palpate to the sacrum.

- Positioning: move the sacrum into the position of somatic dysfunction (Table 8.4).
- Hold: remain still and hold all forces and positions until release occurs or for up to 2 minutes.

- Optional: add respiratory cooperation.
- Release forces.
- Retest the sacrum for changes in position and/or passive range of motion.

Table 8.4 Indirect techniques: sacrum positioning

Somatic dysfunction	Positioning
Torsions	Position the sacrum with your fingers and thenar and hypothenar eminences and in the direction of the sacral rotation, rotating the sacrum around the named oblique axis.
Shears	Apply superiorly directed force with the thenar or hypothenar eminence that is contacting the inferior lateral angle on the same side of the anterior sacral base. Inferior shears will require inferior traction by the finger pads on the same side as the shear.

Upper Extremity, Clavicle

This technique is useful for cases of acromioclavicular pain and minor shoulder/arm injuries. It also eliminates myofascial tension around the thoracic outlet, which improves lymphatic fluid circulation. Because the clavicles attach to the sternum and are connected through the interclavicular ligament, it is often the case that both clavicles have somatic dysfunction and benefit from OMT (Fig. 8.6).

Key Elements

- Somatic dysfunction corrected: clavicle— internal/external rotation, anterior/posterior, superior/inferior.
- End goal: to position a clavicle in order to restore sternoclavicular and acromioclavicular joint alignment and resolve associated myofascial tensions.

WATCH ▷ ► ▷

▶ *Video 8.6 Upper Extremity, Clavicle— Narrated*

Example Somatic Dysfunction: Left Clavicle Inferior and Posterior

Positioning and Preparation

▶ Patient: supine.

▶ Physician: sitting at the head of the table.

Tissue Contact

- Both hands contact the clavicle.

Fig. 8.6 Clavicle, superior view.

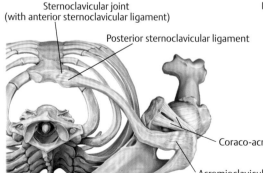

Sternoclavicular joint (with anterior sternoclavicular ligament)

Posterior sternoclavicular ligament

Coraco-acromial ligament

Acromioclavicular joint (with acromioclavicular ligament)

- Performing hands: contact the clavicle with the fingers and thumbs.
  - Detailed suggestion: contact the superior edge of the clavicle with the pads of both thumbs near the midline of the clavicle. Contact the inferior edge of the clavicle, near the acromion and the sternum, with the pads of the second through fifth digits.

Movements, Barriers, and Forces

Use both hands to do the following:

- Layer palpate to the clavicle.
- Disengagement: apply superior traction forces with the second through fifth digits simultaneously to disengage the clavicle from both the sternoclavicular and acromioclavicular joints articulations.
- Positioning: move the clavicle in the directions of the somatic dysfunction (Table 8.5). Use the fingers to move the clavicle and the thumbs as a fulcrum.
  - For anterior/posterior somatic dysfunctions, reposition the first and second finger pads onto the anterior surface of the clavicle.
- Hold: remain still and hold all forces and positions until release occurs or for up to 2 minutes.
  - Optional: add respiratory cooperation.
- Release forces.
- Retest the clavicle for changes in position.

Table 8.5 Indirect techniques: upper extremity, clavicle positioning	
Somatic dysfunction	**Positioning**
Clavicle superior	Move the sternal end superiorly and the acromion end inferiorly.
Clavicle inferior	Move the sternal end inferiorly and the acromion end superiorly.
Clavicle internally rotated	Torque the clavicle to rotate it inferiorly (internal rotation).
Clavicle externally rotated	Torque the clavicle to rotate it superiorly (external rotation).
Clavicle anterior	Apply anteriorly directed forces at the sternal end.
Clavicle posterior	Apply anteriorly directed forces at the clavicular end.

Upper Extremity, Multiple Joints and Interosseous Membrane

This technique is useful for the entire upper extremity as a whole, when subjected to minor trauma, such as a fall. This is an intermediate-novice technique because forces and positions are "stacked" upon each other. While performing, be mindful to maintain all forces and joint positions (Fig. 8.7).

Key Elements

- Somatic dysfunction corrected: any somatic dysfunction of the radiocarpal, ulnocarpal, radial head, and glenohumeral joints; interosseous membrane somatic dysfunction.
- End goal: to position multiple joint somatic dysfunctions in the upper extremity simultaneously in order to restore joint alignment and resolve associated myofascial tissue tensions.

> **WATCH ▷▶▷**
>
> ▶ *Video 8.7 Upper Extremity: Multiple Joints and Interosseous Membrane—Narrated*
>
> *Example Somatic Dysfunction: Wrist Extension, Forearm Pronation, Interosseous Membrane Tightness and Humerus Internal Rotation*

Positioning and Preparation

- ▶ Patient: supine, with arm by side.
- ▶ Physician: sitting at the level of the elbow facing the patient's head.

Tissue Contact

- Both hands contact the upper extremity, create disengagement forces, and position multiple joints.

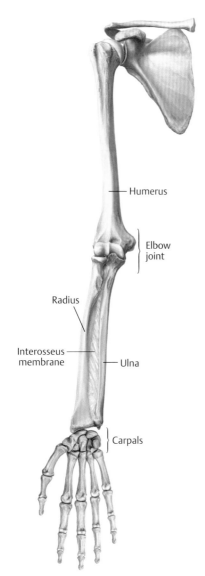

Fig. 8.7   Upper extremity.

- Performing hands: with one hand, grasp, as if shaking, the patient's hand. The other hand contacts the elbow and bends it slightly so the elbow is in the palm of the hand.
  - Detailed suggestion: use your right hand to contact the patient's right wrist, and your left hand to contact the patient's left wrist. Contact the elbow at the medial and lateral epicondyles with the fingers and the olecranon with the palm of the hand.

Movements, Barriers, and Forces

With both hands, layer palpate to the bony layer.

Part 1: Radiocarpal and Ulnocarpal Joint

Disengagement: with the hand contacting the wrist:

- Create a compressive force into the wrist joints using the hand contact at the elbow to hold the forearm steady. Hold this force.
- Positioning: move the wrist in the direction(s) of the somatic dysfunction and hold this position.

Part 2: Interosseous Membrane

- Disengagement: add an additional compressive force into the interosseous membrane until the force is felt with your hand contacting the elbow. Hold this force.
- Positioning: move the forearm in the direction of the somatic dysfunction. Hold this position.

Part 3: Glenohumeral Joint

- Disengagement: with the hand contacting the elbow, create a compressive force along the long axis of the humerus toward the glenohumeral joint. Hold this force.
- Positioning: move the humerus in the direction of somatic dysfunction.
- Hold: remain still and hold all forces and positions until release occurs or for up to 2 minutes.
  - Optional: add respiratory cooperation.
- Release forces.
- Retest the affected joints for changes in position, active and/or passive range of motion.

Notes

- Distraction can be used in place of compression as the disengagement force.
- This technique can be performed on the lower extremity with analogous contacts and movements. Contact the ankle and knee instead of the wrist and elbow.

Lower Extremity: Tibiofemoral Joint

Among others, this technique is useful in cases of musculoskeletal knee pain, patella-femoral syndrome, postoperative knee arthroplasty, and osteoarthritis. This technique is safe to perform if mild edema is present and severe pathology has been ruled out. Keep in mind the ligaments, bursae, and menisci that support this joint (**Fig. 8.8**).

Key Elements

- Somatic dysfunction corrected: tibia internally/externally rotated, anterior/posterior, medial/lateral.
- End goal: to position the tibia and femur in order to restore tibiofemoral joint alignment and resolve associated myofascial tensions.

WATCH ▷▶▷

▶ *Video 8.8 Lower Extremity, Tibiofemoral Joint—Narrated*

Example Somatic Dysfunction: Tibia Posterior, Internally Rotated, and Abducted

---

Positioning and Preparation

▶ Patient: supine.
▶ Physician: standing on the side of the dysfunctional knee, facing the knee.

Tissue Contact

- Both hands create disengagement forces. One hand moves the femur and the other moves the tibia.
- Superior performing hand: contact the medial femoral condyle with the fingertips of the second and third fingers, and the lateral femoral condyle with the thumb. Wrap the remaining fingers and hand around the contour of the femur.
- Inferior performing hand: contact the medial condyle of the tibia with the fingertips of the second and third fingers and the lateral condyle of the tibia with the thumb. Wrap the remaining fingers and hand around the contour of the tibia.

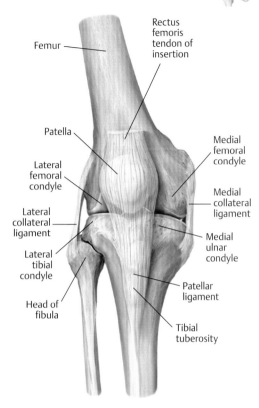

Femur — Rectus femoris tendon of insertion

Patella

Lateral femoral condyle

Medial femoral condyle

Lateral collateral ligament

Medial collateral ligament

Lateral tibial condyle

Medial ulnar condyle

Head of fibula

Patellar ligament

Tibial tuberosity

Fig. 8.8 Knee joint.

Movements, Barriers, and Forces

Use both hands to do the following:

- Layer palpate to the bony layer.
- Disengagement: apply compressive forces into the tibiofemoral joint by drawing both hands together.
- Positioning: move the tibia and femur in all directions of the somatic dysfunction.
- Hold: remain still and hold all forces and positions until release occurs or for up to 2 minutes.
  - Optional: add respiratory cooperation.
- Release forces.
- Retest the tibiofemoral joint for changes in position, active and/or passive range of motion.

Lower Extremity, Fibula and Interosseous Membrane

Classically used as part of OMT for minor ankle sprains, this technique is also useful for cases of shin splints and musculoskeletal pain of the foot and knee. OMT to the fibula is also recommended as part of a comprehensive approach to improving or resolving postural imbalance (**Fig. 8.9**).

Key Elements

- Somatic dysfunction corrected: anterior/posterior fibular head, interosseous membrane restriction.
- End goal: to position the fibula in order to restore proximal and distal tibiofibular joint alignments and resolve associated interosseous membrane and ligamentous tensions.

> **WATCH ▷ ▶ ▷**
>
> ▶ *Video 8.9 Lower Extremity, Fibula and Interosseus Membrane—Narrated*
>
> *Example Somatic Dysfunction: Right Fibular Head Anterior*

Positioning and Preparation

▶ Patient: supine.

▶ Physician: sitting beside the affected fibula, facing the patient.

Tissue Contact

- Both hands are used simultaneously for disengagement and positioning.
- Superior performing contact: Fibular head: use your hand that is nearer the patient's head. Contact the posterior aspect of the fibular head with the thumb pad.
- Inferior performing contact: lateral malleolus: use your hand that is nearer the patient's foot. Contact the posterior aspect of the lateral malleolus with your thumb pad.
- Ask the patient to keep the leg relaxed in order for you to bend the hip and knee.
- Lift the leg so the hip and knee are both at 90 degrees of flexion.

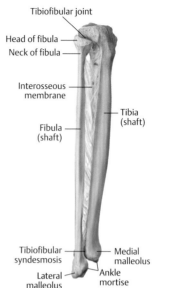

Fig. 8.9   Tibiofibular joints and interosseous membrane.

- Place your elbows on the edge of the table. Allow the weight of the patient's leg to rest on both of your thumbs. If necessary due to the weight, support the calcaneus with the palm or heel of your hand.

Movements, Barriers, and Forces

Use both hands to do the following:

- Layer palpate to the bony layer.
- Disengagement: gravity and the weight of the patient's leg upon the thumbs create the disengagement forces (essentially moving the fibula anteriorly).
- Positioning: move the fibula into the direction of the somatic dysfunction until tissue tensions decrease (Table 8.6).
- Hold: remain still and hold all forces and positions until release occurs or for up to 2 minutes.
  - Optional: add respiratory cooperation.
- Release forces.
- Retest the fibular head and/or interosseous membrane for changes in tension, position, active and/or passive range of motion.

Table 8.6 Indirect techniques: lower extremity, fibula and interosseus membrane positioning	
Somatic dysfunction diagnosis	**Positioning**
Fibular head anterior	Move the fibular head further anteriorly.
Fibular head posterior	Move the lateral malleolus further anteriorly.

Lower Extremity: Talonavicular and Calcaneocuboid

These techniques are invaluable in cases of plantar fasciitis and symptomatic pes planus. Proceed slowly, but be sure to use sufficient force to position the affected bone. Remember that the foot is subject to many pounds of pressure per square inch. These technique steps can also be modified to address the cuneiforms and metatarsals.

Key Elements

- Somatic dysfunction corrected: any cuboid or navicular somatic dysfunction.
- End goal: to position the cuboid or navicular to restore joint alignment and resolve associated plantar fascial and ligamentous tensions.

> **WATCH** ▷▷▷
>
> ▶ *Video 8.10 Lower Extremity, Calcaneocuboid—Narrated*
>
> ***Example Somatic Dysfunction: Dropped Cuboid***

Positioning and Preparation

- ▶ Patient: supine.
- ▶ Physician: standing near the foot with the somatic dysfunction, facing the patient's foot.

Tissue Contact

- One hand positions the dysfunctional bone while the other hand stabilizes the articulation nearer the ankle.
- Performing hand: contact the dysfunctional bone on the side of the foot with the thumb and second and third fingers so as to grasp it.
- Assisting contact: contact the bone of the proximal joint.
  - For a navicular dysfunction, contact the anterior and medial talus with the thumb and second and third fingers.
  - For a cuboid dysfunction, contact the anterior and lateral calcaneus with the thumb and second and third fingers.

Movements, Barriers, and Forces

Use both hands to do the following:

- Layer palpate to the bones.
- Disengagement: compress hands together to compress the affected joint. Hold forces.
- Positioning: move the affected bone in the direction of the somatic dysfunction (Table 8.7).
- Hold: remain still and hold all forces and positions until release occurs or for up to 2 minutes.
- Release forces.
- Retest the cuboid or navicular bone for changes in position.

Table 8.7 Indirect techniques: lower extremity: talonavicular and calcaneocuboid positioning	
Somatic dysfunction diagnosis	**Positioning**
Dropped navicular	Rotate the navicular medially around the long axis of the foot.
Dropped cuboid	Rotate the cuboid laterally around the long axis of the foot

Chapter Summary

Indirect techniques are original osteopathic techniques, well tolerated by patients and applicable for every joint in the body. They gently reestablish normal joint motions, tissue tensions, and arterial, venous, and lymphatic fluid flow. In this chapter, specific IND techniques are detailed to emphasize the principles while permitting adaptability of each technique for unique joint configurations.

Clinical Cases and Review Questions

Case 1

A 75-year-old man presents to the clinic with chronic back pain. He has a history of an L5 compression fracture 1 year ago and mild spinal stenosis. He is monitored regularly for his spinal stenosis by his neurologist. On examination you find diffuse tenderness to palpation over the lumbar paraspinal muscles and moderately decreased range of motion with flexion and rotation. Strength is a 4 out of 5 in both lower extremities, and reflexes are intact bilaterally in the upper and lower extremities. L3 is ER_RS_R, the right sacroiliac joint has decreased passive range of motion, and the right innominate is anteriorly rotated.

Q1. Which of the following is a contraindication for performing indirect technique on this patient's innominate?
   A. The patient's age.
   B. The history of compression fracture at L5.
   C. Exam findings of decreased muscle strength.
   D. The history of mild spinal stenosis.
   E. There are no contraindications.

Q2. What directions(s) would you position his L3 vertebra to perform an indirect technique?
   A. Flexion, rotation left, and side-bending left.
   B. Extension, rotation left, and side-bending left.
   C. Flexion, rotation right, and side-bending right.
   D. Extension, rotation right, and side-bending right.
   E. Extension only.

Q3. You also correct his innominate somatic dysfunction with indirect technique. You disengage the appropriate joint by
   A. Applying anteriorly directed force into the sacrum near the sacroiliac joint.
   B. Applying posteriorly directed force into both sacroiliac joints.
   C. Asking the patient to bend both of his knees.
   D. Asking the patient to take a deep breath and hold it.
   E. Rotating the innominate anteriorly.

Case 2

A 32-year-old woman complains of anterior and medial knee pain. The pain is worse when walking up stairs. Physical exam is positive for patellar grind. Structural exam reveals that the tibia is internally rotated, flexed, and resists medial translation.

Q4. After making appropriate tissue contact with the tibia and femur and layer palpating, what is the next step for performing indirect technique in this patient?
   A. Apply a medial disengagement force into the joint. Lift the patient's leg so the tibia is resting on your fingers.
   B. Request that the patient take three deep breaths for respiratory cooperation.
   C. Position the tibia in internal rotation.
   D. Position the tibia in external rotation.
   E. Apply a compressive force into the tibiofemoral joint.

Q5. What is the corrective force that resolves the somatic dysfunction in this patient, using indirect technique?
   A. The patient's inherent physiological mechanisms.
   B. The patient's popliteus muscle contraction effort.
   C. The physician holding the tibia in a position of ease.
   D. The physician's use of a thrust force.
   E. The physician's use of gentle, repetitive forces at the tibiofemoral joint.

Q6. In the clinic, you have just examined a 19-year-old man for viral upper respiratory symptoms, including cough. The patient complains of pain in his right lateral rib cage with inhalation. Exam reveals that his right rib 6 has an exhalation somatic dysfunction. The correct directions to position his rib are

A. Anterior and posterior shafts anteriorly.

B. Anterior and posterior shafts posteriorly.

C. Anterior shaft inferior, posterior shaft superior.

D. Anterior shaft superior, posterior shaft inferior.

Answers to Review Questions

Q1. The correct answer is **E**: There are no contraindications.

A is incorrect. Indirect techniques can be used safely in all ages.

B is incorrect. The fracture is old and we are not doing OMT directly over the area of injury. Indirect technique may be applied to L5 if healed and well tolerated by the patient.

C is incorrect. There are no red flags on exam preventing indirect treatment at this time. If he had an acute change in his findings then further workup may be warranted before treating with OMT.

D is incorrect. History of mild spinal stenosis is not a contraindication to indirect technique if symptoms are stable.

Q2. The correct answer is **D**. For indirect techniques the dysfunctional segment is positioned to the ease. Therefore the treatment position is the same as the somatic dysfunction diagnosis (ERSR).

Q3. The correct answer is **A**: Applying anteriorly directed force into the sacrum near the sacroiliac joint.

B is incorrect. Applying posteriorly directed force is not the correct direction of force.

C is incorrect. Asking the patient to bend both of his knees is not disengagement.

D is incorrect. Asking the patient to take a deep breath and hold it describes respiratory cooperation, not disengagement.

E is incorrect. Rotating the innominate anteriorly describes the correct positioning, not disengagement.

Q4. The correct answer is **E**. The first step of any indirect technique is to apply a disengagement force to the joint. After the joint is disengaged, the tissues can be taken into the direction of the diagnosis (i.e., away from the restrictive barrier and toward the ease) to a balance point.

Q5. The correct answer is **A**: The patient's inherent physiological mechanisms.

B is incorrect. The patient's popliteus muscle contraction effort is used in muscle energy techniques.

C is incorrect. The physician holding the tibia in a position of ease is not a corrective force; it is an assisting force.

D is incorrect. The physician's use of a thrust force is used in high velocity, low amplitude techniques.

E is incorrect. The physician's use of gentle, repetitive forces at the tibiofemoral joint is used in articulatory techniques.

Q6. The correct answer is **C**: Anterior shaft inferior, posterior shaft superior describes the positioning for an exhalation rib somatic dysfunction.

A is incorrect. Anterior and posterior shafts anteriorly describes the positioning for an anterior rib somatic dysfunction.

B is incorrect. Anterior and posterior shafts posteriorly describes the positioning for a posterior rib somatic dysfunction.

D is incorrect. Anterior shaft superior, posterior shaft inferior describes the positioning for an inhalation rib somatic dysfunction.

Reference

1. Kimberly PE, Dickey J, Halma KD. Outline of Osteopathic Manipulative Procedures: The Kimberly Manual. Kirksville, MO: AT Still University of Health Sciences, Kirksville College of Osteopathic Medicine, Department of Osteopathic Manipulative Medicine; 2009

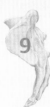

9 Articulatory Techniques

LEARNING OBJECTIVES

1. Explain the goals of performing articulatory techniques.
2. Identify the clinical considerations, including indications, contraindications, and precautions for performing articulatory techniques.
3. Outline the general movements, barriers, and forces used when performing articulatory techniques.
4. Visualize, verbalize, and identify the preparation, positioning, tissue contact, movements, barriers, and forces for each articulatory technique.
5. Perform articulatory techniques using appropriate somatic dysfunction diagnosis, preparation, positioning, tissue contact, movements, barriers, forces, retest for effectiveness, communication, and safe tissue handling.

Articulatory Techniques Introduction

Articulatory (ART) techniques are some of the earliest osteopathic techniques directed at increasing joint range of motion. ART techniques are presented here as a general technique because a specific positional somatic dysfunction diagnosis is not required. Initiation of the technique steps and the end points can, in many cases, be chosen at the discretion of the physician. Despite the apparent lack of specificity, ART techniques are widely applicable across a range of patients and conditions because of the gentle forces used. Thus, ART techniques are clinically useful, especially when other techniques that correct joint somatic dysfunction are contraindicated, as evidenced by reports that ART techniques for the sacrum and pelvis are commonly performed.[1]

ART techniques can also be applied to joints in which the joint architecture has been slightly altered by arthritic or degenerative changes. Joints most amenable to ART techniques are those with larger ranges of motion, such as synovial joints.

ART techniques can be used as a primary treatment or following soft tissue or myofascial release techniques, to do the following:

- Increase or restore joint range of motion.
- Improve local arterial, venous, and lymph circulation.
- Normalize autonomic nervous system tone (costal and sacroiliac joint techniques).

Background

Most ART techniques have been performed since the inception of osteopathic medicine. The version presented here is one of three types of exaggeration techniques derived from the original techniques of Dr. Still. ART techniques are classified as an exaggeration technique because tissue ranges of motion are exaggerated with the assistance of a force vector.

Research

ART techniques are often included as a part of osteopathic manipulative treatment research protocols for clinical trials, especially costal and sacral techniques. A short research bibliography is included at the end of this chapter.

Clinical Considerations

Some common clinical things to consider when using ART techniques are listed in Table 9.1. Always acquire adequate data in the form of an appropriate history, a thorough physical exam that includes an exam for somatic dysfunction, and relevant diagnostic tests to exercise best clinical judgment before performing OMT.

Somatic Dysfunction Corrected

- ART techniques correct joint somatic dysfunction. ART techniques can be performed when passive range of motion somatic dysfunction is identified in a joint. Additionally, because ART techniques are general techniques, active range of motion

restrictions are also an acceptable somatic dysfunction diagnosis substitute. In the spine and in other joints, multiple plane positional diagnosis is not required.

Positioning and Preparation

- ▶ Patient: the patient must be comfortable and relaxed for the duration of the technique.
- ▶ Physician: the physician must also be comfortable and able to ensure his or her own safety as well as the safety of the patient.

Tissue Contact

Tissue contact is made with the finger pads, thenar or hypothenar eminences of one or both hands. Contact is relatively firm because bones are being mobilized.

- Performing contact: the performing contact creates the force vector and range of motion movements.
- Monitoring/stabilizing contact: one hand monitors and/or stabilizes the joint so the performing hand can perform the technique. Some techniques are unmonitored.

Movements, Barriers, and Forces

ART techniques described in this manual are classified as combined techniques that use both indirect and direct methods for correction of somatic dysfunction. Because a joint is moved through its full range of physiological motions, some motions move the joint toward, and some away from, the restrictive barriers. The end goal of ART techniques

Table 9.1 Clinical considerations		
Indications	**Contraindications**	**Precautions**
Mechanical neck and back pain	Fracture or suspected fracture	Use when performing on joints with
Sacroiliac joint pain/sacroiliitis	Joint dislocation	mild effusion.
Postural imbalance	Joint infection	Discontinue or modify technique if
Osteoarthritis	Moderate–severe or full-thickness	it causes pain.
Chronic pain conditions	tendon, ligament, or meniscal	
Adhesive capsulitis	tear	
Somatovisceral and viscerosomatic	Vertebral disk or spinal nerve	
reflexes	compression	
Carpal tunnel syndrome		

is to increase joint range of motion and articular surface alignment.

The joint is first disengaged using a force vector that is either compression or traction. A compressive force is directed in a linear fashion from a distant point into the articular surfaces. Compressive forces loosen the surrounding myofascial structures that enables the physician to move the joint. Traction forces can also be performed, but these are directed away from the joint and create a little space in an articulation, again enabling the physician to move the joint. The physician can choose to create compression or traction force vectors. Each technique guides the physician as to a recommended force vector to use. The amount of force to use to create the force vector is the amount that causes the myofascial tissues around the joint to change in tension (loosen or stretch slightly).

When a force vector is applied, the force is held and movements are created to move one bone of the joint. The other bone of the joint is stabilized, either with the monitoring/stabilizing contact or the surface of the treatment table. The corrective forces are the movements, which are performed at a moderate speed in multiple directions of the full anatomical range of motion. ART techniques are thus sometimes referred to as low velocity, medium amplitude (LVMA), and sometimes also called springing techniques. The physician creates joint movements in one direction in a planar, circular, or figure-eight fashion as the articular surface permits. The initial direction is chosen arbitrarily (remember this is a general technique) because the joint will be moved through its entire range of motion in at least two directions. After one or two movements in one direction of range or motion, the direction can be reversed and one or two movements performed in the reversed directions. This alternating directional pattern can be performed for a few cycle until the joint range of motion is increased.

Joint articular surfaces often realign either at the beginning of the range of motion movements or at the end. This makes intuitive sense. When moving the joint in the direction of the somatic dysfunction (indirect method), ligamentous recoil repositions the joint. When moving the joint in the direction of the restrictive barrier (direct method), the barrier is approached and overcome.

Retest for Effectiveness

Correction of somatic dysfunction is often palpated as joint movement during technique performance. If palpated, the technique can be stopped and the joint retested for changes in range of motion and/or position. In addition, correction can be palpated as increased range of motion. However, because ART is a general technique, it may not fully correct the somatic dysfunction. If resolution of somatic dysfunction is not achieved, recheck the patient's diagnosis, assess for other related somatic dysfunctions, and consider performing an alternate technique.

ART Technique Summary Steps

- Identify active or passive range of motion somatic dysfunction in a joint.
- Stabilize and monitor the dysfunctional joint.
- Apply a disengagement force (force vector) directed at the articular surfaces and hold this force throughout the rest of the technique.
  - The disengagement force can be compression or distraction.
- Move the joint through its full range of motion in one direction. Keep the force vector directed at the articular surfaces.
- Repeat this movement two or three times.
- Reverse directions and move the joint through its full range of motion.
- Repeat this movement two or three times.
  - Continue alternating directions of movements as necessary two or three more times until range of motion increases.
- Release the disengagement force.
- Retest the joint for improvements in position, active, and/or passive range of motion.

Note: The steps for techniques Costal, Ribs 2–10; Sacrum; and Upper Extremity, Glenohumeral Joint vary slightly from these steps.

Cervical C2–C7

This technique is especially useful as a diagnostic aid and in cases of cervical spondylosis. Perform slowly at first, increasing speed as the patient can tolerate it (**Fig. 9.1**).

Key Elements

- Somatic dysfunction corrected: any articular C2–C7 somatic dysfunction, including active and passive range of motion restrictions.
- End goal: to reposition a cervical vertebra at the inferior articulations by moving the vertebra through ranges of motion using the head and neck as a lever.

> **WATCH** ▷ ► ▷
>
> ► *Video 9.1a Cervical C2–7—Real-Time*
>
> ► *Video 9.1b Cervical C2–7—Narrated*
>
> **Example Somatic Dysfunction: C3 passive range of motion restrictions**

Positioning and Preparation

- ► Patient: supine, without a pillow under the head and neck.
- ► Physician: sitting at the head of the table.

Tissue Contact

One hand performs the technique, using the head and superiorly located vertebra to create the vector force and movements. The other assists by stabilizing and monitoring the vertebra below. It does not matter which hand makes which contact.

- Assisting hand: contact each side of the vertebral arch, of the vertebra inferior to the dysfunctional one, with the thumb on one side and the second and/or third fingers on the other side.
- Performing hand: contact the vertex of the head with the palm. Wrap your fingers around the contour of the head to hold and move it.
  - Suggestion for creating the disengagement force: place your elbow into the side of your abdomen or on your anterior superior iliac spine, so that as you lean forward, you create additional force through your forearm.

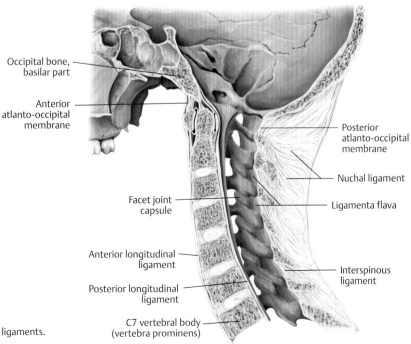

Occipital bone, basilar part

Anterior atlanto-occipital membrane

Facet joint capsule

Anterior longitudinal ligament

Posterior longitudinal ligament

C7 vertebral body (vertebra prominens)

Posterior atlanto-occipital membrane

Nuchal ligament

Ligamenta flava

Interspinous ligament

Fig. 9.1   Cervical spine ligaments.

Movements, Barriers, and Forces

Note: if at any time a release is palpated, the technique can be discontinued.

- With the assisting hand, layer palpate to the vertebral arches. Grasp the vertebra between your contacting fingers and thumb.

Use the performing hand to do the following:

- Apply a compressive force from the vertex of the patient's head to the inferior articular surfaces of the dysfunctional vertebra. Hold this force.
- Move the head and neck (superior to the dysfunctional vertebra) as a lever to move the inferior articular surfaces of the

dysfunctional vertebra. Move in the shape of an infinity sign (a figure-of-eight on its side).
  - Start in one direction and complete the loop, ending where you began.
- Repeat this movement two or three times.
- Reverse directions and move the joint through its full range of motion, again in the shape of an infinity sign.
- Continue altering directions of movements two or three more times until range of motion increases.
- Release the disengagement force and tissue contacts.
- Retest the vertebra for improvements in range of motion.

Costal, Rib 1

This technique is an excellent way to correct stubborn somatic dysfunctions of the first rib, especially superior shears (**Fig. 9.2**). Be sure that the patient's elbow, shoulder, and clavicle are without significant pathology and can withstand the force vector and movement through range of motion.

Key Elements

- Somatic dysfunction corrected: any first rib articular somatic dysfunction.
- End goal: to reposition the first rib at the costovertebral joint by moving the rib through range of motion using the humerus as a lever.

> **WATCH ▷ ▶ ▷**
>
> ▶ *Video 9.2a Costal Rib 1—Real-Time*
>
> ▶ *Video 9.2b Costal Rib 1—Narrated*
>
> ***Example Somatic Dysfunction: Left 1st rib superior shear***

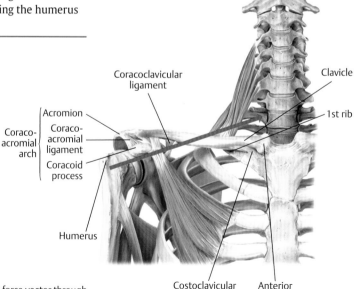

Fig. 9.2 Rib 1. The arrow depicts the force vector through the humerus to the first rib.

Positioning and Preparation

▶ Patient: supine, with the shoulder on the side of the dysfunctional rib near the edge of the table.

▶ Physician: standing on the side of the table nearer the patient's dysfunctional rib, at the level of the patient's torso, facing the patient's head.

Tissue Contact

One hand creates the disengagement and corrective forces, and the other hand monitors the first rib. Stabilization of the rib is created by the force vector.

• Monitoring hand: use the hand that is nearer the patient. Contact the superior aspect of the first rib near the costotransverse articulation with the pad of the second or third finger.

• Performing hand: bend the patient's elbow, and contact the humerus with the palm of the hand. Wrap your fingers and thumb around the elbow joint to firmly grasp it.

Movements, Barriers, and Forces

• With the monitoring hand, layer palpate to the head of the first rib.

Use the performing hand to do the following:

• Abduct the patient's elbow until it is horizontally in line with the long axis of the first rib.

• Apply a compressive disengagement force vector from the elbow in the direction of the head of the first rib. Hold this force.
  – The force vector begins at the elbow and continues through the soft tissues, not the clavicle (although the clavicle will no doubt be subject to the force). Be sure the vector reaches the rib head.

• Move the humerus in relatively large circular motions starting in one direction, keeping the force vector directed at the costal articulation.

• Repeat this movement two or three times.

• Reverse directions and move the humerus again in relatively large circular motions.

• Repeat this movement two or three times.
  – Continue altering directions of movements two or three more times until range of motion increases.

• Release the disengagement force and tissue contacts.

• Retest the first rib for improvements in position and range of motion.

Costal, Ribs 2–12

Traditionally called rib raising, this technique improves rib range of motion. It also affects autonomic reflexes mediated by the sympathetic nervous system. The sympathetic chain ganglia lie anterior to the rib heads, and forces are transmitted from the rib heads toward the fascias that surround the chain ganglia (**Fig. 9.3**). This helps eliminate fascial restrictions around the ganglia.

Key Elements

• Somatic dysfunction corrected: sympathetically mediated somatovisceral or viscerosomatic reflexes (typically this involves a group of ribs).

• End goal: to influence sympathetic nervous system activity (or tone) using the ribs as long levers.

> **WATCH** ▷▶▷
> _____
> ▶ *Video 9.3 Costal, Ribs 2–12—Narrated*
>
> *Example Somatic Dysfunction: Left Ribs 2–6 decreased ROM related to viscerosomatic reflex activity from pulmonary disease (such as asthma or pneumonia)*

Positioning and Preparation

▶ Patient: supine.

▶ Physician: seated at the side of the table near the affected ribs, facing the patient.

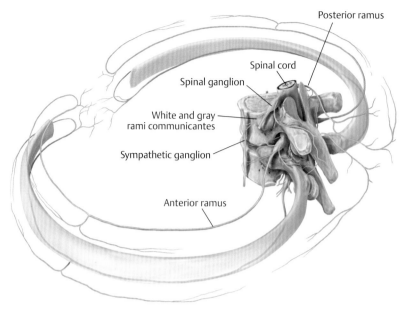

Fig. 9.3 Spinal nerve branches.

Tissue Contact

Both hands create the corrective and disengagement forces simultaneously.

- Performing hands: contact each affected rib angle with the pads of the fingers. One or two fingers can contact each rib. Do this by supinating your hands and sliding them under the patient.

Movements, Barriers, and Forces

Use both hands to do the following:

- Layer palpate to the rib head.
- Apply anteriorly directed forces to move the head of the rib until a restrictive barrier is felt. Hold this force.

- After a few seconds, release forces and repeat in a gentle rhythmic fashion until rib motion is improved or for 30 seconds, up to 2 minutes.
  - Alternatively, forces can be sustained in a fashion similar to thoracic inhibitory pressure technique.
- Release forces.
- Retest the ribs for improvements in somatic dysfunction.

Note: For rib somatic dysfunction due to a viscerosomatic reflex, full resolution of the reflex will not occur until the underlying visceral disease is treated.

Pelvis, Innominate

This technique is useful to perform in patients who cannot lie prone (**Fig. 9.4**). Be sure that the patient's hip does not have significant pathology and can both withstand the force vector and be moved through range of motion.

Key Elements

- Somatic dysfunction corrected: any innominate somatic dysfunction at the sacroiliac joint.
- End goal: to reposition the innominate bone at the sacroiliac joint by moving the femur as a long lever.

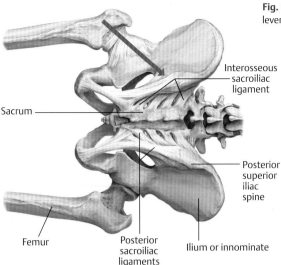

Fig. 9.4   Sacroiliac joint. The arrow depicts the femur as a lever to move the sacroiliac joint.

Interosseous sacroiliac ligament

Sacrum

Posterior superior iliac spine

Femur

Posterior sacroiliac ligaments

Ilium or innominate

WATCH ▷▶▷

▶   *Video 9.4a Pelvis Innominate—Real-Time*

▶   *Video 9.4b Pelvis Innominate—Narrated*

Example Somatic Dysfunction: Left innominate anteriorly rotated

Positioning and Preparation

▶   Patient: supine, with the knee on the side of the dysfunctional innominate bent and foot on the table.

▶   Physician: standing on the side of the dysfunctional innominate at the level of the patient's bent knee, facing the head of the table.

Tissue Contact

One hand creates the disengagement and corrective forces and the other hand monitors the sacroiliac joint. Stabilization comes from the treatment table.

- Performing hand: contact the patient's bent knee with the palm of your near hand. Flex the patient's hip. Bend forward at your waist.
  - Optional: place the patient's knee in the space between your humerus and chest wall. Your hand may be in between the patient's knee and your chest wall or hooked under the knee for control.
- Monitoring hand: use the hand that is farther from the table and patient. Contact the sacroiliac joint with the pads of the second, third, and fourth fingers.

- Detailed/ergonomic suggestion: push the patient's knee medially until the pelvis rolls up off of the table. Locate the posterior superior iliac spine and the sacroiliac joint, and roll the patient's pelvis back onto the table and your hand.

Movements, Barriers, and Forces

- With the monitoring hand, layer palpate to the sacroiliac joint.

Use the performing hand to do the following:

- Apply a compressive disengagement force from the knee to the sacroiliac joint. Hold this force.
  - The force vector is through the head of the femur and continues through the innominate to the sacroiliac joint.
- Move the femur in circular motions in one direction through the femoroacetabular range of motion.
- Repeat this movement two or three times.
- Reverse direction, and again move the femur through the femoroacetabular range of motion.
- Repeat this movement two or three times.
  - Continue altering directions of movements two or three more times until range of motion increases.
- Release the disengagement force and tissue contacts.
- Retest the innominate for improvement in position and/or range of motion.

Sacrum

Traditionally called sacral rocking, this technique has commonly been used to affect parasympathetic nervous system activity in nerves S2–S4. Therefore, it is useful for cases of constipation, dysmenorrhea, or cystitis. Note the proximity of sympathetic nerves, and although less described in the literature, this technique may also influence sympathetic tone (**Fig. 9.5**).

Key Elements

- Somatic dysfunction corrected:
  - Any sacral articular somatic dysfunction, including range of motion restrictions associated with thoracolumbar breathing.
  - Parasympathetically mediated somatovisceral or viscerosomatic reflexes.
- End goals:
  - To improve sacral motion associated with thoracolumbar breathing by taking the sacrum through range of motion.
  - To affect parasympathetic nervous system activity (or tone).

WATCH ▷ ▶ ▷

- ▶ *Video 9.5a Sacrum—Real-Time*
- ▶ *Video 9.5b Sacrum—Narrated*

Example Somatic Dysfunction: Posterior sacral base (sacral motion limited with exhalation)

Positioning and Preparation

- ▶ Patient: prone, head resting in head rest or turned to either side, whichever is more comfortable for the patient.
- ▶ Physician: standing at one side of the table at the level of the sacrum, facing the patient.

Tissue Contact

The physician uses both hands to create the corrective forces. One hand contacts the sacral base and the other hand is placed over it. Stabilization comes from the treatment table.

- Performing hand: use the hand that is closer to the patient's head. Contact the sacral base with the heel of the hand, in between the posterior superior iliac spines. Your metacarpophalangeal joints should be about at the level of the inferior lateral angles.
  - To avoid palpating and applying pressure directly on and below the coccyx lift the fingertips off of the patient by extending the metacarpophalangeal joints.
- Assisting hand: use the hand that is closer to the patient's feet. Place this hand on top of the performing hand, so the heel of this hand is resting on the metacarpophalangeal joints (approximately at the level of the inferior lateral angles).

Note: Do not reverse hand placements, because excessive force may be applied over the coccyx.

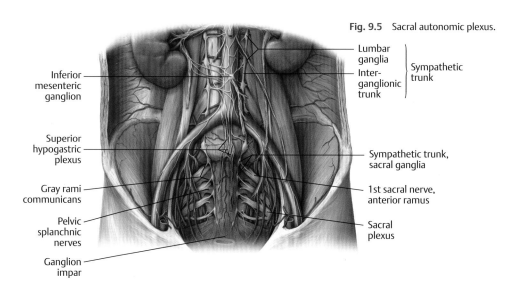

Fig. 9.5 Sacral autonomic plexus.

Inferior mesenteric ganglion

Superior hypogastric plexus

Gray rami communicans

Pelvic splanchnic nerves

Ganglion impar

Lumbar ganglia

Inter-ganglionic trunk

Sympathetic trunk

Sympathetic trunk, sacral ganglia

1st sacral nerve, anterior ramus

Sacral plexus

Movements, Barriers, and Forces

Performing and assisting hand movements must be coordinated with each other and synchronized with the patient's breathing efforts. Allow your hands to move with the sacrum. You may ask the patient to take slow, full (but not deep) breaths, or simply perform with the patient's normal breathing.

Use both hands to do the following:

- Layer palpate to the sacrum.
- On the patient's inhalation, follow the anterior movement of the inferior lateral angles. Near the end of inhalation, apply an anteriorly directed force with the heel of the assisting hand, through the contacting metacarpophalangeal joints, to augment this motion.

  - This is best done by keeping the arms relatively stiff and leaning body weight.
- On the patient's exhalation, release the anterior force and follow the sacrum as the base moves anteriorly.
- Just before the end of the patient's exhalation, apply an anteriorly directed force with the heel of the performing hand to augment this motion.
- Repeat the steps of the technique for up to 2 minutes, or until sacral movements become symmetrical and smooth.

  - Use more force on the sacral motion that is more restricted.
- Release forces and tissue contacts.
- Retest the sacrum for changes in range of motion and/or position.

Upper Extremity, Glenohumeral Joint (Fig. 9.6)

This technique was first described in 1916 by Charles H. Spencer, DO, and is commonly called the Spencer Technique.[2] The original technique was written with eight steps, but was abbreviated to seven. All eight steps are included here. Step 6, adduction with external rotation, has been reintroduced. Commonly used in cases of minor shoulder injuries and adhesive capsulitis, this technique is performed sequentially with gentle motions. The last step of this technique is a combination lymphatic pump and soft tissue longitudinal stretch.

Key Elements

- Somatic dysfunction corrected: glenohumeral joint passive range of motion restrictions in one or more directions: flexion/extension/internal rotation/external rotation/abduction/adduction; anterior/posterior humeral head.
- End goal: to improve glenohumeral joint range of motion and fluid circulation.

> **WATCH** ▷▶▷
>
> ▶ *Video 9.6a Upper Extremity, Glenohumeral Joint—Real Time*
>
> ▶ *Video 9.6b Upper Extremity, Glenohumeral Joint—Narrated*
>
> *Example Somatic Dysfunction: Left Glenohumeral Joint: Extension, Abduction, and External Rotation Restrictions*

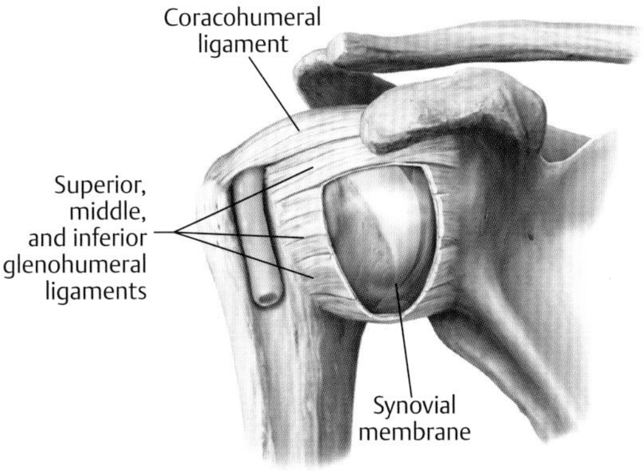

Fig. 9.6 Glenohumeral joint.

Positioning and Preparation

▶ Patient: laterally recumbent, with the affected shoulder off of the table and the head supported by a pillow or the patient's arm.

▶ Physician: standing and facing the front of the patient, at the level of the humerus.

  - Alternatively, the physician stands facing the back of the patient. However, to perform step 6, the physician moves to the front.

Tissue Contact

- The physician uses one hand to create the disengagement forces and move the humerus. The other hand assists by stabilizing the anterior and posterior shoulder girdle (glenoid fossa).
- Performing hand: this hand contacts the humerus at different locations. Refer to each step for the description.
- Assisting hand: contact the top of the shoulder with the palm of the hand, the clavicle with the thumb, and the scapula with the fingers for all steps except the last (step 8). Create an inferiorly directed force to hold and stabilize the glenoid fossa to move the humerus. Hold this force until the last step (step 8).

Movements, Barriers, and Forces

Because this technique has numerous steps that are performed sequentially, it is helpful to memorize a summary list of the key positions and movements created by the physician.

Spencer Technique Summary Steps

1. Extension.
2. Flexion.
3. Compression with circumduction.
4. Distraction with circumduction.
5. Abduction.
6. Adduction with external rotation.
7. Internal rotation with abduction.
8. Lymphatic pump and longitudinal stretch.

- Extension.
  - Performing hand: bend the patient's elbow and grasp the arm at the olecranon. Move the humerus into extension until a restrictive barrier is felt.
  - Create gentle, repetitive, springing motions against the restrictive barrier five to seven times, until motion increases.
  - Return the humerus to neutral position.
- Flexion.
  - Move the humerus into flexion until a restrictive barrier is felt.
  - Create gentle, repetitive, springing motions against the restrictive barrier five to seven times, until motion increases.
  - Return the humerus to neutral position.

- Compression with circumduction.
  - Move the humerus into 90 degrees of abduction.
  - Apply a gentle compressive force from the elbow in the direction of the glenohumeral fossa. Hold this force.
  - Move the humerus in circular motions, first in one direction then the other. Start with small circles and progress to larger ones.
  - Return the humerus to 90 degrees of abduction.
- Distraction with circumduction.
  - Performing hand: bend the patient's elbow and now contact the humerus so that the elbow drapes over the fingers.
  - Apply a gentle traction force away from the glenohumeral fossa. Hold this force.
  - Move the humerus in circular motions, first in one direction then the other. Start with small circles and progress to larger ones.
  - Return the humerus to neutral position.
- Abduction.
  - Performing hand: use the same tissue contact for flexion, extension steps.
  - Move the humerus into full abduction until a restrictive barrier is felt.
  - Create gentle, repetitive, springing motions against the restrictive barrier five to seven times until motion increases.
  - Return the humerus to neutral position.
- Adduction with external rotation.
  - Performing hand: move the humerus into adduction and external rotation until a restrictive barrier is felt.
  - Patient positioning: place the patient's hand on your forearm and ask the patient to gently grasp your forearm.
  - Create gentle, repetitive, springing motions against the restrictive barrier five to seven times, until motion increases.
  - Return the humerus to neutral position.
- Internal rotation with abduction.
  - Patient positioning: place the back of the patient's hand on the ilium to create internal rotation. Slowly increase the amount of internal rotation by sliding the arm superiorly and posteriorly, until a restrictive barrier is felt.
  - Tissue contact: contact the patient's medial epicondyle.

- Create gentle, repetitive, springing motions against the restrictive barrier five to seven times, until motion is increased.
- Return the humerus to neutral position.
- Lymphatic pump and longitudinal stretch.
  - Patient positioning: place the patient's hand on your shoulder.
  - Performing hands: contact the proximal humerus with the pads of all fingers and thumbs, grasping the arm.
  - Layer palpate to the musculature.

- Apply longitudinal traction forces in a repetitive fashion to create a very slight stretch in the glenohumeral ligaments and musculature. The distance of the stretch is ~ 0.5 cm or less. Perform on all glenohumeral musculature for 30 seconds, up to 2 minutes.
  - Return the humerus to neutral position.
- Retest the glenohumeral joint for improvements in range of motion.

Upper Extremity, Radiocarpal Joint

This technique is useful for wrist pain, range of motion restrictions due to repetitive use activities, and symptoms of carpal tunnel syndrome (**Fig. 9.7**).

Key Elements

- Somatic dysfunction corrected: any radiocarpal somatic dysfunction.
- End goal: to reposition the scaphoid, lunate, and/or triquetrum at the radiocarpal articulation.

> **WATCH** ▷ ▶ ▷
>
> ▶ *Video 9.7a Upper Extremity, Radiocarpal Joint—Real-Time*
>
> ▶ *Video 9.7b Upper Extremity, Radiocarpal Joint—Narrated*

Positioning and Preparation

▶ Patient: seated.

▶ Physician: seated in front of the patient, facing the patient, at eye level.

Tissue Contact

Both hands contact the radiocarpal joint and create the disengagement and corrective forces.

- Performing hands: contact the patient's proximal carpal joint with the heels of both hands so that your wrists and the patient's wrist are parallel. Interlace your fingers.

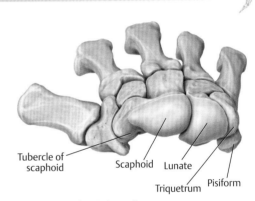

Tubercle of scaphoid   Scaphoid   Lunate

Triquetrum   Pisiform

Fig. 9.7 Carpal articular surfaces.

Movements, Barriers, and Forces

Use the heels of both hands to do the following:

- Apply a compressive disengagement force into the radiocarpal joints.
  - Do this by squeezing the wrists together.
- Move the wrist in the shape of a figure-of-eight on its side starting in one direction.
- Repeat this movement two or three times.
- Reverse directions and move the wrist through its full range of motion, again in a figure-of-eight.
- Repeat this movement two or three times.
- Continue altering directions two or three more times until range of motion increases.
- Release the disengagement force.
- Retest the radiocarpal joint for changes in range of motion.

Chapter Summary

ART techniques are generalized joint mobilizers, incorporating both direct and indirect principles while using repetitive physiological motions. Among the techniques offered in this chapter are the foundational osteopathic techniques of rib raising and sacral rocking. Included also is a standard for the shoulder, the Spencer Technique, in its original form. Greater than simple structural corrections, ART techniques are dynamic in functional range of motion and autonomic reregulation.

Clinical Cases and Review Questions

Case 1

A 65-year-old woman presents for evaluation of neck pain. The pain has been slowly worsening over several years. She takes calcium for mild osteopenia and has a history of osteoarthritis. Examination reveals no neurological deficits, but significant restriction of cervical motion in left rotation. On somatic dysfunction diagnosis you find C2 FRS$_R$. You elect to try an articulatory technique for this patient.

Q1. Which of the following is considered a goal for performing articulatory technique in this patient?
   A. Treatment of osteopenia.
   B. Treatment of osteoporosis.
   C. Removal of somatic dysfunction of the cervical spine using an indirect approach.
   D. Improved range of motion of the cervical spine.
   E. Articulatory technique is contraindicated in this patient.

Q2. Which of the following history and physical exam findings would be a contraindication for using an articulatory technique on the cervical spine in this patient?
   A. Moderate restriction of motion with side bending and rotation.
   B. Osteoporosis.
   C. History of whiplash 3 months prior.
   D. Moderate tenderness of the cervical paraspinal muscles.
   E. Suspected compression fracture in the neck.

Case 2

A 45-year-old man presents to the clinic with complaints of right-hand numbness. He states the numbness affects his first, second, and third digits and that it is worse after working many hours at the computer. Physical exam reveals normal upper extremity reflexes, but a positive Tinel's sign at the transverse carpal ligament. Osteopathic exam reveals an anterior lunate bone somatic dysfunction. A tender point in the pronator teres and fascial tensions around the carpal tunnel are also noted.

Q3. What is the goal of performing an articulatory technique on this patient's radiocarpal articulations?
   A. Restore normal position of the lunate bone.
   B. Remove fascial restrictions around the carpal tunnel.
   C. Directly mobilize the median nerve.
   D. Reset the muscle spindle organs in the hypertonic musculature.
   E. Prevent further irritation of the nerve during computer work.

Q4. Which of the following best describes the movements used when performing articulatory technique on the radiocarpal joint?
   A. A high velocity, low amplitude thrust into the restrictive barrier.
   B. A figure-of-eight motion repeatedly mobilizing the joint in all planes.
   C. A repetitive movement directly into the barrier of motion.
   D. Taking the joint indirectly and then directly one time.
   E. Taking the joint to the balance point and holding for a release.

Answers to Review Questions

Q1. The correct answer is **D**: Improve range of motion of the cervical spine.

   A is incorrect. OMT does not treat osteopenia; it treats somatic dysfunction.

   B is incorrect. OMT does not treat osteopenia; it treats somatic dysfunction.

   C is incorrect. Articulatory is both direct and indirect.

   E is incorrect. There are no contraindications to articulatory technique mentioned in the case presentation.

Q2. The correct answer is **E**: Suspected compression fracture in the neck.

A is incorrect. Moderate restriction of motion with side bending and rotation is an indication for OMT.

B is incorrect. Osteoporosis is not a contraindication for articulatory technique.

C is incorrect. History of whiplash 3 months prior is not a contraindication for articulatory technique.

D is incorrect. If no other red flags, moderate tenderness of the cervical paraspinal muscles is an indication for OMT.

Q3. The correct answer is **A**: Restore normal position of the lunate bone. Articulatory techniques are focused on restoring normal joint position and biomechanics.

B is incorrect. Myofascial release technique would more directly describe this answer choice.

C is incorrect. Direct mobilization of the median nerve is not the direct focus of this technique. The goal is to restore normal position of the lunate, and this may decrease pressure on the median nerve.

D is incorrect. Resetting the muscle spindle organs in the hypertonic musculature describes counterstrain or muscle energy techniques, but not articulatory techniques.

E is incorrect. Altering ergonomics may be necessary to prevent repeat irritation.

Q4. The correct answer is **B**: A figure-of-eight motion repeatedly mobilizing the joint in all planes.

A is incorrect. A high velocity, low amplitude thrust into the restrictive barrier describes high velocity, low amplitude.

C is incorrect. A repetitive movement directly into the barrier of motion describes challenging the barrier technique.

D is incorrect. Taking the joint indirectly and then directly one time describes the Still Technique, and articulatory technique is performed multiple times rather than once.

E is incorrect. Taking the joint to the balance point and holding for a release describes balanced ligamentous tension.

References

1. Fryer G, Morse CM, Johnson JC. Spinal and sacroiliac assessment and treatment techniques used by osteopathic physicians in the United States. Osteopath Med Prim Care 2009;3(1):4
2. Patriquin DA. The evolution of osteopathic manipulative technique: the Spencer technique. J Am Osteopath Assoc 1992;92(9):1134–1136, 1139–1146

Bibliography

Gosling C, Williams KA. Comparison of the effects of thoracic manipulation and rib raising on lung function of asymptomatic individuals. J Osteopath Med 2004;7:103

Henderson AT, Fisher JF, Blair J, Shea C, Li TS, Bridges KG. Effects of rib raising on the autonomic nervous system: a pilot study using noninvasive biomarkers. J Am Osteopath Assoc 2010;110(6):324–330

Hensel KL, Buchanan S, Brown SK, Rodriguez M, Cruser A. Pregnancy Research on Osteopathic Manipulation Optimizing Treatment Effects: the PROMOTE study. Am J Obstet Gynecol 2015;212(1):108.e1–108.e9

Lopez D, King HH, Knebl JA, Kosmopoulos V, Collins D, Patterson RM. Effects of comprehensive osteopathic manipulative treatment on balance in elderly patients: a pilot study. J Am Osteopath Assoc 2011;111(6):382–388

Noll DR, Degenhardt BF, Johnson JC, Burt SA. Immediate effects of osteopathic manipulative treatment in elderly patients with chronic obstructive pulmonary disease. J Am Osteopath Assoc 2008;108(5):251–259

O-Yurvati AH, Carnes MS, Clearfield MB, Stoll ST, McConathy WJ. Hemodynamic effects of osteopathic manipulative treatment immediately after coronary artery bypass graft surgery. J Am Osteopath Assoc 2005;105(10):475–481

Snider KT, Snider EJ, DeGooyer BR, Bukowski AM, Fleming RK, Johnson JC. Retrospective medical record review of an osteopathic manipulative medicine hospital consultation service. J Am Osteopath Assoc 2013;113(10):754–767

Snider KT, Snider EJ, Johnson JC, Hagan C, Schoenwald C. Preventative osteopathic manipulative treatment and the elderly nursing home resident: a pilot study. J Am Osteopath Assoc 2012;112(8):489–501

Swender DA, Thompson G, Schneider K, McCoy K, Patel A. Osteopathic manipulative treatment for inpatients with pulmonary exacerbations of cystic fibrosis: effects on spirometry findings and patient assessments of breathing, anxiety, and pain. J Am Osteopath Assoc 2014;114(6):450–458

Wheatley A, Gosling C, Gibbons P. Investigation of the effects of using a rib raising technique on FEV1 and FVC outcomes in people with asthma: a clinical investigation. J Osteopath Med 2000;3(2):60–64

Wieting JM, Beal C, Roth GL, et al. The effect of osteopathic manipulative treatment on postoperative medical and functional recovery of coronary artery bypass graft patients. J Am Osteopath Assoc 2013;113(5):384–393

10 Challenge the Barrier Techniques

LEARNING OBJECTIVES

1. Explain the goals of performing challenge the barrier techniques.
2. Identify the clinical considerations, including indications, contraindications, and precautions for performing challenge the barrier techniques.
3. Outline the general movements, barriers, and forces for performing challenge the barrier techniques.
4. Define a force vector.
5. Visualize, verbalize, and identify the preparation, positioning, tissue contact, movements, barriers, and forces for each challenge the barrier technique.
6. Perform the techniques using appropriate somatic dysfunction diagnosis, preparation, positioning, tissue contact, movements, barriers, forces, retest for effectiveness, communication, and safe tissue handling.

Challenge the Barrier Technique Introduction

Challenge the barrier (CBR) is one of three types of exaggeration techniques performed by Dr. Still. CBR technique relies on the use of disengagement forces along with repetitive, rhythmic movements, which are directed at a joint that has restricted motion and tissue texture changes. In contrast with other joint-focused techniques, the surrounding fascias and supporting ligaments are also considered and addressed. Because of this holistic, fascial, and articular approach, CBR techniques are direct-method techniques and can be especially useful for treating chronic joint somatic dysfunctions. Also, because most CBR techniques are performed with the patient seated, these techniques are appropriate for patients who cannot lie prone or supine and for those times when a treatment table is not available.

Similar to other techniques aimed at correcting joint and fascial somatic dysfunctions, CBR techniques can:

- Decrease pain.
- Improve local and regional range of motion.
- Increase local arterial, venous, and lymph circulation.
- Restore normal myofascial tissue tensions of a joint.

Background

Although originally performed by Dr. Still, these are perhaps considered his "lost" techniques because they were not commonly taught by his students. It is suspected that this was due to the difficulty in translating the method into discrete steps with precise directional instructions. The term used by Dr. Still was "exaggerate the lesion," which is itself ambiguous, as were the directional movements. However, after much study, three modern-day osteopathic physicians have revived and reinterpreted exaggeration techniques.

Jerry Dickey, DO, FAAO, is among those who present a version of the direct exaggeration techniques, and his interpretation serves as the foundation of this chapter. Karen Steele, DO, FAAO, describes the techniques that Dr. Still's son, Richard Still, DO, performed as seated facet release techniques. Richard VanBuskirk, DO, PhD, FAAO, describes his interpretation of Dr. Still's techniques, also historically based, as Still techniques. Together, these three variations of direct exaggeration techniques provide a great insight into Dr. Still's original methods of treatment.

Clinical Considerations

Some common clinical things to consider when using CBR techniques are listed in Table 10.1. Always acquire adequate data in the form of an appropriate history and a thorough physical exam, including an exam for somatic dysfunction and relevant diagnostic tests in order to exercise best clinical judgment before performing osteopathic manipulative treatment.

Somatic Dysfunction Corrected

CBR techniques correct joint somatic dysfunction with a focus on passive range of motion. Because of this, CBR techniques can be performed as soon as passive range of motion restriction in a joint is identified on physical examination. It is clinically useful to examine all the joints in one region, such as all the cervical vertebrae, then to perform the technique on the joint with the most restricted motion first. Often, correcting the most restricted joint results in correction of the others.

Positioning and Preparation

▶ Patient: most techniques are performed with the patient seated. The patient should remain relaxed throughout the duration of the technique performance.

▶ Physician: the physician stands or sits, using appropriate ergonomics, which includes adjustment of the table height in order to dynamically move the joint and to move with the patient. A stable, wide-based stance helps to both control and create patient movements.

Tissue Contact

- Both hands are used to perform CBR techniques. One hand monitors the tissues around the dysfunctional joint while the other one creates disengagement force vectors and moves the patient.
- Monitoring contact: the pad of the thumb or fingers monitors a dysfunctional joint on the side or aspect that has the most restricted motion or tissue texture changes.
- Performing contact: the palm of the hand, upper arm/axilla, and/or abdomen creates the force vectors. The patient is also moved with this contact.

Movements, Barriers, and Forces

CBR is a direct technique that requires the patient to remain passive during the technique performance. The end goal is to restore joint motion with focused attention on the ligaments and fascia surrounding the joint. The physician can take generous liberties in terms of the number of force vectors created and the directions of the physician-created corrective movements. However, precision in the direction of the force vectors is required.

Table 10.1 Clinical considerations		
Indications	**Contraindications**	**Precautions**
Mechanical neck and back pain	Fracture or suspected fracture	Use care when performing on joints with mild effusion.
Sacroiliac joint pain/sacroiliitis	Joint dislocation	Discontinue or modify technique if it causes pain.
Postural imbalance	Joint infection	
Osteoarthritis	Moderate–severe or full-thickness tendon, ligament or meniscal tear	
Chronic pain conditions	Vertebral disk or spinal nerve compression	
Somatovisceral and viscerosomatic reflexes		

The preparation for the corrective movements is perhaps more essential than creating the movements themselves. Patients must first be positioned such that they can be easily moved. This is accomplished by asking the seated patient to lean the body backward, usually onto the physician's body, then to slump forward. This decreases ligamentous and fascial tensions. The physician may turn to one side so the patient is leaning on the side of the physician's rib cage. Alternatively, a firm but small pillow may be placed between the patient and the physician's abdomen for modesty.

The physician then moves the relaxed patient into a position that "exaggerates the lesion" or tightens the tissues further into the restrictive barriers. The restrictive barriers are approached by palpatory feel. This means that the physician does not have to consider specifically which directions to move the patient, only to move the patient into whatever directions create the most tissue tension at the affected joint.

After the patient is positioned, the physician creates as many force vectors as possible with the performing contact(s). Force vectors are compressive or traction forces, made from a distant site on the patient's body, and directed into or away from, in the case of traction forces, the restricted area of the joint. However, the force vectors are not forces that further loosen or tighten the tissues. They are assisting forces, like keys that unlock a door, they disengage the joint to permit further movement. Similar to indirect techniques, either traction or compression forces may be used, but all the techniques in this manual are written with compression. Both types of force vectors permit increased joint movement, or creation of the corrective forces. The type of disengagement force vectors to create is determined by the physician's judgment, taking into account ergonomics, tissue feel, and psychomotor skills.

Recall that multiple force vectors, named A and B, summate into a new force vector with a different magnitude and direction, named R (**Fig. 10.1**). The force vector, R, in the figure, is exaggerated for visualization. Force vector R is directed into the affected joint surfaces and surrounding fascias. The amount of force created at each separate vector can be minimal because force vectors summate. Only enough force should be applied so that it can be felt with the monitoring contact at the joint. The forces are held throughout the duration of the technique.

The last step in performing CBR techniques is to move the patient. Coordination on the part of the physician is necessary to simultaneously cre-

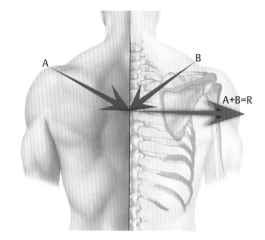

Fig. 10.1 Vectors.

ate and hold vector forces and to introduce motion at the dysfunctional barrier of the patient. While holding all force vectors directed at the affected joint, the physician creates rhythmic, oscillatory motions that move the affected joint further in the direction of the restrictive barriers to "challenge the barrier." These movements are the corrective forces that gently nudge the restrictive barriers such that total range of physiological motion is restored. At some point during the physician-created movements, the tissues palpated with the monitoring hand will soften, and often the gliding return of normal joint alignment can be palpated. Either or both of these tissue changes indicate that the technique is complete. It can take as little as a few seconds or up to 2 minutes to achieve correction of somatic dysfunction. With practice the movements become more fluid and expedient.

Retest for Effectiveness

If a release is not palpated, retest the joint for passive range of motion and/or position to determine if the somatic dysfunction has corrected. The technique can be performed again from beginning to end, and an additional force vector can be added if possible. A common reason that the technique may be ineffective is that the force vectors were not held for the duration of the technique. As with all other osteopathic techniques, if there is little to no change in the somatic dysfunction, the patient should be reexamined and the technique reattempted, or an alternate technique may be tried.

CBR Technique Summary Steps

- Identify a joint with passive range of motion restrictions, including any somatic dysfunction diagnosis.
- With the monitoring hand, layer palpate to the dysfunctional joint.
- With the performing hand, move the patient so that the tissues surrounding the joint are tightened to "exaggerate the lesion."
- Apply as many compressive/traction force vectors as possible with the performing contacts to the dysfunctional joint. Hold these forces.

- Create slow, rhythmic, springing movements in the direction of the restrictive barrier, or "challenge the barrier."
- Stop movements when the tissue tension resolves and/or passive motion is increased, or after about 2 minutes.
- Return the patient to a neutral position and release force vectors.
- Retest the joint for changes in passive range of motion.

Head, Occipitoatlantal Joint

Unlike other techniques for the occipitoatlantal (OA) joint, this technique specifically treats one portion, anterior or posterior, of one occipital condyle (**Fig. 10.2**). In cases where the OA joint is more restricted in gliding anteriorly (in extension), use the anterior technique. In cases where the OA joint is more restricted in gliding posteriorly (in flexion), use the posterior technique. If undeterminable, perform both variations.

Key Elements

- Somatic dysfunction corrected: any OA joint somatic dysfunction.
- End goal: to release the tissues around the OA joint using a force vector and repetitive, springing movements to restore joint alignment.

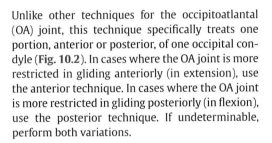

WATCH ▷ ► ▷

▶ *Video 10.1 Head, OA Joint—Narrated*

Example Somatic Dysfunction: Right anterior OA passive range of motion restriction

---

Positioning and Preparation

▶ Patient: seated.
▶ Physician: standing behind the patient, with the table height adjusted so the physician can easily contact the vertex of the head.

Tissue Contact

- Monitoring hand: contact the posterior arch of the atlas with the thumb and index finger. This hand also stabilizes the neck so the occipital bone can be moved.
- Performing contact:
  - Anterior occiput: contact the middle of the forehead with the palm of the hand, avoiding the eyes.
  - Posterior occiput: contact the side of the forehead on the side opposite the condyle with somatic dysfunction.

Movements, Barriers, and Forces

- With the monitoring hand, layer palpate to the suboccipital musculature and then firmly contact the posterior arch of the atlas to stabilize it.
- Ask the patient to relax the head forward, and with the performing hand, allow the head to flex at the OA joint.

Use the performing hand to do the following:

- Move the head into a position that tightens the tissues further to exaggerate the lesion.
  - This may be any combination of rotation/ side bending.

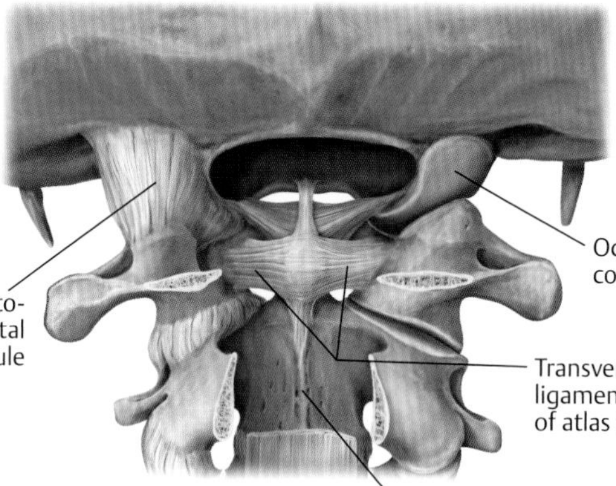

Fig. 10.2   Occipitoatlantal joint.

Occipito-
atlantal
capsule

Occipital
condyle

Transverse
ligament
of atlas (C1)

C1

- Apply a compressive force vector from your performing hand to the dysfunctional condyle. Hold this force.
- Slowly create rhythmic, springing, rocking movements from anterior to posterior along the plane of the condylar articular surface to challenge the barrier.
  - Anterior: the direction is directly posterior.

- Posterior: the direction is oblique, at an angle from your performing to your monitoring hand.
- Stop movements when the tissue tension resolves, joint motion increases, or after about 2 minutes.
- Return the patient's head and neck to a neutral position and release the force vectors.
- Retest the OA joint for changes in passive range of motion.

Thoracic Spine

This technique is a great exercise for the physician to use to practice creating multiple vectors with one arm and the abdomen (**Fig. 10.3**). Clinically, it helps loosen or even resolves long-standing thoracic somatic dysfunction.

Key Elements

- Somatic dysfunction corrected: any passive range of motion restriction and/or joint somatic dysfunction of the thoracic spine.
- End goal: to release the tissues around a vertebral facet joint using multiple force vectors and repetitive, springing movements to restore joint alignment.

> **WATCH ▷ ▶ ▷**
>
> ▶ *Video 10.2 Thoracic Spine*
>
> ***Example Somatic Dysfunction: Right T6 facet joint passive range of motion restriction***

Positioning and Preparation

▶ Patient: seated, positioned so the pelvis is near the back edge of the table.

  - Ask the patient to cross both arms in front of the chest.

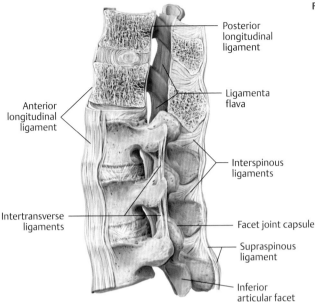

Fig. 10.3   Ligaments of the vertebral column.

Posterior longitudinal ligament

Ligamenta flava

Anterior longitudinal ligament

Interspinous ligaments

Intertransverse ligaments

Facet joint capsule

Supraspinous ligament

Inferior articular facet

– Ask the patient to flex the knees so they hook around the front edge of the table. This helps the patient to remain stable during the technique performance.
▶ Physician: standing behind the patient, turned slightly to one side, in an ergonomic posture, including a wide-based stance, in order to control and move your body and that of the patient.

Tissue Contact

• Monitoring hand: contact the inferior facet joint of the dysfunctional vertebra with the thumb or second or third finger pad.
   – Keep in mind that this contact does not create a force vector.
• Performing contacts: contact the patient's shoulders so as to firmly hold the torso. Wrap your arm on top of the patient's crossed arms so that your hand is on top of the patient's shoulder and your humerus, near your axilla, is on top of the patient's other shoulder.

Movements, Barriers, and Forces

• With the monitoring hand, layer palpate to the dysfunctional joint.
• Ask the patient to lean backward onto your abdomen or trunk and slump forward.

Use the performing contacts to do the following:

• Move the patient so that the joint and surrounding ligaments are tight to exaggerate the lesion.
   – This may be rotation, side bending, and/or increased or decreased flexion.
• Apply compressive force vectors from your performing contacts to the dysfunctional joint. Hold these forces.
   – An additional force vector can be generated from the abdomen.
• Create slow, rhythmic, springing, side-swaying movements along the articular surfaces to challenge the barrier.
   – Move your hips and knees to created side-swaying movements.
• Stop movements when the tissue tension resolves, joint motion increases, or after about 2 minutes.
• Return the patient to a neutral position and release forces.
• Retest the vertebra for changes in passive range of motion.

Pelvis, Innominate

This technique uses an additional force on the innominate to create disengagement with the monitoring hand (**Fig. 10.4**). It is useful for conditions in which patients have limited sacroiliac joint mobility or an inability to lie supine or prone.

Key Elements

- Somatic dysfunction corrected: any mechanical innominate somatic dysfunction.
  - In addition to, or in lieu of, the standing flexion test, perform a variation of the sacroiliac joint compression test with the patient seated. Do this by creating anteriorly directed springing forces on each posterior superior iliac spine. Perform the technique on the innominate that has the more restricted motion.
- End goal: to release the tissues around the sacroiliac joint using multiple force vectors and repetitive, springing movements to restore innominate alignment.

> ### WATCH ▷ ▶ ▷
> ▶ **Video 10.3 Pelvis, Innominate—Narrated**
> **Example Somatic Dysfunction: Right innominate anterior rotation**

Positioning and Preparation

- ▶ Patient: seated, positioned so the pelvis is near the back edge of the table.
  - Ask the patient to flex the knees so they hook around the front edge of the table. This helps the patient to remain stable during the technique performance.
- ▶ Physician: standing behind the patient, turned slightly to one side, in an ergonomic posture, including a wide-based stance, to control and move your body and that of the patient.

Tissue Contact

- Monitoring and assisting hand: contact the inferior aspect, or under slope, of the posterior superior iliac spine (PSIS) on the dysfunctional side with the thumb or fingers. Use your right hand if contacting the patient's right PSIS and your left hand to contact the left PSIS.
- Performing contacts: contact the patient's shoulders so as to firmly hold the torso. Wrap your arm so that your hand is on top of the patient's shoulder on the side of the dysfunctional innominate and your humerus, near your axilla, is on top of the patient's other shoulder.

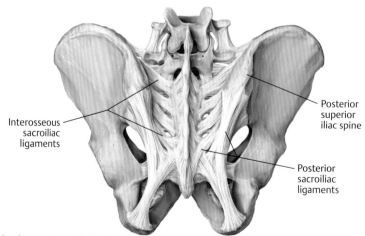

Fig. 10.4 Sacroiliac ligaments, posterior view.

Interosseous sacroiliac ligaments

Posterior superior iliac spine

Posterior sacroiliac ligaments

Movements, Barriers, and Forces

- With the monitoring hand, layer palpate to the bony layer.
- Ask the patient to lean backward onto your abdomen or trunk and slump forward.
- With the monitoring hand, superiorly lift the PSIS to disengage the sacroiliac joint.

Use the performing hand to do the following:

- Move the patient so that the tissues surrounding the sacroiliac joint are tight to exaggerate the lesion.
  - This is often side bending toward the side of the dysfunctional innominate.

- Apply compressive force vectors from your performing contacts to the dysfunctional joint. Hold these forces.
  - An additional force vector can be generated from the abdomen.
- Create slow, rhythmic, springing, side-swaying movements directed at the dysfunctional sacroiliac joint, to challenge the barrier.
  - Move your hips and knees to created side-swaying movements. Stop movements when the tissue tension resolves, or after about 2 minutes.
- Return the patient to a neutral position and release the forces.
- Retest the sacroiliac joint for changes in passive range of motion.

Sacrum

Sacral somatic dysfunctions can be challenging to correct, especially if a patient cannot lie supine or prone. Use this technique for pregnant patients, patients who have limited mobility, or even small children who prefer to sit upright (**Fig. 10.5**).

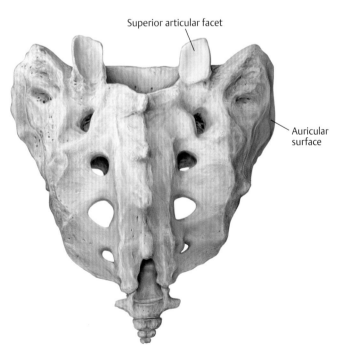

Superior articular facet

Auricular surface

Fig. 10.5   Sacral articular surfaces.

Key Elements

- Somatic dysfunction corrected: any articular sacral or sacroiliac (SI) joint somatic dysfunction.
  - In addition to or in lieu of performing a seated flexion test, test both sides of the sacral base for passive range of motion. With a patient seated, contact the sacral base near the SI joint and apply anteriorly directed springing forces. Monitor and direct force vectors toward the more restricted side.
- End goal: to release the tissues around the SI joint using one force vector and repetitive, springing movements to restore the alignment of the sacrum.

WATCH ▷ ► ▷

► *Video 10.4 Sacrum—Narrated*

Example Somatic Dysfunction: Left sacroiliac joint passive range of motion restriction

Positioning and Preparation

► Patient: seated, positioned so the pelvis is near the back edge of the table.
  - Ask the patient to flex the knees so they hook around the front edge of the table. This helps the patient to remain stable during the technique performance. The patient can also place one or both hands on the table near the pelvis for additional stabilization.
► Physician: sitting behind the patient.

Tissue Contact

- Monitoring hand: contact the dysfunctional sacral sulcus or SI joint. Use your right hand if contacting the patient's right side and your left if contacting the patient's left side.
- Performing contact: contact the shoulder on the side opposite of the dysfunctional sacroiliac joint with the entire hand.

Movements, Barriers, and Forces

- With the monitoring hand, layer palpate to the sacroiliac joint.

Use the performing hand to do the following:

- Move the patient so that the tissues surrounding the SI joint are tight to exaggerate the lesion.
  - This is often side bending toward the side of the restricted SI joint.
- Apply a compressive force vector from your performing contact to the dysfunctional SI joint. Hold this force.
- Create slow, rhythmic, springing motions directed posteriorly and diagonally at the dysfunctional joint to challenge the barrier.
- Stop movements when the tissue tension resolves, or after about 2 minutes.
- Return the patient to a neutral position and release the forces.
- Retest the SI joint for changes in passive range of motion.

Chapter Summary

Challenge the barrier is classified as an exaggeration technique, original to Dr. Still. This chapter describes the exaggeration, or tightening, of a restricted joint, followed by the use of multiple vector forces directed to the restricted joint. The technique culminates in physiological movements directed at the maximally restricted, multiply vectored joint. Though standard positional joint diagnosis is not required, coordinated compression, traction, and safe oscillatory movements must be achieved. CBR techniques require physician creativity, fluidity of movements, and adaptability. This allows a physician to apply the principles of disengagement using force vectors, and to create movements that integrate fascial, ligamentous, and tendinous components of joint biomechanics with articular shape.

Clinical Case and Review Questions

Case

A 50-year-old woman presents to the clinic with chronic pelvic pain. She manages the pain with massage therapy, home exercises, and a vegan diet and would like to try osteopathic manipulative medicine. The pain began after a fall during her last pregnancy, 20 years ago. She denies bowel or bladder dysfunction.

Physical examination is positive for the following:

- Right iliac crest superior.
- Standing flexion test positive on the right.
- Sacroiliac joint compression test positive on the right.

Q1. You decide to perform a direct exaggeration technique to correct her innominate somatic dysfunction. To disengage the joint, you

A. Apply pressure to the right sacral base.
B. Compress the anterior superior iliac spines medially.
C. Lift the right posterior superior iliac crest superiorly.
D. Side-sway the patient toward the left.
E. Side-sway the patient toward the right.

Q2. If present, which of the following would be a contraindication to performing a direct exaggeration technique?

A. A history of a sacral fracture.
B. A hysterectomy 6 weeks ago.
C. An implanted sacral nerve stimulator 2 weeks ago.
D. The chronicity of the condition.
E. The patient's age.

Q3. Which of the following best classifies challenge the barrier techniques?

A. Indirect and active.
B. Direct and active.
C. Indirect and passive.
D. Direct and passive.
E. Active and passive.

Answers to Review Questions

Q1. The correct answer is C.

Q2. The correct answer is C.

Q3. The correct answer is D. CBR techniques are direct because a barrier is being engaged and passive because patient effort is not required.

LEARNING OBJECTIVES

1. Explain the goals of performing muscle energy techniques.
2. Identify the clinical considerations, including indications, contraindications, and precautions for performing muscle energy techniques.
3. Compare and contrast the various muscle energy technique methods.
4. Outline the general movements, barriers, and forces required to perform muscle energy techniques.
5. Identify and avoid common errors made when performing muscle energy techniques.
6. Identify the end goal of each muscle energy technique.
7. Visualize, verbalize, and identify the preparation, positioning, tissue contact, movements, barriers, and forces for each muscle energy technique.
8. Perform muscle energy techniques using appropriate somatic dysfunction diagnosis, preparation, positioning, tissue contact, movements, barriers, forces, retest for effectiveness, communication, and safe tissue handling.

Muscle Energy Techniques Introduction

Muscle energy (ME) techniques correct joint and muscle somatic dysfunctions in a dynamic fashion. The physician and patient interact and work together to perform the technique. Patients participate by using their own "energy," or muscle contraction. There are different types of muscle contractions, useful in several ways, depending on the biomechanics of the region to be addressed.

Therefore, physician knowledge of muscle anatomy, particularly attachment sites and actions, is essential because that knowledge guides the performance of ME techniques. In addition, physicians must guide patient participation using clear and precise instructions. When first learning ME techniques, movements are often hesitant, and the technique may take a bit of time owing to the need for precise positioning and patient instructions. As with other techniques, movements become fluid, and instructions become easier to communicate with practice.

By restoring normal joint position and muscle tone, ME techniques achieve the following:

- Restore muscle balance of agonist/antagonist muscles.
- Improve muscle contraction efficiency.
- Increase joint range of motion.
- Improve local arterial, venous, and lymphatic circulation.

Background

ME is a relatively modern osteopathic technique. It may have multiple origins, but is credited to Fred Mitchell, Sr., DO, who credited T.K. Ruddy, DO, and Clark Kettler, DO. Dr. Mitchell published an initial description in an article in the Yearbook of the American Academy of Osteopathy in 1958.[1] His work was further developed and published by his son Fred Mitchell, Jr., DO. Sally Sutton, DO, FAAO, and Phillip Greenman, DO, FAAO, among others, were taught this new model by Dr. Mitchell, Sr., and shared it with the profession, where it ultimately became a part of standard osteopathic medical school curricula.

Research

The effects and mechanisms of ME techniques are frequently researched, and ME techniques are often incorporated into clinical research protocols. A short reference bibliography is provided at the end of this chapter.

Clinical Considerations

Some common clinical things to consider when using ME techniques are listed in Table 11.1. Always acquire adequate data in the form of an appropriate history, a thorough physical exam that includes an exam for somatic dysfunction, and relevant diagnostic tests to exercise best clinical judg-

ment before performing osteopathic manipulative treatment.

Somatic Dysfunction Corrected

ME techniques correct joint and/or muscular somatic dysfunction, which must be identified using standard positional joint diagnosis based on the barrier concept. Muscular somatic dysfunction may also be identified, but should be correlated to the joint diagnosis. For example, in the case of a right hamstring muscle restriction, the joint correlate is knee extension restriction/hip flexion restriction, or knee flexion/hip extension somatic dysfunction. Learners should attain proficiency in using the varied terminology.

Positioning and Preparation

- ▶ Patient: the patient can be positioned as supine, prone, laterally recumbent, or seated.
- ▶ Physician: the physician is positioned to effectively perform the technique as well as to safely control the patient movements with appropriate mechanical advantage. Therefore, proper ergonomics are essential.

Tissue Contact

There are two primary tissue contacts used in ME techniques: performing and monitoring. One or both of these contacts may be used as counterforce to the patient's muscle effort.

- Monitoring hand: the dysfunctional joint should be monitored at all times. The monitoring hand palpates joint motion and tissue tension to detect when the patient has been initially positioned at the restrictive barrier(s). A second function is to palpate the musculature to ensure that the patient is

Table 11.1 Clinical considerations		
Indications	**Contraindications**	**Precautions**
Mechanical back and neck pain	Fracture or suspected fracture	Not suitable for patients who
Tension headache	Joint dislocation	cannot follow precise instructions
Postural imbalance	Joint infection	or who can't move voluntarily
Scoliosis	Joint effusion	Avoid performing on acutely or
As a component of a	Oculocephalogyric reflex: do not	chronically ill patients who do not
comprehensive rehabilitation	perform after recent eye trauma	have the metabolic reserves to
program	or surgery.	perform repetitive muscle efforts.

performing an appropriate muscular action. Third, the monitoring hand may also help to create a counterforce that the patient pushes against when performing a muscle contraction effort. The joint space, attached musculature, or a portion of one bone can be contacted for monitoring, and each technique identifies the suggested contact. Physicians can make adjustments to the monitoring contact to maintain proper ergonomics.

- Performing Contact: this is the contact that creates a counterforce that the patient pushes against when performing a muscle contraction effort. The patient must be instructed as to the amount of force to use (usually minimal) before making the muscle effort to avoid injury to either the physician or the patient.

Movements, Barriers, and Forces

Muscle energy is a direct, active technique. There are five ME technique methods: (1) postisometric relaxation, (2) reciprocal inhibition, (3) respiratory assistance, (4) direct muscle action, and (5) crossed-extensor reflex. The naming of the method is related to the type of muscle effort performed by the patient.

All ME methods begin with the physician moving a dysfunctional joint or muscle into the directions of the restrictive barriers, to the point where tissue tensions increase and motion restriction is first appreciated. The term "feather edge of the barrier" is used colloquially to describe this positioning. This is referred to as initial positioning in the technique steps. The joint can either be moved directly, such as moving the femur to correct hip (femoroacetabular) somatic dysfunction, or from a distance using a lever, such as moving the trunk to correct vertebral somatic dysfunction. The patient should remain relaxed so the physician can accurately identify and palpate when the restrictive barriers are first encountered.

When positioned in all directions of the restrictive barriers, the patient is asked to create a muscle effort, or contraction. The patient's muscle effort will be either isometric or isotonic. It is referred to as patient activity in the technique steps. The muscle effort should be produced for 3 to 5 seconds to ensure appropriate activation. Then the patient is asked to stop the muscle effort, and a 1-second pause is taken to allow for the postisometric relaxation phase. The postisometric relaxation phase is key because this is when the musculature can be stretched, and the joint "repositioned" in the directions of the restrictive barriers, nudging the joint closer to the physiological barrier. One patient muscle effort is usually not sufficient to correct the somatic dysfunction, so the steps of the technique should be repeated at least twice more, up to four times, for a total of three to five patient muscle efforts–repositioning cycles.

Table 11.2 compares and contrasts ME technique methods. However, this manual does not include any specific techniques that use the reciprocal inhibition or crossed extensor reflex methods. A variation of respiratory assistance has been incorporated into chapter 6, Thoracoabdominal Diaphragm and Pelvic Diaphragm Techniques.

In the upper cervical spine, there is an oculocephalogyric reflex whereby eye movement and head movement are linked. Through a brain stem connection, eye movements cause reflex activation of the suboccipital muscles. Thus the patient's looking in one direction is a substitute for contraction of the suboccipital musculature. The oculocephalogyric reflex can be used in lieu of gross head and neck movement when performing ME technique on the occipitoatlantal (OA) and atlantoaxial (AA) joints.

Retest for Effectiveness

Retest the dysfunctional joint for changes in tissue texture and normalization of joint position and active and/or passive range of motion. Because ME techniques require performing numerous steps sequentially, precise positioning, and patient cooperation, it can be challenging for beginners to achieve full correction. Therefore, if a step isn't followed, full correction of the somatic dysfunction may not be achieved. It is therefore acceptable to perform the technique again, from beginning to end, taking care to complete every step.

ME Technique Summary Steps

These steps are for the postisometric relaxation method, which includes all of the techniques except the ME technique for the pubic symphysis. The pubic symphysis technique uses a direct muscle action method, which is described in the steps of the technique.

Be sure to remember to briefly describe the steps of the technique, including the patient's participation, before performing.

- With the monitoring hand, layer palpate to the muscle or joint tissue layer.

Table 11.2 Muscle energy methods

Muscle energy method	Patient activity	Corrective force	Physiology
Post-isometric relaxation	An isometric contraction of the agonist, which is hypertonic and shortened. Usually, the directions of the contraction are in the directions of the somatic dysfunction.	Repositioning by the physician to move the restrictive barrier closer to the physiological barrier	Contraction of an agonist results in a post-isometric relaxation phase. This transient relaxation permits stretching of that muscle, and subsequent joint movement.
Reciprocal inhibition	An isometric contraction of the antagonist muscle(s)	Repositioning by the physician to move the restrictive barrier closer to the physiological barrier	Contraction of an antagonist muscle group reflexively relaxes its agonist. This transient relaxation permits stretching of the agonist, and subsequent joint movement.
Respiratory assistance	Contraction of the thoracoabdominal diaphragm (TAD) by breathing deeply	Repositioning by the physician, during exhalation, the structures moved by the TAD during inhalation	Relaxation of the TAD (exhalation) permits stretching of the TAD and/or movement of structures attached to it.
Direct muscle action	An isotonic contraction of the antagonist muscle(s)	The patient's muscle effort restores joint alignment.	The muscle contraction moves a bone or joint in the direction of the restrictive barrier(s).
Crossed extensor reflex	An isometric contraction of the extremity without somatic dysfunction. This is used when an extremity is immobilized or significantly injured that voluntary muscle contraction is contraindicated.	The patient's muscle effort	Voluntary contraction in one extremity causes a reflex relaxation of the same muscle in the opposite extremity and relaxation of the antagonist.

Initial Positioning

- Move the dysfunctional joint or muscle in the direction(s) of the restrictive barrier(s) until tissue resistance is felt.
  - Hold the patient steady to prepare for the muscle effort.

Patient Activity

- Ask the patient to perform a muscle effort in the directions of the somatic dysfunction, away from the restrictive barrier(s), for 3 to 5 seconds.
  - Produce a counterforce to the patient's muscle effort.
- After 3 to 5 seconds, ask the patient to stop the muscle effort.
- Pause for 1 second.

Repositioning

- Move the dysfunctional joint or muscle further in the directions of the new restrictive barrier(s), which should now be closer to the physiological barrier.
- Repeat steps 3–6 two to four more times until the restrictive barrier is eliminated and physiological motion is restored.
- Return the patient to a neutral position.
- Retest the somatic dysfunction for improvement in range of motion and position.

For ease, and because most muscle energy techniques are performed the same way, tables are provided that outline the initial positioning, muscle effort/patient activity, and repositioning for each somatic dysfunction. Narrations include these specific directions.

Method: Head, Occipitoatlantal Joint

Postisometric Relaxation

Superficial and deep muscles attach to the occiput to direct and stabilize a heavy cranium on a relatively narrow cervical spine (**Fig. 11.1**). These muscles become hypertonic, and ME technique can simultaneously stretch the muscles and reposition the joint.

Key Elements

- Somatic dysfunction corrected: OA joint: NS_XR_Y, ER_XS_Y, FR_XS_Y.
- End goal: to create relaxation in the suboccipital muscles for repositioning the OA joint.

> **WATCH** ▷ ▶ ▷
>
> ▶ *Video 11.1a Head, OA Joint—Real-Time*
> ▶ *Video 11.1b Head, OA Joint—Narrated*
> *Example Somatic Dysfunction: OA ESLRR*

Positioning and Preparation

- ▶ Patient: supine.
- ▶ Physician: seated at the head of the table.

Tissue Contact

- Both hands contact the head to move and to hold it steady during the patient's muscular effort. Some fingers of one hand monitor the OA joint.
- Monitoring hand: with the hand on the same side of the posterior occiput (the side of occipital rotation), contact the suboccipital musculature with the tips or pads of the second and/or third fingers. Depending on your hand size, contact the zygoma, or temporal bone, superior and posterior to the ear with the thumb, avoiding the temporomandibular joint. This thumb will be used to oppose the patient's muscle effort.
- Assisting hand: with the thenar eminences and thumbs, contact the (opposite) lateral side of the head.
- Wrap both hands around the contour of the head so that you can lift and move it.

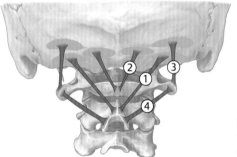

Fig. 11.1 Schematic of suboccipital muscles. 1, rectus capitis posterior major; 2, rectus capitis posterior minor; 3, obliquus capitis superior; 4, obliquus capitis inferior.

Muscle	Origin	Insertion	Innervation	Action
① Rectus capitis posterior major	Spinous process of the axis	Middle third of the inferior nuchal line	Posterior ramus of C1 (suboccipital nerve)	*Bilateral:* extends the head *Unilateral:* rotates the head to the same side
② Rectus capitis posterior minor	Posterior tubercle of the atlas	Inner third of the inferior nuchal line	Posterior ramus of C1 (suboccipital nerve)	*Bilateral:* extends the head *Unilateral:* rotates the head to the same side
③ Obliquus capitis superior	Transverse process of the atlas	Above the insertion of the rectus capitis posterior major or middle third of nuchal line	Posterior ramus of C1 (suboccipital nerve)	*Bilateral:* extends the head *Unilateral:* tilts the head to the same side and rotates it to the opposite side
④ Obliquus capitis inferior	Spinous process of the atlas	Transverse process of the atlas	Posterior ramus of C1 (suboccipital nerve)	*Bilateral:* extends the head *Unilateral:* rotates the head to the same side

Note: The prevertebral muscles are not included among the intrinsic back muscles as they are innervated by the anterior rami of the spinal nerves.

Movements, Barriers, and Forces

Use the monitoring hand to do the following:

- Layer palpate to the occiput.

Use both hands to do the following:

- Position the OA joint by moving the head in the directions of the restrictive barriers until tissue resistance is felt (Table 11.3).
  - Hold the patient steady to prepare for the muscle effort.
- Ask the patient to move the head in the direction of the somatic dysfunction, away from the restrictive barrier(s), for 3 to 5 seconds.

- Produce a counterforce to the patient's muscle effort.
- After 3 to 5 seconds, ask the patient to stop the muscle effort.
- Pause for 1 second.
- Move the OA joint further in the directions of the new restrictive barriers.
- Repeat steps 3–6 two to four more times until the restrictive barrier is eliminated and physiological motion is restored.
- Return the patient to a neutral position.
- Retest the OA joint for improvement in range of motion and position.

Table 11.3   ME: head, occipitoatlantal joint steps

Step	OA FS$_X$R$_Y$	OA ES$_X$R$_Y$	OA NS$_X$R$_Y$
2. Initial positioning	ES$_Y$R$_X$	FS$_Y$R$_X$	NS$_Y$R$_X$
3. Patient activity Option—head Option—eyes	FS$_X$R$_Y$ Look in the direction of Y	ES$_X$R$_Y$ Look in the direction of Y	NS$_X$R$_Y$ Look in the direction of Y
6. Repositioning	ES$_Y$R$_X$	FS$_Y$R$_X$	NS$_Y$R$_X$

Thoracic, T1–T5

Postisometric Relaxation

Somatic dysfunction in the upper thoracic vertebrae can be challenging to correct. The head and neck are used as a lever for positioning and moving the upper thoracic vertebrae (Fig. 11.2).

Key Elements

- Somatic dysfunction corrected: T1–T5: NS$_X$R$_Y$, FR$_X$S$_X$, ER$_X$S$_X$.
- End goal: to restore normal motion and position of the upper thoracic vertebrae.

WATCH ▷ ► ▷

- ► *Video 11.2a Thoracic, T3 E S$_R$R$_R$—Real Time*
- ► *Video 11.2b Thoracic, T3 E S$_R$R$_R$—Narrated*

Example Somatic Dysfunction: T3 E S$_R$R$_R$

- ► *Video 11.2c Thoracic, T3 N S$_L$R$_R$—Real Time*
- ► *Video 11.2d Thoracic, T3 F S$_R$R$_R$—Real Time*

Positioning and Preparation

- ► Patient: seated, so that the patient's shoulders are at or below the physician's shoulder level.
- ► Physician: standing or seated closely behind the patient on the side that is opposite the direction of vertebral rotation.

Tissue Contact

- One hand contacts the head to move it and to hold it steady during the patient's muscular effort. The other hand monitors the dysfunctional vertebra.
- Performing contact: contact the vertex of the patient's head with the palm of your hand. Allow fingers to wrap around the contour of the head.
  - Move this hand as necessary to control the head position and to create the counter force for the patient's muscle effort.
- Monitoring hand: contact the posterior transverse process of the dysfunctional vertebra.

Muscle		Origin	Insertion	Innervation	Action
Semispinalis	① Semispinalis capitis	C4–T7 (transverse and articular process)	Occipital bone (between superior and inferior nuchal lines)	Spinal nn. (posterior rami)	*Bilateral:* Extends thoracic and crevical spines and head (stabilizes craniovertebral joints) *Unilateral:* Bends head, cervical, and thoracic spines to same side, rotates to opposite side
	② Semispinalis cervicis	T1–T6 (transverse process)	C2–C5 (spinous processes)		
	③ Semispinalis thoracis	T6–T12 (transverse process)	C6–T4 (spinous processes)		

Abbreviation: nn, nerves.

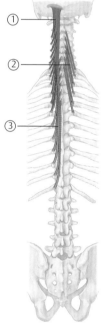

Fig. 11.2 Schematic of upper thoracic musculature. 1, semispinalis capitis; 2, semispinalis cervicis; 3, semispinalis thoracis.

Movements, Barriers, and Forces

- With the monitoring hand, layer palpate to the transverse process.
- With the performing contact, position the dysfunctional vertebra by moving the patient's head and neck in the directions of the restrictive barriers until tissue resistance is felt in the monitoring hand (Table 11.4).
  - Prepare for the muscle effort, moving your performing contact if necessary, for the patient to create a muscle effort against it.
- Ask the patient to turn the head in the directions of the somatic dysfunction, away from the restrictive barrier(s), for 3 to 5 seconds.
  - Produce a counterforce to the patient's muscle effort.
- After 3 to 5 seconds, ask the patient to stop the muscle effort.
- Pause for 1 second.
- Move the vertebra by moving the head and neck further in the directions of the restrictive barriers.
- Repeat steps 3–6 two to four more times until the restrictive barrier is eliminated and physiological motion is restored.
- Return the patient to a neutral position.
- Retest the vertebra for improvement in range of motion and position.

Table 11.4 ME: thoracic, T1–T5 steps			
	T1–T5 NS$_X$R$_Y$	**T1–T5 FR$_X$S$_X$**	**T1–T5 ER$_X$S$_X$**
2. Initial positioning	NS$_Y$R$_X$	ER$_Y$S$_Y$	FR$_Y$S$_Y$
3. Patient activity—head movement	NS$_X$R$_Y$	FR$_X$S$_X$	ER$_X$S$_X$
6. Repositioning	NS$_Y$R$_X$	ER$_Y$S$_Y$	FR$_Y$S$_Y$

Thoracic and Lumbar, T6–L5

Postisometric Relaxation

This technique uses torso positioning to mobilize the lower thoracic and lumbar vertebrae (**Fig. 11.3**). Using this approach, diagnosis and treatment can occur in the same position. This saves time and the patient avoids frequent position changes.

Key Elements

- Somatic dysfunction corrected: T6–L5: NS_XR_Y, FR_XS_X, ER_XS_X.
- End goal: to incrementally correct vertebral somatic dysfunction using sequential paraspinal muscle contractions/relaxations by the patient.

WATCH ▷ ▶ ▷

- ▶ *Video 11.3a Thoracic and Lumbar, L1 E S_RR_R—Real Time*
- ▶ *Video 11.3b Thoracic and Lumbar, L1 E S_RR_R—Narrated*

Example Somatic Dysfunction: L1 E R_RS_R

- ▶ *Video 11.3c Thoracic and Lumbar, L1 N S_RR_L—Real Time*

Positioning and Preparation

- ▶ Patient: seated, so that the patient's shoulders are at or below the physician's shoulder level, and with both arms crossed in front of the chest.
- ▶ Physician: standing or seated behind the patient on the side that is opposite to the direction of vertebral rotation, and with body contact between the physician and the patient to provide better body control during the treatment.

Tissue Contact

- One hand positions the trunk to position and move the dysfunctional vertebra. The other hand monitors the dysfunctional joint.

- Performing contact: contact the patient's shoulders so as to firmly hold the torso. Wrap your arm on top of the patient's crossed arms so that your hand is on top of the patient's shoulder and your humerus, near your axilla, is on top of the patient's other shoulder.
- Monitoring contact: contact the posterior transverse process of the dysfunctional vertebra with the second and/or third finger and/or thumb.

Movements, Barriers, and Forces

- With the monitoring hand, layer palpate to the transverse process.
- With the performing hand, position the dysfunctional vertebra by moving the trunk in the directions of the restrictive barriers until tissue resistance is felt in the monitoring hand (Table 11.5).
  - Prepare for the patient's muscle effort by using proper ergonomics and bracing your legs against the table if necessary.
- Ask the patient to move the trunk in the directions of the somatic dysfunction, away from the restrictive barrier(s), for 3 to 5 seconds.
  - Produce a counterforce to the patient's muscle effort.
- After 3 to 5 seconds, ask the patient to stop the muscle effort.
- Pause for 1 second.
- Move the vertebra by moving the trunk further in the directions of the restrictive barriers.
- Repeat steps 3–6 two to four more times until the restrictive barrier is eliminated and physiological motion is restored.
- Return the patient to a neutral position.
- Retest the vertebra for improvement in range of motion and position.

Table 11.5 ME: thoracic and lumbar, T6–L5 steps			
	T6–L5 NS_XR_Y	**T6–L5 FR_XS_X**	**T6–L5 ER_XS_X**
2. Initial positioning	NS_YR_X	ER_YS_Y	FR_YS_Y
3. Patient activity—torso movement	NS_XR_Y	FR_XS_X	ER_XS_X
6. Repositioning	NS_YR_X	ER_YS_Y	FR_YS_Y

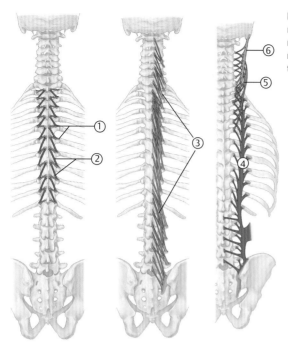

Fig. 11.3 Schematic of thoracic and lumbar spine musculature. 1, rotatores breves; 2, rotatores longi; 3, multifidus; 4, ilicostalis lumborum; 5, iliocostalis thoracis seventh to twentieth ribs; 6, iliocostalis cervicis: third to seventh ribs.

Muscle		Origin	Insertion	Innervation	Action
Rotatores	① Rotatores breves	T1–T12 (between transverse and spinous processes of adjacent vertebrae)		Spinal nn. (posterior rami)	*Bilateral:* Extends thoracic spine *Unilateral:* Rotates spine to opposite side
	② Rotatores longi	T1–T12 (between transverse and spinous processes, skipping one vertebra)			
Multifidus ③		C2–sacrum (between transverse and spinous processes, skipping two to four vertebrae)			*Bilateral:* Extends spine *Unilateral:* Flexes spine to same side, rotates to opposite side
Iliocostalis muscles		④ Iliocostalis lumborum: sacrum, iliac crest, superficial layer of the thoracolumbar fascia ⑤ Iliocostalis thoracis: seventh to twelfth ribs ⑥ Iliocostalis cervicis: third to seventh ribs	• Iliocostalis lumborum: sixth to twelfth ribs, deep layer of thoracolumbar fascia, transverse processes of upper lumbar vertebrae • Iliocostalis thoracis: first to sixth ribs • Iliocostalis cervicis: transverse processes of C4–C6 vertebrae	Lateral branches of posterior rami of spinal nerves C8–L1	*Entire muscle:* bilateral contraction extends the spine, unilateral contraction bends the spine laterally to the same side

Abbreviation: nn, nerves.

Costal, Rib 1

Postisometric Relaxation

The first rib can easily become elevated from muscle tension of the anterior and middle scalene muscles due to carrying heavy bags, working at a desk, or sleeping in a draft. This technique stretches the scalene muscles, permitting restoration of normal joint position of the first rib (**Fig. 11.4**).

Key Elements

- Somatic dysfunction corrected: first rib superior shear or inhalation somatic dysfunction.
- End goal: to relax anterior and middle scalene muscles to resolve dysfunctional positioning of first rib.

> **WATCH** ▷ ▶ ▷
>
> ▶ *Video 11.4a Costal, Rib 1—Real Time*
>
> ▶ *Video 11.4b Costal, Rib 1—Narrated*
>
> **Example Somatic Dysfunction: Left 1st Rib Superior Shear**

Positioning and Preparation

- ▶ Patient: supine.
- ▶ Physician: seated at the head of the table.

Tissue Contact

One hand monitors and positions the first rib. The other hand positions the head and neck for effective scalene contraction.

- Performing and monitoring hand: contact the superior, posterior aspect of the rib with the thumb.
- Assisting hand: contact the posterior occiput and upper cervical spine so as to hold and cradle the head and neck.

Movements, Barriers, and Forces

- With the monitoring hand, layer palpate to the head of the first rib.
- With the assisting hand, position the head and neck by side bending away from the side of the dysfunctional rib, in the directions of the restrictive barriers, until scalene muscle tightness is felt in the monitoring hand.
  - Prepare for the patient's muscle effort. Adjust assisting hand position if necessary.
- Ask the patient to side bend the head in the directions of the somatic dysfunction, away from the restrictive barrier(s), for 3 to 5 seconds (Table 11.6).
  - Produce a counterforce to the patient's muscle effort.
- After 3 to 5 seconds, ask the patient to stop the muscle effort.
- Pause for 1 second.
- Move the head further in the directions of the new restrictive barriers, which should now be closer to the physiological barriers.
  - Additional repositioning can be done with the thumb on the rib head by creating an inferior force on the rib head.
- Repeat steps 3–6 two to four more times until the restrictive barrier is eliminated and physiological motion is restored.
- Return the patient to a neutral position.
- Retest the rib for improvement in range of motion and position.

Table 11.6 ME: costal, rib 1 steps	Right first rib superior shear or inhalation somatic dysfunction	Left first rib superior shear or inhalation somatic dysfunction
2. Initial positioning	Side bend and rotate the head and neck to the left.	Side bend and rotate the head and neck to the right.
3. Patient activity—neck movement	Side bend to the right.	Side bend to the left.
6. Repositioning	Side bend and rotate the head and neck to the left.	Side bend and rotate the head and neck to the right.

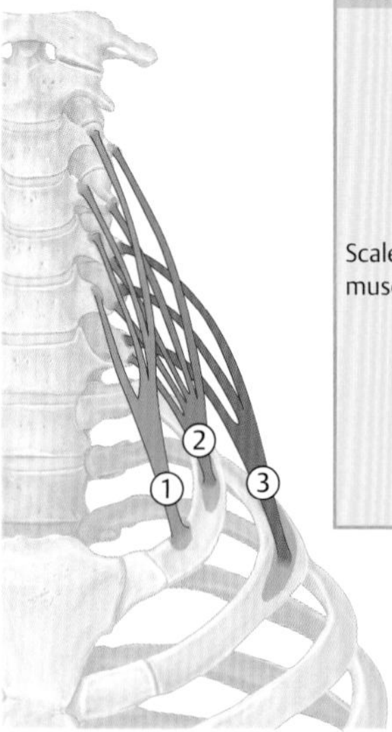

Muscle		Origin	Insertion	Innervation	Action
Scalene muscles	① Anterior scalene muscle	C3–C6 (transverse processes, anterior tubercles)	1st rib (anterior scalene tubercle)	Direct branches from cervical and brachial plexus (C3–C6)	*With ribs mobile:* raises upper ribs (inspiration) *With ribs fixed:* bends cervical spine to same side (unilateral); flexes neck (bilateral)
	② Middle scalene muscle	C3–C7 (transverse processes, posterior tubercles)	1st rib (posterior to groove for subclavian artery)		
	③ Posterior scalene muscle	C5–C7 (transverse processes, posterior tubercles)	2nd rib (outer surface)		

Fig. 11.4 Schematic of scalene muscles. 1, posterior scalene muscle; 2, middle scalene muscle; 3, anterior scalene muscle.

Pelvis, Innominate

Postisometric Relaxation

Innominate rotations are very common somatic dysfunctions of the pelvis due to the normal rotations that occur during the gait cycle. Because these dysfunctions are often compensatory, it is important to find and treat pubic and innominate shears, as well as sacral dysfunction, before addressing rotations (**Fig. 11.5**).

Key Elements

- Somatic dysfunction corrected: anterior and posterior innominate rotations.
- End goal: to restore normal symmetry of the innominate bones by using the leg as a long lever to move the ilium.

> **WATCH ▷ ▶ ▷**
>
> ▶ *Video 11.5a Pelvis, Left Anterior Innominate Rotation—Real Time*
>
> ▶ *Video 11.5b Pelvis, Left Anterior Innominate Rotation—Narrated*
>
> ***Example Somatic Dysfunction: Right anterior innominate rotation***
>
> ▶ *Video 11.6a Pelvis, Left Posterior Innominate Rotation—Real Time*
>
> ▶ *Video 11.6b Pelvis, Left Posterior Innominate Rotation—Narrated*

Positioning and Preparation

▶ Patient: supine.
  - Anterior innominate rotation: ask the patient to bend the knee and place foot on the table.
  - Posterior innominate rotation: ask the patient to move so that the hip is at the edge of the table.

▶ Physician: standing on the side of the innominate somatic dysfunction, facing the head of the table.

Tissue Contact

Anterior Innominate Rotation

- Monitoring hand: contact the posterior superior iliac spine and sacroiliac joint with the fingertips of one hand. Use the hand that is farther from the patient.
- Performing contact: contact the tibia just below the knee with the palm of the other hand. The hip may be flexed so the foot is off the table and the knee may be placed on the physician's anterior shoulder just lateral to the coracoid process.

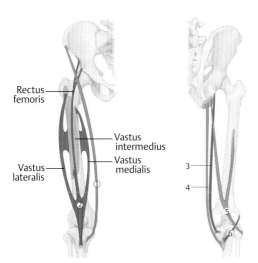

Fig. 11.5 Schematic of hip flexors and extensors. 1, sartorius; 2, quadriceps femoris; 3, biceps femoris; 4, semimenbranosus.

Rectus femoris

Vastus intermedius

Vastus medialis

Vastus lateralis

Muscle	Origin	Insertion	Innervation	Action
① Sartorius	Anterior superior iliac spine	Medial to the tibial tuberosity (together with gracilis and semitendinosus)	Femoral nerve (L2, L3)	*Hip joint:* flexion, abduction, and external rotation *Knee joint:* flexion and internal rotation
② Quadriceps femoris	• Rectus femoris: anterior inferior iliac spine (straight head), acetabular roof of the hip joint (reflected head) • Vastus medialis: medial lip of the linea aspera, distal part of the intertrochanteric line • Vastus lateralis: lateral lip of the linea aspera, lateral surface of the greater trochanter • Vastus intermedius: anterior side of the femoral shaft • Articularis genus (distal fibers of the vastus intermedius): anterior side of the femoral shaft at the level of the suprapatellar recess	• On the tibial tuberosity via the patellar ligament (entire muscle) • Both sides of the tibial tuberosity on the medial and lateral condyles via the medial and lateral longitudinal patellar retinacula (vastus medialis and lateralis) • The suprapatellar recess of the knee joint capsule (articularis genus)	Femoral nerve (L2–L4)	*Hip joint:* flexion (rectus femoris) *Knee joint:* extension (all parts), prevents entrapment of the capsule (articularis genus)
③ Biceps femoris	Long head: ischial tuberosity, sacrotuberous ligament (common head with semitendinosus) Short head: lateral lip of the linea aspera in the middle third of the femur	Head of fibula	Tibial nerve, L5–S2 (long head) Common fibular nerve, L5–S2 (short head)	*Hip joint (long head):* adduction, extends the hip, stabilizes the pelvis in the sagittal plane *Knee joint (entire muscle):* flexion and external rotation
④ Semimembra-nosus	Ischial tuberosity	Medial tibial condyle, oblique popliteal ligament, popliteus fascia	Tibial nerve (L5–S2)	*Hip joint:* adduction, extends the hip, stabilizes the pelvis in the sagittal plane *Knee joint:* flexion and internal rotation
⑤ Semitendinosus	Iscial tuberosity and sacrotuberous ligament (common head with long head of biceps femoris)	Medial to the tibial tuberosity in the pes anserinus (along with the tendons of gracilis and sartorius)	Tibial nerve (L5–S2)	*Hip joint:* adduction, extends the hip, stabilizes the pelvis in the sagittal plane *Knee joint:* flexion and internal rotation
⑥ Popliteus	Lateral femoral condyle, posterior horn of the lateral meniscus	Posterior tibial surface (above the origin of soleus)	Tibial nerve (L4–S1)	Flexes and unlocks the knee by internally rotating the femur on the fixed head of the tibia 5°

Posterior Innominate Rotation

This technique is performed unmonitored.

- Assisting hand: contact the anterior superior iliac spine on the opposite side of the somatic dysfunction with the palm of the hand that is nearer the patient to stabilize the pelvis.
- Performing contact: contact the patient's anterior thigh just above the knee with the palm of the other hand. The thigh may extend off of the table, and the knee will naturally flex.

Movements, Barriers, and Forces

- With the performing hand, position the innominate by moving the leg in the directions of the restrictive barriers until the tissues tighten.
  - Prepare for the patient's muscle effort.

- Ask the patient to push the leg in the directions of the somatic dysfunction (away from the restrictive barrier(s)) for 3 to 5 seconds (Table 11.7).
  - Produce a counterforce to the patient's muscle effort.
- After 3 to 5 seconds, ask the patient to stop the muscle effort.
- Pause for 1 second.
- Move the leg and innominate further in the directions of the new restrictive barriers.
- Repeat steps 2–5 two to four more times until the restrictive barrier is eliminated and physiological motion is restored.
- Return the patient to a neutral position.
- Retest the innominate for changes in position.

Table 11.7 ME: pelvis, innominate steps		
	Anterior innominate rotation	**Posterior innominate rotation**
1. Initial positioning	Rotate the innominate posteriorly by flexing the hip.	Rotate the innominate anteriorly by extending the thigh.
2. Patient activity— hip/thigh movement	Hip extension (to rotate innominate anteriorly)	Hip flexion (to rotate innominate posteriorly)
5. Repositioning	Rotate the innominate further posteriorly by flexing knee and hip and pulling the posterior superior iliac spine inferiorly.	Rotate the innominate further anteriorly by extending the hip.

Pelvis, Pubic Symphysis

Direct Muscle Action

Other pelvic and sacral somatic dysfunctions can be more difficult to diagnose and effectively correct when the pubic bone is not properly aligned, so consider correcting pubic shears first. This technique is useful for cases of cystitis, chronic postural imbalance, and dysmenorrhea (**Fig. 11.6**).

This technique varies from the steps of other ME techniques, in that the technique as written, corrects both superior and inferior pubic shears.

Key Elements

- Somatic dysfunction corrected: pubic shears.
- End goal: to realign the two pubic rami.

> **WATCH ▷▶▷**
>
> ▶ *Video 11.7a Pelvis, Pubic Shear—Real Time*
> ▶ *Video 11.7b Pelvis, Pubic Shear—Narrated*
>
> *Example Somatic Dysfunction: Right Superior Pubic Shear*

Positioning and Preparation

▶ Patient: supine with knees and hips flexed and feet flat on the table.

▶ Physician: standing on one side of the patient.

Tissue Contact

- The pubic symphysis is not monitored during this technique.
- Both hands and arms are used to resist the patient's abduction/adduction at the patient's knees. Specific tissue contacts are written in the steps of the technique because they shift.

Movements, Barriers, and Forces

- Bring the patient's knees together.
- Contact the lateral aspects of the knees with your hands.
  - Alternatively, wrap your arms around the patient's knees.
  - Hold the knees together firmly.
- Ask the patient to push the knees apart for 3 to 5 seconds.
- After 3 to 5 seconds, ask the patient to stop the muscle effort.
- Pause for 1 second.
- Repeat steps 3–5 two more times.
- Now ask the patient to relax the knees and allow them to fall open.
- Contact the medial aspect of the knees with your fist.
- Ask the patient to push the knees together for 3 to 5 seconds.
- After 3 to 5 seconds, ask the patient to stop the muscle effort.
- Pause for 1 second.
- Widen the knees such that the knees are bridged by your forearm.
  - Do this by contacting the medial aspect of the knee joint that is closer to you with your elbow of one arm. Contact the patient's other medial knee joint with your palm.
- Ask the patient to push the knees together for 3 to 5 seconds.
- After 3 to 5 seconds, ask the patient to stop the muscle effort.
- Pause for 1 second.
- Retest the pubic bone for somatic dysfunction.

Note: It is possible that the pubic bone, when corrected, will make a popping sound, similar to when performing high velocity, low amplitude. If this occurs, the technique can be stopped and the pubic bone retested.

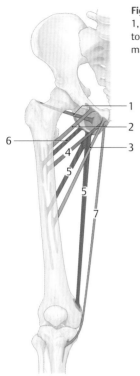

Fig. 11.6 Schematic of thigh adductors. 1, obturator externus; 2, pectineus; 3, adductor longus; 4, adductor brevis; 5, adductor magnus; 6, adductor minimus; 7, cracilis.

Muscle	Origin	Insertion	Innervation	Action
① Obturator externus	Outer surface of the obturator membrane and its bony boundaries	Trochanteric fossa of the femur	Obturator nerve (L3, L4)	Adduction and external rotation of the hip joint Stabilizes the pelvis in the sagittal plane
② Pectineus	Pectin pubis	Pectineal line and the proximal linea aspera of the femur	Femoral nerve, obturator nerve (L2, L3)	Adduction, external rotation, and slight flexion of the hip joint Stabilizes the pelvis in the coronal and sagittal planes
③ Adductor longus	Superior pubic ramus and anterior side of the symphysis	Linea aspera: medial lip in the middle third of the femur	Obturator nerve (L2–L4)	Adduction and flexion (up to 70°) of the hip joint (extends the hip past 80° of flexion) Stabilizes the pelvis in the coronal and sagittal planes
④ Adductor brevis	Inferior pubic ramus	Linea aspera: medial lip in the upper third of the femur	Obturator nerve (L2, L3)	Adduction and flexion (up to 70°) of the hip joint (extends the hip past 80° of flexion) Stabilizes the pelvis in the coronal and sagittal planes
⑤ Adductor magnus	Inferior pubic ramus, ischial ramus, and ischial tuberosity	Deep part ("fleshy insertion"): medial lip of linea aspera Superficial part ("tendinous insertion"): adductor tubercle of femur	Deep part: obturator nerve (L2–L4) Superficial part: tibial nerve (L4)	Adduction, extension, and slight flexion of the hip joint (tendinous insertion is also active in internal rotation) Stabilizes the pelvis in the coronal and sagittal planes
⑥ Adductor minimus (upper division of adductor magnus)	Inferior pubic ramus	Medial lip of the linea aspera	Obturator nerve (L2–L4)	Adduction, external rotation, and slight flexion of the hip joint
⑦ Gracilis	Inferior pubic ramus below the pubic symphysis	Medial border of the tibial tuberosity (along with the tendons of sartorius and semitendinosus)	Obturator nerve (L2, L3)	Hip joint: adduction and flexion Knee joint: flexion and internal rotation

Upper Extremity, Radial Head

Postisometric Relaxation

The radial head is often dysfunctional in elbow pain, especially after a fall onto an outstretched hand. Assuming there is no fracture, treating the radial head can provide great pain relief (**Fig. 11.7**).

Key Elements

- Somatic dysfunction corrected: anterior/ posterior radial head.
- End goal: to correct positional dysfunction of the radial head and restore normal tension across the interosseous membrane.

WATCH ▷ ▶ ▷

- ▶ *Video 11.8a Upper Extremity, Left Anterior Radial Head—Real-Time*
- ▶ *Video 11.8b Upper Extremity, Left Anterior Radial Head—Narrated*
- ▶ *Video 11.9a Upper Extremity, Left Posterior Radial Head—Real-Time*
- ▶ *Video 11.9b Upper Extremity, Left Posterior Radial Head—Narrated*

Positioning and Preparation

- ▶ Patient: seated with the arm flexed to 90 degrees at the elbow on the side of dysfunction.
- ▶ Physician: standing or seated in front of the patient so that the patient's elbow is about at the level of your waist.

Tissue Contact

One hand performs the technique while the other hand monitors the radial head.

- Performing hand: use your right hand to contact the patient's right wrist and vice versa. With one hand, grasp the patient's hand as or a handshake.
- Monitoring hand: use the other hand to contact the anterior aspect of the radial head with your thumb and the posterior aspect with your index finger.

Movements, Barriers, and Forces

- With the monitoring hand, layer palpate to the radial head.
- With the performing hand, position the radial head in the direction of the restrictive barrier until tightness is felt in the monitoring hand.
  - Prepare for the patient's muscle effort.
- Ask the patient to turn the arm in the directions of the somatic dysfunction, away from the restrictive barrier(s), for 3 to 5 seconds (Table 11.8).
  - Produce a counterforce to the patient's muscle effort.
- After 3 to 5 seconds, ask the patient to stop the muscle effort.
- Pause for 1 second.
- Move the radial head further in the directions of the new restrictive barrier.
- Repeat steps 3–6 two to four more times until the restrictive barrier is eliminated and physiological motion is restored.
- Return the patient to a neutral position.
- Retest the radial head for changes in position and range of motion.

Table 11.8 ME: upper extremity, radial head steps

	Radial head anterior	Radial head posterior
2. Initial positioning	Forearm pronation	Forearm supination
3. Patient activity	Supination	Pronation
6. Repositioning	Forearm pronation	Forearm supination

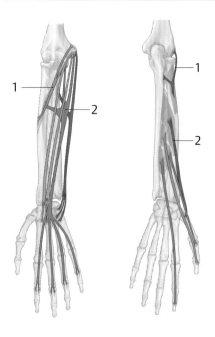

Fig. 11.7 Schematic of pronator teres and supinator muscles. 1, pronator teres; 2, supinator.

Muscle	Origin	Insertion	Innervation	Action
① Pronator teres	Humeral head: medial epicondyle of the humerus Ulnar head: coronoid process of the ulna	Lateral surface of the radius (distal to the supinator insertion)	Median nerve (C6, C7)	Elbow joint: weak flexion Forearm joints: pronation
② Supinator	Olecranon of the ulna, lateral epicondyle of the humerus, radial collateral ligament, anular ligament of the radius	Radius (between the radial tuberosity and the insertion of pronator teres)	Radial nerve (C7, C8)	Radioulnar joint: supination

Lower Extremity, Hamstring Muscle

Postisometric Relaxation

Hamstring muscle restriction is analogous to hip flexion restriction or hip extension somatic dysfunction. The muscle is identified here because this technique, in particular, nicely demonstrates how easy it is to stretch a muscle after postisometric contraction. Also, the hamstring is prone to tightness, and stretching it is often clinically beneficial for treatment of conditions that affect pelvic, sacral, or lower extremity biomechanics. Apply the principles of this technique to any tight and shortened muscle, such as the hip abductors (iliotibial band), or biceps (**Fig. 11.8**).

Key Elements

• Somatic dysfunction corrected: hip flexion restriction, hamstring musculature tightness.

• End goal: to restore normal length and tone to the hamstring musculature.

> **WATCH ▷▶▷**
>
> ▶ *Video 11.10a Lower Extremity, Hamstring Muscle—Real Time*
>
> ▶ *Video 11.10b Lower Extremity, Hamstring Muscle—Narrated*
>
> *Example Somatic Dysfunction: Left Hip Flexion Restriction/Left Hamstring Tightness*

Positioning and Preparation

▶ Patient: supine.

▶ Physician: standing on the side of the tight hamstring musculature, at the level of the thigh, facing the head of the table.

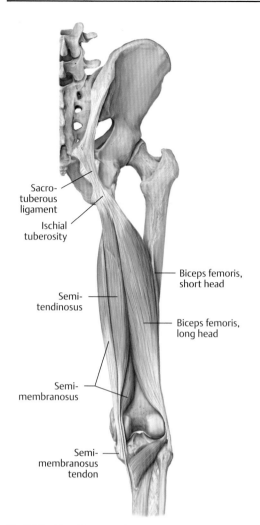

Sacro-
tuberous
ligament

Ischial
tuberosity

Semi-
tendinosus

Semi-
membranosus

Semi-
membranosus
tendon

Biceps femoris,
short head

Biceps femoris,
long head

Fig. 11.8   Hamstring muscles.

Tissue Contact

- This technique is performed unmonitored.
- Lift the patient's leg off of the table and flex the hip. Place the patient's posterior leg on top of your shoulder that is nearer the patient.
- Contact the anterior thigh just superior to the patella with the palms of both hands and gently grasp the thigh.

Movements, Barriers, and Forces

- With the shoulder, gently extend the knee until tissue resistance is appreciated.
  - This position should not hurt the patient. If it does, decrease the amount of extension.
  - Prepare for the patient's muscle effort.
- Ask the patient to very gently push the thigh down into the table for 3 to 5 seconds.
  - Your shoulder provides the counterforce to the patient's muscle effort.
- After 3 to 5 seconds, ask the patient to stop the muscle effort.
- Pause for 1 second.
- Flex the thigh and/or extend the knee further until tissue resistance is felt at the new restrictive barrier, by taking a small step forward.
- Repeat steps 2–5 two to four more times until the restrictive barrier is eliminated and physiological motion is restored.
- Return the patient to a neutral position.
- Retest the hamstring muscle for improvements in tone and range of motion.

Lower Extremity, Fibular Head

Postisometric Relaxation

This technique is useful as part of a comprehensive rehabilitative plan after minor ankle and knee injuries, especially due to sports that require running. This technique is performed slightly differently than most postisometric relaxation techniques because the physician applies pressure directly onto the fibular head during the patient's muscle effort. This is partly because of the small caliber of the muscles used, which are not designed to actively move the fibular head but serve more as joint stabilizers (**Fig. 11.9**).

Key Elements

- Somatic dysfunction corrected: anterior/posterior fibular head.
- End goal: to correct positional dysfunction of the fibular head and restore normal tension across the interosseous membrane.

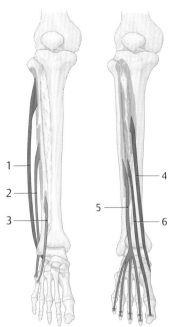

Fig. 11.9 Schematic of the anterior and lateral compartment of the leg. 1, fibularis longus; 2, fibularis brevis; 3, tibialis anterior; 4, extensor digitorumlongus; 5, extensor hallucis longus; 6, fibularis tertius.

Muscle	Origin	Insertion	Innervation	Action
① Fibularis longus	Head of the fibula, proximal two-thirds of the lateral surface of the fibula (arising partly from the intermuscular septa)	Plantar side of the medial cuneiform, base of the first metatarsal	Superficial fibular nerve (L5, S1)	Talocrural joint: plantar flexion Subtalar joint: eversion (pronation) Supports the transverse arch of the foot
② Fibularis brevis	Distal half of the lateral surface of the fibula, intermuscular septa	Tuberosity at the base of the fifth metatarsal (with an occasional division to the dorsal aponeurosis of the fifth toe)	Superficial fibular nerve (L5, S1)	Talocrural joint: plantar flexion Subtalar joint: eversion (pronation)
③ Tibialis anterior	Upper two-thirds of the lateral surface of the tibia, the crural interosseous membrane, and the highest part of the superficial crural fascia	Medial and plantar surface of the medial cuneiform, the medial base of the first metatarsal	Deep fibular nerve (L4, L5)	Talocrural joint: dorsiflexion Subtalar joint: inversion (supination)
④ Extensor digitorum longus	Lateral tibial condyle, head of the fibula, medial surface of the fibula, and the crural interosseous membrane	By four slips to the dorsal aponeuroses of the second through fifth toes and the bases of the distal phalanges of the second through fifth toes	Deep fibular nerve (L4, L5)	Talocrural joint: dorsiflexion Subtalar joint: eversion (pronation) Extends the metatarsophalangeal and interphalangeal joints of the second through fifth toes
⑤ Extensor hallucis longus	Middle third of the medial surface of the fibula, the crural interosseous membrane	Dorsal aponeurosis of the great toe and the base of its distal phalanx	Deep fibular nerve (L4, L5)	Talocrural joint: dorsiflexion Subtalar joint: active in both eversion and inversion (pronation/supination), depending on the position of the foot Extends the metatarsophalangeal and interphalangeal joints of the great toe
⑥ Fibularis tertius (part of extensor digitorum longus)	Anterior border of the distal fibula	Base of the fifth metatarsal	Deep fibular nerve (L5, S1)	Talocrural joint: dorsiflexion Subtalar joint: eversion (pronation)

WATCH ▷ ▶ ▷

▶ *Video 11.11a Lower Extremity, Right Anterior Fibular head—Real Time*

▶ *Video 11.11b Lower Extremity, Right Anterior Fibular Head—Narrated*

Example Somatic Dysfunction: Anterior Fibular Head

▶ *Video 11.12a Lower Extremity, Right Posterior Fibular Head—Real Time*

▶ *Video 11.12b Lower Extremity, Right Posterior Fibular Head—Narrated*

Example Somatic Dysfunction: Posterior Fibular Head

Positioning and Preparation

▶ Patient: supine with knee bent and the heel on the table *or* the patient seated with legs hanging off the table.

▶ Physician: standing at the foot of the table *or* seated on a stool in front of the patient with the fibular head at chest level.

Tissue Contact

One hand monitors the fibular head, and the other hand positions the fibula.

- Monitoring hand: use the hand opposite the side of dysfunction to contact the fibular head. Contact the anterior aspect of the fibular head with your thumb and the posterior aspect with your index finger.
- Performing hand: use the hand on the same side of the dysfunction to contact the foot. Contact the foot at the talus with the palm of the hand. Allow the fingers and thumb to wrap around the contour of the foot and grasp it.

Movements, Barriers, and Forces

- With the monitoring hand, layer palpate to the fibular head.
- With the performing hand, slightly invert the ankle. This helps disengage the fibular head for easier positioning and repositioning.
- With the monitoring hand, position the fibular head by moving it into the direction of the restrictive barrier.
- With the performing hand, move the ankle and foot into the directions of the restrictive barriers until tightness is felt in the monitoring hand.
    - Prepare for the patient's muscle effort.
- Ask the patient to move the ankle in the directions of the somatic dysfunction, away from the restrictive barrier(s), for 3 to 5 seconds (Table 11.9).
    - With the performing hand, produce a counterforce to the patient's muscle effort.
- Concurrently, continue moving the fibular head in the direction of the restrictive barrier.
- After 3 to 5 seconds, ask the patient to stop the muscle effort.
- Pause for 1 second.
- Concurrently move the fibular head further with the monitoring hand while moving the ankle in the direction of the new restrictive barrier.
- Repeat steps 5–9 two to four more times until the restrictive barrier is eliminated and physiological motion is restored.
- Return the patient to a neutral position.
- Retest the fibular head for changes in position and range of motion.

Table 11.9 ME: lower extremity, fibular head steps		
	Fibular head anterior	**Fibular head posterior**
4. Initial positioning	Ankle: plantar flexion Foot: supination	Ankle: dorsiflexion Foot: pronation
5. Patient activity	Ankle: dorsiflexion Foot: pronation	Ankle: plantar flexion Foot: supination
9. Repositioning	Ankle: plantar flexion Foot: supination	Ankle: dorsiflexion Foot: pronation

Chapter Summary

Muscle energy is a versatile, patient-assisted technique that is ideal for the novice learner. This chapter offers examples of muscle energy used throughout the body to correct different types of joints with somatic dysfunction. Muscle energy affords the opportunity to practice not only with different degrees of applied force but also with precise patient communications.

Clinical Cases and Review Questions

Case 1

A 76-year-old woman with a history of arthritis presents to the clinic with neck pain. There is no history of trauma, and the patient denies radiation of pain into the arms. On osteopathic exam of the OA joint, you find that the OA moves easier into flexion and resists extension. Furthermore, you can translate the OA easily from left to right, but it resists translation from right to left.

Q1. What is the proper initial position when correcting this patient's somatic dysfunction using the muscle energy technique?
  A. Flexion, side bending right, rotation left.
  B. Extension, side bending right, rotation left.
  C. Flexion, side bending left, rotation right.
  D. Extension, side bending left, rotation right.
  E. Flexion, side bending right, rotation right.

Q2. After initially positioning the patient's head to perform the muscle energy technique, you ask the patient to look to the right with her eyes. This patient effort is an example of
  A. Reciprocal inhibition.
  B. Cross extensor reflex.
  C. Indirect approach.
  D. Oculocephalogyric reflex.
  E. Direct muscle action.

Q3. Which of the following is a contraindication to asking the patient to look to the right with her eyes when performing the muscle energy technique?
  A. History of arthritis.
  B. Presence of neck pain.
  C. Recent eye surgery.
  D. Use of corrective lenses.
  E. Poor eyesight.

Case 2

A 42-year-old man presents with low back pain. The pain started 2 weeks ago after cleaning up the yard after a hail storm. Physical exam is positive for decreased left hip extension and a left posterior innominate rotation.

Q4. You decide to perform the muscle energy technique using the postisometric relaxation method. After initially positioning his innominate, you ask the patient to perform this muscle contraction effort:
  A. Left hip flexion.
  B. Left hip extension.
  C. Left knee flexion.
  D. Left hip adduction.
  E. Left hip abduction.

Q5. The goal of performing the muscle energy technique in this patient is to
  A. Incrementally move the hip in the direction of the extension physiological barrier.
  B. Stretch the rectus femoris and psoas muscles.
  C. Reposition the hip past the anatomical barrier in flexion.
  D. Restore normal sacroiliac joint alignment by positioning the innominate in posterior rotation.
  E. Progressively rotate the innominate anteriorly after the patient performs the muscle contraction effort.

Answers to Review Questions

Q1. The correct answer is **B**. The diagnosis for the OA is flexed, side bending left, rotation right. Remember to name somatic dysfunction for the ease of motion and that translation from left to right is the same as left side bending. In the OA joint, side bending and rotation move in opposite directions, therefore the OA is rotated right since side bending is to the left. Since muscle energy is a direct technique, the setup should be into the barrier: extension, side bending right, rotation left.

Q2. The correct answer is **D**. The oculocephalogyric reflex can be used in the upper cervical spine because of the connection between eye movements and the suboccipital muscles. This allows the use of eye movements in lieu of head and neck movements in the OA and AA regions.

A is incorrect. Reciprocal inhibition uses the contraction of an antagonist muscle to relax the agonist (e.g., contract the bicep to relax the tricep).

B is incorrect. Voluntary contraction of the muscle in one extremity is used to relax the same muscle in the opposite extremity.

C is incorrect. Muscle energy is a direct technique.

E is incorrect. Direct muscle action is a muscle contraction that directly moves a bone into the restrictive barrier.

Q3. The correct answer is **C**: Recent eye surgery.

A is incorrect. History of arthritis is not a contraindication to muscle energy with the oculocephalogyric reflex.

B is incorrect. Mechanical neck pain is an indication for muscle energy.

D is incorrect. Use of corrective lenses is not a contraindication because you are not directly putting pressure on the eye.

E. Poor eyesight is not a contraindication because it is eye movement that is necessary for the reflex to work and not the vision itself.

Q4. The correct answer is **A**. Muscle energy is a direct technique. Correction of a left posteriorly rotated innominate first involves initially positioning the innominate in the direction of the restrictive barrier of anterior rotation by extending the hip. The patient is then asked to create a muscle effort by moving the hip in flexion while counterforce is applied by the physician.

Q5. The correct answer is **E**: Progressively rotate the innominate anteriorly after the patient performs the muscle contraction effort.

A is incorrect. Incrementally moving the hip in the direction of the extension physiological barrier is the opposite of what is desired.

B is incorrect. The rectus femoris and psoas muscles are being used, but ultimately the goal in this case is to restore normal position of the innominate.

C is incorrect. Never attempt to move tissue past its anatomical barrier. The goal is to progressively move the joint to and through its restrictive barrier to restore normal motion.

D is incorrect. Restoring normal sacroiliac joint alignment by positioning the innominate in posterior rotation is the goal when performing the indirect technique.

References

1. Mitchell FL, Kai Galen Mitchell P. The Muscle Energy Manual. MET Press; 1999

Bibliography

Ballantyne F, Fryer G, McLaughlin P. The effect of muscle energy technique on hamstring extensibility: the mechanism of altered flexibility. J Osteopath Med 2003;6(2):59–63

Burns DK, Wells MR. Gross range of motion in the cervical spine: the effects of osteopathic muscle energy technique in asymptomatic subjects. J Am Osteopath Assoc 2006;106(3):137–142

Eisenhart AW, Gaeta TJ, Yens DP. Osteopathic manipulative treatment in the emergency department for patients with acute ankle injuries. J Am Osteopath Assoc 2003;103(9):417–421

Franke H, Fryer G, Ostelo RW, Kamper SJ. Muscle energy technique for non-specific low-back pain. Cochrane Database Syst Rev 2015;(2):CD009852. doi: 10.1002/14651858

Fryer G, Ruszkowski W. The influence of contraction duration in muscle energy technique applied to the atlanto-axial joint. J Osteopath Med 2004;7(2):79–84

Fryer G. Muscle energy technique: An evidence-informed approach. Int J Osteopath Med 2011;14(1):3–9

Küçükşen S, Yilmaz H, Sallı A, Uğurlu H. Muscle energy technique versus corticosteroid injection for management of chronic lateral epicondylitis: randomized controlled trial with 1-year follow-up. Arch Phys Med Rehabil 2013;94(11):2068–2074

Lenehan, KL, Fryer G, McLaughlin P. The effect of muscle energy technique on gross trunk range of motion. J Osteopath Med 2003;6(1):13–18

Moore SD, Laudner KG, McLoa TA, Shaffer MA. The immediate effects of muscle energy technique on posterior shoulder tightness: a randomized controlled trial. J Orthop Sports Phys Ther 2011;41(6):400–407

Selkow NM, Grindstaff TL, Cross KM, Pugh K, Hertel J, Saliba S. Short-term effect of muscle energy technique on pain in individuals with non-specific lumbopelvic pain: a pilot study. J Manual Manip Ther 2009;17(1):E14–E18

Tanwar R, Moitra M, Goyal M. Effect of muscle energy technique to improve flexibility of gastro-soleus complex in plantar fasciitis: a randomised clinical, prospective study design. Indian Journal of Physiotherapy and Occupational Therapy-An International Journal 2014;8(4):26–30

Wilson E, Payton O, Donegan-Shoaf L, Dec K. Muscle energy technique in patients with acute low back pain: a pilot clinical trial. J Orthop Sports Phys Ther 2003;33(9):502–512

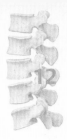

12 High Velocity, Low Amplitude Thrust Techniques

LEARNING OBJECTIVES

1. Explain the goals of performing high velocity, low amplitude thrust techniques.
2. Identify the clinical considerations, including indications, contraindications, and precautions for performing high velocity, low amplitude thrust techniques.
3. Outline the general movements, barriers, and forces for performing high velocity, low amplitude thrust techniques.
4. Describe the thrust force used in high velocity, low amplitude thrust techniques, including direction(s), distance, and magnitude of the thrust force(s).
5. Identify the end goal of performing each high velocity, low amplitude technique.
6. Visualize, verbalize, and identify the preparation, positioning, tissue contact, movements, barriers, and forces for each high velocity, low amplitude thrust technique.
7. Perform high velocity, low amplitude thrust techniques using appropriate somatic dysfunction diagnosis, preparation, positioning, tissue contact, movements, barriers, forces, retest for effectiveness, communication, and safe tissue handling.

High Velocity, Low Amplitude Thrust Techniques Introduction

Performed correctly, high velocity, low amplitude (HVLA) thrust techniques are safe, effective, and relatively fast techniques to perform to correct joint somatic dysfunction. Patients often feel immediate relief. HVLA techniques require that the physician create a short, quick corrective thrust force directed at the articular surfaces of a joint. Although the thrust force is quickly performed, the preparation and adjustment of patients into appropriate positions takes time, as does the development of psychomotor skill proficiency. Visualizing the three-dimensional joint anatomy and practicing the required coordinated body movements are essential for achieving precise technique performance. At its finest, HVLA is an elegant technique, such that when accurate positioning is obtained, only a minimal and short-distanced thrust force is necessary.

HVLA techniques can achieve the following:

- Restore normal joint alignment.
- Improve active and passive joint range of motion.
- Improve local arterial, venous, and lymphatic circulation.

Background

This manual credits Earle Willard, DO, with developing some of the earliest of what are now called HVLA techniques, around 1921. They were first named low table with speed techniques because they were performed on a McManis low table (invented by John McManis, DO). There are some accounts that Dr. Andrew Taylor Still, in his early years as a "lightning bone setter," may have used some high-speed techniques. However, it is clear that he did not teach these high-speed techniques, yet his early students did. Historical accounts suggest that HVLA techniques were easier to teach and perform compared with Dr. Still's early exaggeration techniques. Therefore, HVLA was taught as curriculum at osteopathic medical schools by the mid-20th century. Today, HVLA remains a useful tool in the toolbox of osteopathic techniques.

Clinical Considerations

Some common clinical things to consider when using HVLA techniques are listed in Table 12.1. Always perform an appropriate history, a thorough physical exam that includes an exam for somatic dysfunction, and relevant diagnostic tests, and exercise clinical judgment before performing osteopathic manipulative treatment (OMT).

Research and Safety of HVLA Techniques

HVLA techniques have been used as part of OMT research protocols, including as a stand-alone technique. A sample research bibliography is provided at the end of this chapter. Research on general thrust techniques is included here because the literature includes other manual therapy professions that likely use similar, but not exactly the same, types of thrust techniques as HVLA techniques. Therefore, it is important to use clinical judgment and thoughtful translation of research into practice.

Presumably, one of the most controversial osteopathic manipulative techniques is the cervical HVLA technique. Significant injury, disability, and even death have been reported with the use of cervical thrust techniques.[1] Numerous investigations have been undertaken, and when performed with precision, minimal thrust forces, and minimal neck extension, cervical HVLA technique is safe and is endorsed by the American Osteopathic Association. A position paper can be found at the American Academy of Osteopathy website, issued by the American Association House of Delegates[2]:

Estimates indicate that risks of cervical high-velocity, low-amplitude (HVLA) manipulation are very low—with serious adverse events such as death being rare and adverse reactions being self-limiting, usually resolving spontaneously within a few days. The American Osteopathic Association House of Delegates' position paper on this matter states that benefits outweigh the risks for osteopathic manipulative treatment, including HVLA, in osteopathic clinical practice and education.[1]

Table 12.1 Clinical considerations		
Indications	**Contraindications**	**Precautions**
Mechanical neck and back pain	Fracture or suspected fracture	Exercise care in patients with joint hypermobility.
Postural imbalance	Joint dislocation	
Chronic pain conditions	Joint infection	
Minor sprains/ strains	Tendon, ligament, or meniscal tear	
	Conditions that predispose patients to fractures and/or joint instability such as the following:	
	Osteoporosis	
	Rheumatoid arthritis	
	Osteogenesis imperfecta	
	Osseous malignancies	
	Down syndrome (occipitoatlantal and atlantoaxial joints)	
	Acute disk herniation	
	Myelopathy	
	Cervical high velocity, low amplitude: do not perform if the patient has, or if at any time during technique develops, signs or symptoms of transient vertebrobasilar artery insufficiency	

Somatic Dysfunction Corrected

HVLA corrects joint somatic dysfunction. Because the corrective thrust is precisely directed along a plane of an articulation, a specific positional joint somatic dysfunction diagnosis is required.

Positioning and Preparation

▶ Patient: the patient must be comfortable and should remain relaxed for the duration of most techniques. Some patient assistance for initial positioning is acceptable when necessary (e.g., for lumbar HVLA techniques). HVLA techniques can be performed with the patient seated, supine, prone, or laterally recumbent.

▶ Physician: the physician must be comfortable and positioned to ensure safety, using the best ergonomic posture and movements possible.

Tissue Contact

Both hands are used to perform HVLA techniques. The hands may operate independently or together. Thoracic, patient supine position, and costal HVLA techniques also require physicians to use their abdomen to create the thrust force.

- Monitoring hand: one hand monitors the affected joint for changes in tissue tensions and movement throughout the duration of the technique performance. Monitoring ensures that the joint is moved into the direction of the appropriate restrictive barrier. The monitoring contact sometimes transitions into the performing contact.
- Performing contact: the corrective thrust is made with this contact. One or both hands or the physician's abdomen can be used.
- Assisting contact: this contact helps move the patient into position and may assist in creating the corrective thrust.
- Fulcrum contact: this contact is used as a fulcrum against which a thrust force is applied to reposition a bone. It does not perform the thrust.

Movements, Barriers, and Forces

HVLA is a direct technique. The end goal is to quickly, with very little force, reposition the articular surfaces of a joint with somatic dysfunction.

The joint is positioned, and a thrust force created, in the direction of at least one restrictive barrier. To best accomplish this, body structures above and/or below the joint with somatic dysfunction are moved and positioned prior to creating the thrust force in one of the following ways:

- Structures are positioned in all directions of the restrictive barriers. The rationale for this should be obvious—as a direct technique, all structures are positioned at the restrictive barriers.
- Structures are positioned so that a small space is created in the affected joint. This small space, or gap, permits the articular surfaces to glide more easily during the corrective thrust.
- Structures above and/or below the dysfunctional joint are moved to limit motion of these structures. This eliminates "joint play" or joint motions in various planes so that the thrust force is more precisely directed along the articular surfaces.

Individual technique instructions explain the intended purpose of positioning.

The corrective thrust is made along the plane or planes of the articular surfaces of the affected joint. The thrust should be created with the minimum amount of force necessary to move a bone within its physiological barriers. Joints with somatic dysfunction have moved very little, perhaps a millimeter or less, so the distance of the thrust should be the same. Sometimes the thrust is performed directly on one part of a bone with the performing hand, such as in HVLA technique for the talus. But sometimes the thrust is created using levers, or adjacent bones or body regions. The lumbar spine serves as a good example because the shoulders and pelvis of the patient are used as levers to move a lumbar vertebra.

Because the thrust is performed at a high speed, it is possible that local tissues are excited or activated, instead of relaxed, making precision in performing the technique paramount. Transient activation usually resolves quickly. However, loosening tight soft tissues and fascia as preparation and postthrust can lessen the muscle excitation. Some techniques that can be used include soft tissue, myofascial release, and muscle energy (for preparation only) techniques.

Sometimes a characteristic popping sound is heard when the thrust force returns the joint to its normal position. The sound is attributed to changes in volume, and therefore pressure, in the joint cavity and is also called joint cavitation.[3] Cavitation is an effect, but not an essential or reliable indicator that a joint has been repositioned.

The motions required for performing the corrective thrust may be practiced with hands in the air, or by moving the patient without positioning exactly at the restrictive barriers. Some students find that asking faculty to perform the technique with the faculty member's hands over the student's hands is also beneficial.

Technique Enhancement

Patient respiratory cooperation can be useful when performing HVLA techniques. The thrust should be performed at the end of a patient's exhalation effort to help the patient stay fully relaxed, thereby preventing muscle contraction and guarding. This is essential when performing HVLA in the thoracic and costal regions. Thrust on the thoracic spine or ribs when the patient is inhaling will cause breathing obstruction, essentially "knocking the wind out" of the patient.

Retest for Effectiveness

Elimination of asymmetry and restoration of passive range of motion are indicators that the somatic dysfunction has resolved. If a correction is not made after the first thrust attempt, the technique can be repeated, from the very beginning to the end, once more. After that, the somatic dysfunction should be reevaluated, considering other possible causes of the somatic dysfunction. Another technique can be attempted, such as an indirect, myofascial release, or muscle energy technique.

Clinically, it is reported that a rubbery endfeel, or an absence of a firm restrictive barrier, is sometimes palpated in costal and spinal somatic dysfunctions that do not correct with HVLA techniques. These tissue findings are related to viscerosomatic reflex activity. Therefore, in cases where the thrust in costal and spinal HVLA somatic dysfunctions is either difficult to perform due to an inability to feel tissue tightening, or is not corrective, the patient's clinical condition should be reevaluated with a high index of suspicion for visceral disease.

HVLA Technique Summary Steps

- Identify articular somatic dysfunction.
  - Recollect contraindications and precautions to performing HVLA technique. Do not perform if contraindicated.
- Monitor the dysfunctional bone and/or joint space.
- With the performing hand, layer palpate to the dysfunctional bone and/or joint.
- Move the affected joint in the direction(s) of the restrictive barrier (s) until the tissues feel tight and no further movement is possible.
- Use additional movements in different directions to make the technique more effective.
  - Make minor adjustments in movements as necessary to ensure a discrete restrictive barrier, or end-feel of tissue tightness.
- Perform a high velocity, low amplitude thrust along the plane of the articular surfaces of the dysfunctional joint.
  - Optional: use respiratory cooperation.
- Retest the joint for improvements in position and/or passive range of motion.

Cervical, Atlantoaxial Joint

Use this technique when significant C1 range of motion restrictions are identified, such as in cases of mechanical neck pain, tension-type headache, and temporomandibular joint dysfunction (**Fig. 12.1**). Perform a suboccipital inhibitory pressure technique first to loosen the soft tissues. Avoid rotating and creating thrusting forces on the lower cervical vertebrae.

Key Elements

- Somatic dysfunction corrected: atlantoaxial (AA) joint rotated right or left.
- End goal: to reposition the AA joint using a short, quick rotational thrust, using the head as a lever to move C1.

WATCH ▷ ► ▷

- ► *Video 12.1a Cervical, AA—Real time*
- ► *Video 12.1b Cervical, AA—Narrated*

Example Somatic Dysfunction: AA Rotated Left

Positioning and Preparation

- ► Patient: supine.
- ► Physician: standing at the head of the table facing the patient.

Tissue Contact

- Monitoring and performing hand: use the hand that is on the same side as the atlantoaxial (AA) rotation. Contact the vertebral arch of C1 with the pad of your second or third finger. Point the fingers inferiorly. Wrap the remaining fingers and hand around the contour of the head.
- Assisting hand: contact the other side of the head at the occiput with your other hand and fingers. Wrap the hand and fingers around the contour of the head to hold and move it.

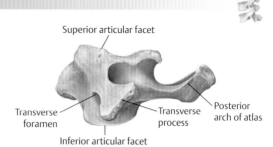

Superior articular facet

Transverse foramen

Transverse process

Posterior arch of atlas

Inferior articular facet

Fig. 12.1 First cervical vertebra.

Movements, Barriers, and Forces

- With the monitoring hand, layer palpate to the C1 vertebral arch.

Use both hands to do the following:

- Flex the head to the AA joint.
  - Flexion localizes and limits forces to the AA joint.
- Rotate the patient's head to rotate C1 in the direction of the rotational restrictive barrier until the tissues tighten and no further movement is possible.
  - Keep the arms relatively stiff, with elbows flexed and wrists neutral.
- Perform an HVLA rotatory thrust in the direction of the rotational restrictive barrier, along the plane of the C1 inferior articular surfaces. Do this by rotating the head.
  - Optional: add respiratory cooperation.
- Return the patient's head and neck to a neutral position and release tissue contact.
- Retest the AA joint for improvements in passive rotational motion.

Cervical, C2–C7

This technique varies from traditional "rotation or side bending only" thrust techniques. Instead, the thrust is performed using a combination of rotation and translation (side bending), which is along the plane of the obliquely oriented articular facets (**Fig. 12.2**). Recall that side bending and rotation motions are coupled and move in the same direction in the cervical spine. Keep forces to a minimum, remembering to be mindful of any contraindications.

Key Elements

- Somatic dysfunction corrected: C2–C7: NS_XR_X, FR_XS_X, ER_XS_X.
- End goal: to reposition a dysfunctional cervical vertebra using a short, quick rotational and translatory thrust.

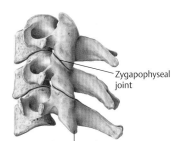

Zygapophyseal joint

Inferior articular process

Fig. 12.2 Cervical vertebrae.

WATCH ▷ ▶ ▷

▶ *Video 12.2a Cervical, C3 FR_LS_L—Real Time*

▶ *Video 12.2b Cervical, C3 R_LS_L—Narrated*

Example Somatic Dysfunction: C3 FR_LS_L

▶ *Video 12.3 Cervical, C3 ER_LS_L—Real Time*

Example Somatic Dysfunction: C3 ER_LS_L

Positioning and Preparation

▶ Patient: supine.

▶ Physician: standing at the head of the table facing the patient.

Tissue Contact

- One hand creates the corrective rotatory and translatory HVLA thrust force. The other hand assists with the movement of the head and neck.
- Monitoring and performing hand: use the hand that is on the same side as vertebral rotation. Contact the vertebral arch of the dysfunctional vertebra with the palmar side of the metacarpophalangeal joint of the second finger. Keep the finger extended. Wrap the remaining fingers around the back of the head. The thumb may gently rest on the face or not touch the patient.
- Assisting hand: use the other hand to contact the posterior and lateral neck on the opposite side. Wrap the hand and fingers around the contour of the head to hold and move it.

Movements, Barriers, and Forces

- With the performing hand, layer palpate to the vertebral arch and inferior joint space.

Use both hands to do the following:
- Flex the neck at the level of the dysfunctional vertebra. Flexion localizes and limits forces to the dysfunctional joint.
  - If flexion or extension dysfunction is present, use slight motions to move the vertebra in the direction of the flexion or extension restrictive barrier. Do not hyperextend.
- Side bend the head and neck in the direction of the side bending somatic dysfunction at the inferior articulation of the dysfunction vertebra. Hold this position.
  - Side bending in this case prevents excessive movement of the dysfunctional vertebra and tightens the tissues further at the rotational restrictive barrier.
- Rotate the patient's head and neck in the direction of the rotational restrictive barrier until the tissues feel tight and no further movement is possible.
  - The performing hand should move with the vertebra and remain on the posterior vertebral arch. Keep the arms relatively stiff, with elbows flexed and wrists in neutral.
- Perform a high velocity, low amplitude, obliquely oriented, rotatory thrust in the direction of the rotation restrictive barrier.
  - The thrust is made mostly with the performing hand along the plane of the zygapophyseal articular surfaces.
  - The assisting hand should remain firm in the side bending position but should rotate with the performing hand.
  - Optional: add respiratory cooperation.
- Return the patient to a neutral position and release tissue contacts.
- Retest the vertebra for improvements in position and passive range of motion.

Thoracic, T3–T12, Prone Patient Position

It is easy to transition to this technique after performing a soft tissue technique on the paraspinal muscles. Beginners often find this technique easier than other HVLA techniques because of the relatively straightforward positioning and the uniplanar direction of the thrust (**Fig. 12.3**).

Key Elements

- Somatic dysfunction corrected: T3–T12: NS_XR_Y FR_XS_X.
- End goal: to reposition a dysfunctional thoracic vertebra using a short, quick thrust directed from posterior to anterior.
- Note: this technique is not ideal for correcting extended somatic dysfunctions because the thrust forces create further extension. However, extended somatic dysfunctions are not an absolute contraindication, and we recommend using clinical reasoning and care.

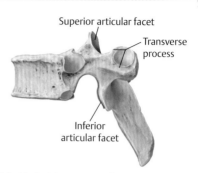

Fig. 12.3 Typical thoracic vertebra (T6).

Labels: Superior articular facet; Transverse process; Inferior articular facet

---

WATCH ▷ ► ▷

- ► **Video 12.4a Thoracic, Prone Patient Position, T9 FR_LS_L—Real Time**
- ► **Video 12.4b Thoracic, Prone Patient Position, T9 FR_LS_L—Narrated**

Example Somatic Dysfunction: T9 FR_LS_L

- ► **Video 12.5 Thoracic, Prone Patient Position, T9 NS_RR_L—Real Time**

Example Somatic Dysfunction: T9 N S_RR_L

Positioning and Preparation

▶ Patient: prone with arms either by the sides or hanging off the table.

▶ Physician: standing at the side of the table, at the level of the dysfunctional vertebra, on the side of the posterior transverse process (side of rotational component of the somatic dysfunction), and facing the patient's torso.

– Tissue contacts vary depending on the type of vertebral somatic dysfunction. Regardless, keep both arms internally rotated, the elbows bent, and the wrists extended to best perform the thrust.

Tissue Contact

- One hand creates the corrective or HVLA thrust. The other hand provides a counterforce.
- Neutral somatic dysfunction:
  – Performing hand: contact the posterior transverse process with the thenar eminence so that your fingers point toward the patient's head.
  – Assisting hand: contact the transverse process of the vertebra inferior to the dysfunctional one with the thenar eminence so that your fingers point toward the patient's feet (**Fig. 12.4**).
- Flexion (non-neutral) somatic dysfunction:
  – Performing hand: contact the posterior transverse process with the thenar eminence so that your fingers point toward the patient's feet.
  – Assisting hand: contact the transverse process of the vertebra superior to the dysfunctional one with the thenar eminence so that your fingers point toward the patient's head (**Fig. 12.5**).

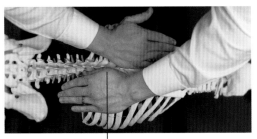

Left transverse process of T9

Fig. 12.4 Hand contact for thoracic high velocity, low amplitude, prone patient position, T9 NS_RR_L.

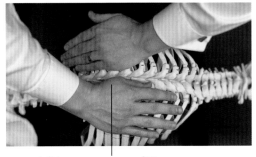

Left transverse process of T9

Fig. 12.5 Hand contact for thoracic high velocity, low amplitude, prone patient position T9 FR_LS_L.

Movements, Barriers, and Forces

Use both hands to do the following:

- Layer palpate to the transverse processes.
- Apply slight anterior pressure with both hypothenar eminences for firm contact.
- Move both hands in the directions your fingers are pointing to move the dysfunctional vertebra in the direction of the side bending restrictive barrier. Hold this force.
- With the performing hand, apply additional anteriorly directed force until the tissues tighten and no further movement is possible. Hold this force.
  - Do this by leaning forward with your body weight.
- Instruct the patient to take a few deep breaths, maintaining forces and hand positions. Move with the breath cycles, but move the vertebra further anteriorly (in the direction of the rotational barrier) during each exhalation effort.

- Perform an HVLA thrust from posterior to anterior (rotation) and in the direction of the side bending restrictive barrier (superior/inferior or inferior/superior) simultaneously near the end of the patient's second or third exhalation effort.
  - The thrust is directed along the plane of the zygapophyseal articular surfaces.
  - Do this by dropping your body weight.
- Release forces and tissue contacts.
- Retest the vertebra for changes in position and passive range of motion.

Note: Regarding alternate positioning and tissue contacts, the physician can stand on either side of the table; the hand positions can change so that the hypothenar eminence is used to thrust upon the posterior transverse process instead of the thenar eminence.

Thoracic, T3–T12, Supine Patient Position

This technique allows correction of thoracic spine somatic dysfunction quickly and effectively, with very little force after correct patient positioning. Despite the whole-body patient positioning and maneuvering, physician corrective forces should remain localized, precisely directed at the vertebral articular surfaces (**Fig. 12.6**).

Key Elements

- Somatic dysfunction corrected: T3–T12: NS_XR_Y, FR_XS_X, ER_XS_X.
- End goal: to reposition a dysfunctional thoracic vertebra using a short, quick thrust directed from anterior to posterior. The thrust is created from the physician's body and forces are through the patient's elbows and torso to reach the vertebra.

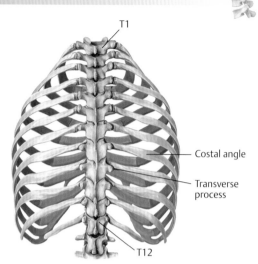

Fig. 12.6 Posterior thoracic cage.

WATCH ▷ ► ▷

► *Video 12.6a Thoracic, Supine Patient Position, T6 NS_RR_L—Real Time*

► *Video 12.6b Thoracic, Supine Patient Position, T6 NS_RR_L—Narrated*

Example Somatic Dysfunction: T6 NS_RR_L

► *Video 12.7 Thoracic, Supine Patient Position, T6 FS_RR_L—Real Time*

Example Somatic Dysfunction: T6 FR_LS_L

► *Video 12.8 Thoracic, Supine Patient Position, T6 ER_LS_L—Real Time*

Example Somatic Dysfunction: T6 ER_LS_L

Positioning and Preparation

▶ Patient: supine

▶ Physician: standing at the side of the table, a few inches inferior to the dysfunctional vertebra, on the side opposite that of the posterior transverse process (therefore, opposite the side of vertebral rotation), facing the patient, with the table lowered so that the patient's thorax is just below the physician's waist level.

▶ Additional patient positioning: cross the patient's arms over the torso, placing the arm on the side of the vertebral rotation anterior to (or on top of) the other arm. Position the elbows so they are midline, and rest the hands on the opposite arm or shoulder.

Tissue Contact

Three contacts are used: your abdomen, which performs the corrective thrust, and both hands.

- Assisting hand: use the hand that is closer to the patient's head. This hand controls and positions the patient's head, neck, and torso into the restrictive barriers.
- Fulcrum hand: use the other hand as a fulcrum for the HVLA thrust.
- Performing contact: use your abdomen to create the corrective thrust by dropping your weight upon your fulcrum hand.

Contact the dysfunctional vertebra (**Fig. 12.7**) as follows:

- Assisting hand: roll the patient's torso toward you by lifting the patient's shoulder on the side opposite from which you are standing, so that you can position your fulcrum hand.

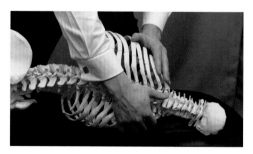

Fig. 12.7 Fulcrum hand contact, thoracic high velocity, low amplitude, supine patient position.

- Fulcrum hand: contact the posterior transverse process with the thenar eminence. Abduct the thumb and contact the musculature with a flat hand to create a firmer fulcrum.
- Assisting hand: place the patient's stacked elbows in your epigastric region or abdomen. Do not place the patient's elbows on your sternum or ribs or you risk fracturing them.
- Roll the patient so the torso is completely flat on the table and on top of your fulcrum hand.

Movements, Barriers, and Forces

- With your assisting hand and arm, flex the patient's torso at the level of the dysfunctional vertebra, shifting hand contact to cradle the head and neck.
  - Flexion helps localize and limit forces to the dysfunctional vertebra. Perform this regardless of the somatic dysfunction sagittal plane position.
- Create a posteriorly directed force from your abdomen, through the patient's elbows and onto your fulcrum hand, until the tissues under your fulcrum hand tighten. Hold this force.

- Side bend the patient's head and torso in the direction of the side bending restrictive barrier until the tissues tighten further.
- Instruct the patient to take a few deep breaths. Create additional force, from anterior to posterior, coordinated with the patient's exhalation as necessary to ensure that the tissues remain tight.
- Near the end of the patient's second or third exhalation effort, perform an HVLA thrust directed posteriorly from your abdomen, through the patient's arms, and onto your fulcrum hand. Use your body weight to generate the thrust force.
  - The thrust is along the plane of the inferior articular surface of the affected vertebra.
  - For somatic dysfunctions with an extension component, direct the thrust posteriorly and superiorly at a 45 degree angle toward the patient's head.
- Return the patient to a neutral position.
- Release tissue contact.
- Retest the vertebra for changes in position and passive range of motion.

Costal, Ribs 2–10

This technique is expedient when thoracic vertebral and rib dysfunctions are found at the same level, since it is a slight modification from thoracic HVLA, supine patient position (**Fig. 12.8**). Perform the thoracic HVLA technique first, then without moving any other contacts, reposition your fulcrum hand laterally onto the affected rib and proceed with the rest of the steps of the costal HVLA technique.

Key Elements

- Somatic dysfunction corrected: ribs 2–10 inhalation, exhalation, or posterior somatic dysfunctions.
- End goal: to reposition a dysfunctional rib using a short, quick thrust.

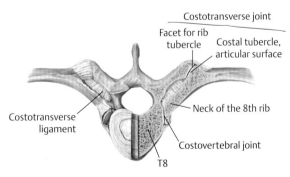

Costotransverse joint
Facet for rib tubercle
Costal tubercle, articular surface
Costotransverse ligament
Neck of the 8th rib
Costovertebral joint
T8

Fig. 12.8   Costovertebral joints.

Note: This technique is not ideal for correcting anterior rib somatic dysfunctions because the thrust forces create further anterior movement. However, anterior somatic dysfunctions are not an absolute contraindication, and we recommend using clinical reasoning and care.

WATCH ▷ ► ▷

► *Video 12.9a Costal, Ribs 2–10—Real Time*

► *Video 12.9b Costal, Ribs 2–10—Narrated*

Example Somatic Dysfunction: Left 4th Rib Posterior

Positioning and Preparation

▶ Patient: supine.

▶ Physician: standing a few inches inferior to the level of the dysfunctional rib, on the side opposite that of the vertebral rotation, facing the patient, with the table lowered so that the patient's thorax is just below the physician's waist level.

▶ Additional patient positioning: cross the patient's arms over the torso, placing the arm on the side of the dysfunctional rib anterior to (or on top of) the other arm. Position the elbows so they are midline, and rest the hands on the opposite arm or shoulder.

Tissue Contact

Three contacts are used: your abdomen, which performs the corrective thrust, and both hands.

- Assisting hand: use the hand that is closer to the patient's head. This hand controls and positions the patient's head, neck, and torso into the restrictive barriers.
- Fulcrum hand: use the other hand as a fulcrum for the HVLA thrust.
- Performing contact: use your abdomen to create the corrective thrust by dropping your weight upon your fulcrum hand.

Contact the dysfunctional rib as follows:

- Assisting hand: roll the patient's torso toward you by lifting the patient's shoulder on the side opposite that on which you are standing, so that you can position your fulcrum hand.
- Fulcrum hand: contact the rib angle with the thenar eminence. Abduct the thumb and contact the musculature with a flat hand to create a firmer fulcrum.
- Assisting hand: place the patient's stacked elbows in your epigastric region or abdomen. To avoid pain or injury, do not place the patient's elbows on your sternum or ribs.
- Roll the patient so the torso is completely flat on the table and on top of your fulcrum hand.

Movements, Barriers, and Forces

- With your assisting hand and arm, flex the patient's head and torso from superior to inferior to the dysfunctional vertebra. Cradle the head and neck. Ask the patient to remain relaxed.
  - Flexion localizes and limits forces to the dysfunctional rib.
- Create a posteriorly directed force from your abdomen, through the patient's elbows, and onto your fulcrum hand until the tissues under your fulcrum hand tighten. Hold this force.
- Side bend the patient's head and torso away from the dysfunctional rib (or toward you).
  - This creates a small gap.
- Instruct the patient to take a few deep breaths. Create additional force from anterior to posterior as necessary to ensure that the tissues remain tight.
- Near the end of the patient's second or third exhalation effort, perform an HVLA thrust directed posteriorly from your abdomen, through the patient's arms, and onto your fulcrum hand. Use your body weight to generate the thrust force.
  - The thrust is along the plane of the costovertebral and costotransverse articulations.
- Return the patient to a neutral position.
- Release tissue contact.
- Retest the rib for changes in position and passive range of motion.

Lumbar

Often called the lumbar roll, this technique is one of the few HVLA techniques in this manual that relies on using two long levers as the patient's body is essentially twisted around the dysfunctional vertebra (**Fig. 12.9**).

Key Elements

- Somatic dysfunction corrected: L1–L5 NS_XR_Y, FR_XS_X or ER_XS_X.
- End goal: to reposition a dysfunctional lumbar vertebra using a short, quick rotatory thrust.

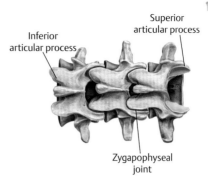

Fig. 12.9   Lumbar zygapophyseal (intervertebral facet) joints.

> **WATCH** ▷ ► ▷
>
> ► *Video 12.10a Lumbar L3 N S_RR_L—Real Time*
> ► *Video 12.10b Lumbar L3 N S_RR_L—Narrated*
> *Example Somatic Dysfunction: L3 NSLRR*
> ► *Video 12.11 Lumbar L3 F R_LS_L—Real Time*
> *Example Somatic Dysfunction: L3 FR_LS_L*

Positioning and Preparation

▶ Patient: laterally recumbent, lying so that the posterior transverse process is "up," or off the table.

▶ Physician: standing in front of the patient at the level of the dysfunctional vertebra.

Tissue Contacts, Movements, Barriers, and Forces

The physician's forearms and torso create the corrective HVLA rotatory thrust force.

Note: Because this technique requires multiple patient positions and contacts, tissue contacts are integrated with movements, barriers, and forces in the steps of the technique.

- Initial monitoring hand: contact the posterior transverse process of the dysfunctional vertebra with the hand that is closer to the patient's head.
- Ask the patient to bend both knees.
- With your free hand, flex the patient's hips and trunk until the dysfunctional vertebra moves.

  – Stop here for neutral somatic dysfunctions. Continue to (a) or (b) for non-neutral somatic dysfunctions.
    (a) Extension somatic dysfunction: continue flexing the patient's hips and trunk until a restrictive barrier is felt.
    (b) Flexion somatic dysfunction: push the patient's knees posteriorly toward the extension barrier.
- Ask the patient to straighten the leg that is on the table. Hook the patient's other foot behind the popliteal fossa of the straightened leg.
- Final monitoring contact: switch monitoring hands and keep this contact throughout the technique.
- Performing hand: rotate the patient's torso until the dysfunctional vertebra is positioned at the restrictive barrier.
  – Do this by asking the patient to grasp your forearm with the arm that is on the table, then grasp the patient's forearm and pull the arm anteriorly to rotate the torso. Do not let go yet.
  – Note that the patient's torso should be rotated to the vertebral level that is superior to the dysfunctional one, to rotate the dysfunctional vertebra in the direction of the restrictive barrier.
- Side bend the patient at the side bending restrictive barrier, using the patient's arm to move the torso.
  – Pulling the arm superiorly creates a curve in the body with the apex of a concave curve (side bending) closer to the table.

Pulling the arm inferiorly creates a convex curvature.

- Place the patient's hand on the waist with a bent elbow. Relax the patient's other arm over her body as well.
- Thread the performing hand just beneath the patient's axilla from anterior to posterior. Rest your arm or forearm on the patient's upper, lateral chest wall just medial to the humeral head. If possible, additionally monitor the dysfunctional vertebra with the fingertips.
- With the forearm that is closer to the patient's pelvis (final monitoring contact), contact the posterior iliac crest that is off the table. Rotate the patient's pelvis until the tissues tighten and no further rotation is possible.

- The patient may be quite rotated at this point. Prevent the patient from falling off the table by bracing the patient's knee or leg against your thigh.
- Perform a rotatory HVLA thrust with both forearms, twisting the patient's body with the dysfunctional vertebra in the middle of the twist.
  - The thrust is along the plane of the inferior vertebral articulations (zygapophyseal joints).
- Release tissue contact and assist the patient with repositioning to a stable position.
- Retest the vertebra for improvements in position and passive range of motion.

Note: Regarding alternate positioning, an acceptable variation is to perform the technique with the posterior transverse process "down" or on the table. In the variation, thrust forces are directed in side bending.

Lower Extremity, Talocrural Joint

This technique is useful after the acute phase of healing of a minor ankle sprain, especially when range of motion is limited (**Fig. 12.10**).

Key Elements

- Somatic dysfunction corrected: talus anterior, talus in plantar flexion, talocrural joint restricted in dorsiflexion.
- End goal: to reposition a dysfunctional talus at the tibiofemoral articulation using a short, quick thrust.

> **WATCH ▷ ▶ ▷**
>
> ▶ *Video 12.12a Lower Extremity, Talocrural Joint—Real Time*
>
> ▶ *Video 12.12b Lower Extremity, Talocrural Joint—Narrated*
>
> ***Example Somatic Dysfunction: Left Talus Anterior***

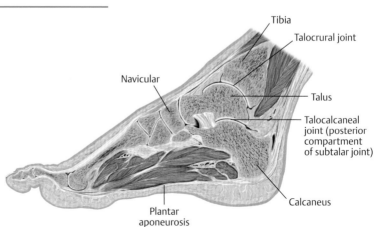

Fig. 12.10 Talocrural joint.

Tibia
Talocrural joint
Navicular
Talus
Talocalcaneal joint (posterior compartment of subtalar joint)
Calcaneus
Plantar aponeurosis

Positioning and Preparation

▶ Patient: supine.

▶ Physician: standing at the end of the table facing the patient's feet, with the table raised ~ 4 to 6 inches from the customary height.

Tissue Contact

Both hands create the corrective thrust force.

- Monitoring and performing hands: with the fourth or fifth metacarpophalangeal joints of both hands, contact the talus near the articulation with the tibia to monitor motion of the tibia. Wrap the remaining fingers and hand around the dorsum of the foot. Wrap the thumbs around the plantar surface of the foot and grasp the foot firmly.

Movements, Barriers, and Forces

Use both hands to do the following:

- Lift the patient's foot and extend the leg so it is off the table ~ 6 to 12 inches.
- Add an inferiorly directed traction force at the talocrural joint to create space for repositioning the talus. Hold this force.
- Dorsiflex the talus into the restrictive barrier.
- Perform an HVLA thrust in dorsiflexion.
- The thrust is along the plane of the curved talocrural articular surfaces.
- Return the foot to a neutral position and release tissue contact.
- Retest the talus for changes in position and passive range of motion.

Chapter Summary

This chapter details the osteopathic HVLA technique, with emphasis on precisely moving patients into a position so that only a minimal thrust force is necessary to restore joint alignment. Mastery of this technique requires careful anatomical study of articular surfaces and visualization and observation of the step-by-step technique performance. When performed properly, the HVLA technique is safe, quick, and beneficial for the patient.

Clinical Cases and Review Questions

Case 1

A 48-year-old man presents to the office with 6 months of neck stiffness. He has pain only with excessive rotation of his neck. He denies trauma or radiation of pain into his arms. Neurological and muscle strength physical examinations are within normal limits. Active range of motion is decreased in right rotation and right side bending. Passive range of motion testing of the C4 vertebra reveals restricted movements in extension, right rotation, and right side bending.

Q1. You chose to perform a high velocity, low amplitude technique on this patient's somatic dysfunction to
  A. Decrease gamma signaling to the intrafusal muscle fibers.
  B. Increase tension on the Golgi tendon organs.
  C. Release the restrictions through indirect positioning of the joint.
  D. Increase motion of the cervical facet joints.
  E. Resolve tissue texture changes, specifically hypertonicity and tenderness.

Q2. When performing a high velocity, low amplitude technique on this patient, which of the following is the appropriate tissue contact?
  A. Contact the left vertebral arch of C4 with your left second digit.
  B. Contact the right vertebral arch of C4 with your right third digit.
  C. Contact the left transverse process of C4 with your left heel of the hand.
  D. Contact the right transverse process of C4 with your left fifth digit.
  E. Contact the spinous process of C4 with your right heel of the hand.

Q3. Which of the following additional history or physical exam findings, if present, would preclude the performance of a high velocity, low amplitude technique in this patient?

A. History of a whiplash injury to the neck 5 years ago.

B. History of rheumatoid arthritis.

C. 2/4 reflexes at the biceps, triceps, and brachioradialis.

D. The presence of multiple anterior and posterior tender points in the cervical spine.

E. Neck pain when reaching the end range of passive motion.

Case 2

A 31-year-old woman presents to the office with generalized low back pain. She works as a cashier, and the pain worsens when she stands for more than 1 hour. She denies paresthesias, radiation of pain, weakness, and loss of bowel or bladder control. The exam is positive for lumbar paravertebral muscle hypertonicity. The right transverse process of L3 is posterior compared with the left, and during lumbar extension, the transverse processes become symmetrical.

Q4. You perform a lumbar high velocity, low amplitude technique on this patient and ask the patient to lie on her right side and position her appropriately. In which directions do you perform the corrective thrust?

A. Extension.

B. Flexion.

C. Left rotation and left side bending.

D. Left rotation only.

E. Left side bending only.

F. Right rotation and right side bending.

Q5. Which of the following is true about high velocity, low amplitude techniques?

A. Correction of somatic dysfunction occurs when the anatomical barrier is thrusted against.

B. High velocity, low amplitude techniques are appropriate to perform in a joint that is not fully formed.

C. High velocity, low amplitude techniques require active patient participation for correction of somatic dysfunction.

D. The corrective thrust should be performed quickly over a short distance.

E. The patient should be positioned in all directions of motion ease.

Answers to Review Questions

Q1. The correct answer is **D**: Increase motion of the cervical facet joints.

A is incorrect. Counterstrain and muscle energy work on the level of the intrafusal muscle fibers (i.e., muscle spindles).

B is incorrect. HVLA is directed at an articulation.

C is incorrect. HVLA is performed into the restrictive barrier in one or more planes.

E is incorrect. Resolve tissue texture changes is not the primary goal of HVLA. This would better describe soft tissue, counterstrain, or myofascial release.

Q2. The correct answer is **A**. The diagnosis is C4 flexed, rotated left, side bent left. The correct tissue contact for cervical HVLA is to contact the vertebral arch of the affected vertebra on the side of rotation (left) with the ipsilateral hand (left).

Q3. The correct answer is **B**: History of rheumatoid arthritis. Rheumatoid arthritis is a contraindication due to possible laxity of the ligaments surrounding the dens.

A is incorrect. History of a whiplash injury to the neck 5 years ago is not a contraindication by itself.

C is incorrect. 2/4 reflexes at the biceps, triceps, and brachioradialis are normal findings and are therefore not contraindications.

D is incorrect. The presence of multiple anterior and posterior tender points in the cervical spine are indications for HVLA.

E is incorrect. Neck pain when reaching the end range of passive motion is an indication for HVLA with muscular preparation.

Q4. The correct answer is **C**. The thrust is in both rotation and side bending, in the direction of the restrictive barriers, which are left rotation and left side bending.

Q5. The correct answer is **D**: The corrective thrust should be performed quickly over a short distance.

A is incorrect. The restrictive barrier is thrusted against, not the anatomical barrier.

B is incorrect. This is a contraindication/precaution.

C is incorrect. HVLA is a passive technique that requires the patient to remain relaxed.

E is incorrect. The patient should be positioned in at least one direction of motion restriction.

References

1. Todd AJ, Carroll MT, Robinson A, Mitchell EK. Adverse events due to chiropractic and other manual therapies for infants and children: a review of the literature. J Manipulative Physiol Ther 2015;38(9):699–712
2. American Academy of Osteopathy. AOA Position Papers List. Accessed May 28, 2016
3. Protopapas MG, Cymet TC. Joint cracking and popping: understanding noises that accompany articular release. J Am Osteopath Assoc 2002;102(5):283–287

Research Bibliography

Boesler D, Warner M, Alpers A, Finnerty EP, Kilmore MA. Efficacy of high-velocity low-amplitude manipulative technique in subjects with low-back pain during menstrual cramping. J Am Osteopath Assoc 1993;93(2):203–208, 213–214

Boesler D, Warner M, Alpers A, Finnerty EP, Kilmore MA. Efficacy of high-velocity low-amplitude manipulative technique in subjects with low-back pain during menstrual cramping. J Am Osteopath Assoc 1993;93(2):203–208, 213–214

Dunning JR, Cleland JA, Waldrop MA, et al. Upper cervical and upper thoracic thrust manipulation versus nonthrust mobilization in patients with mechanical neck pain: a multicenter randomized clinical trial. J Orthop Sports Phys Ther 2012;42(1):5–18

Dunning J, Mourad F, Giovannico G, Maselli F, Perreault T, Fernández-de-Las-Peñas C. Changes in shoulder pain and disability after thrust manipulation in subjects presenting with second and third rib syndrome. J Manipulative Physiol Ther 2015;38(6):382–394

Goertz CM, Pohlman KA, Vining RD, Brantingham JW, Long CR. Patient-centered outcomes of high-velocity, low-amplitude spinal manipulation for low back pain: a systematic review. J Electromyogr Kinesiol 2012;22(5):670–691

Griswold D, Learman K, O'Halloran B, Cleland J. A preliminary study comparing the use of cervical/upper thoracic mobilization and manipulation for individuals with mechanical neck pain. J Manual Manip Ther 2015;23(2):75–83

Guevarra CC, Seffinger MA. High-velocity thrust to the atlantoaxial joint does not increase mechanical stress on the vertebral artery. J Am Osteopath Assoc 2015;115(5):343 doi: 10.7556/jaoa.2015.067

Hamilton L, Boswell C, Fryer G. The effects of high-velocity, low-amplitude manipulation and muscle energy technique on suboccipital tenderness. Int J Osteopath Med 2007;10(2):42–49

Martínez-Segura R, Fernández-de-las-Peñas C, Ruiz-Sáez M, López-Jiménez C, Rodríguez-Blanco C. Immediate effects on neck pain and active range of motion after a single cervical high-velocity low-amplitude manipulation in subjects presenting with mechanical neck pain: a randomized controlled trial. J Manipulative Physiol Ther 2006;29(7):511–517

McReynolds TM, Sheridan BJ. Intramuscular ketorolac versus osteopathic manipulative treatment in the management of acute neck pain in the emergency department: a randomized clinical trial. J Am Osteopath Assoc 2005;105(2):57–68

Vieira-Pellenz F, Oliva-Pascual-Vaca A, Rodriguez-Blanco C, Heredia-Rizo AM, Ricard F, Almazán-Campos G. Short-term effect of spinal manipulation on pain perception, spinal mobility, and full height recovery in male subjects with degenerative disk disease: a randomized controlled trial. Arch Phys Med Rehabil 2014;95(9):1613–1619

Young JL, Walker D, Snyder S, Daly K. Thoracic manipulation versus mobilization in patients with mechanical neck pain: a systematic review. J Manual Manip Ther 2014;22(3):141–153

13. Osteopathic Cranial Manipulative Medicine Techniques

LEARNING OBJECTIVES

1. Explain the goals of performing osteopathic cranial manipulative medicine (OCMM) techniques.
2. Identify the clinical considerations, including indications, contraindications, and precautions for performing OCMM techniques.
3. Recall the unique physiological motions of the cranium.
4. Diagnose cranial and sacral somatic dysfunctions related to inherent cranial motion.
5. Compare and contrast the different OCMM techniques.
6. Outline the general movements, barriers, and forces used to perform OCMM techniques.
7. Identify the end goal for performing each OCMM technique.
8. Visualize, verbalize, and identify the preparation, positioning, tissue contact, movements, barriers, and forces for each OCMM technique.
9. Perform cranial techniques using appropriate somatic dysfunction diagnosis, preparation, positioning, tissue contact, movements, barriers, forces, retest for effectiveness, communication, and safe tissue handling.

Osteopathic Cranial Manipulative Medicine Techniques Introduction

Osteopathic cranial manipulative medicine (OCMM) techniques include those that are specifically applied to the cranial bones, sacrum, and dura mater as first described by William Garner Sutherland, DO. OCMM techniques are performed with respect to the inherent motion of the cranium, which is also described as the physiological, oscillatory cranial motion. The cranium's spherical shape, the intricate nature of the articulations, the delicate nature of the central nervous system, and the circulation of cerebrospinal fluid all compound the complexity of OCMM. It is clear to see the necessity of a strong working knowledge of cranial anatomy, coupled with a well-developed palpatory sensitivity on the part of the physician. This manual offers some clinically useful, yet simple, techniques for beginners to practice.

OCMM techniques assist patients in recovery from disease and injuries in ways that medications and other therapies cannot. OCMM techniques can be used throughout a patient's lifetime, relieving the cranial compression that occurs during birth as well as the effects of subsequent head trauma.

OCMM techniques can achieve the following:

- Improve arterial, venous, lymphatic, and cerebral spinal fluid circulation in the cranium.
- Resolve biomechanical strains in the cranial sutures and dura mater.
- Improve neurological functioning of the central and peripheral nervous systems.

Background

William Garner Sutherland, DO, student of Dr. Andrew Taylor Still, developed the osteopathic cranial concept and shared it in 1939 with the publication *The Cranial Bowl*.[1] Through his studies, Dr. Sutherland identified five phenomena that are found in the cranium and collectively named them the Primary Respiratory Mechanism (PRM). Together, these components provide a contextual framework for understanding the functional anatomy and physiology of the cranium. Much more can be said about Dr. Sutherland's original work, and references for further study are provided at the end of this chapter.

The five components of the PRM[2] are as follows:

- Inherent motility of the brain and spinal cord.
- Fluctuation of the cerebrospinal fluid.
- Mobility of intracranial and intraspinal membranes.

- Articular mobility of the cranial bones.
- Involuntary mobility of the sacrum between the ilia.

Research

There is robust evidence that supports the five components of the PRM. The most comprehensive list can be found on the Cranial Academy website.[3]

Clinical Considerations

Some common clinical applications of OCMM are listed in Table 13.1. Always acquire adequate data in the form of an appropriate history, a thorough physical exam to include cranial nerves, and relevant diagnostic tests to exercise best clinical judgment before performing osteopathic manipulative treatment.

Somatic Dysfunction Corrected

Students should become familiar with basic cranial mechanics and terminology before proceeding to examining the cranium for somatic dysfunction. This manual presents only the steps required to perform the exam. For reference, however, Table 13.2 presents a summary of the physiological cranial movements.

Table 13.1 Clinical considerations		
Indications	**Contraindications**	**Precautions**
Headaches	Recent trauma with significant or serious injury to the brain, blood vessels, cranium, or other related structures	Congenital cranial bone or brain malformations
Cranial nerve entrapment syndromes		Brain or other intracranial tumor
Minor head trauma, including postconcussion	Severe infections, such as meningitis or encephalitis	Shunt, coil, or other intracranial implanted device
Infectious diseases: sinusitis, otitis media, upper respiratory tract infection, labyrinthitis	Elevated intracranial pressure	Use cautiously in patients with orthodontic appliances. Note that orthodontics can restrict cranial motion, rendering cranial techniques less effective. Also, orthodontic appliances may not fit properly after cranial techniques are performed.
Dental-related disorders: trauma after dental work, malocclusions	Cerebral edema	
Temporomandibular joint disorder	Recent shunt surgery or neurosurgery	
Vertigo	Epidural or subdural hematoma	
Tinnitus	Recent hemorrhagic stroke	
Ocular dysfunctions, such as strabismus		
Infants with plagiocephaly, torticollis, colic, latching or nursing difficulties, history of difficult delivery		

Motions	Cranial inhalation	Cranial exhalation
Table 13.2 Inherent cranial motion: cranial rhythmic impulse phases		
Cranial vault	Lengthening of transverse diameter, shortening of anterior-posterior diameter	Shortening of transverse diameter, lengthening of anterior-posterior diameter
Sphenobasilar synchondrosis	Elevates	Descends
Midline cranial bones	Cranial flexion	Cranial extension
Paired cranial bones	External rotation	Internal rotation
Sacrum	Counternutation	Nutation

The term *cranial somatic dysfunction* is used to differentiate those somatic dysfunctions in the head that are correctable with OCMM techniques. Cranial somatic dysfunctions can be classified as follows:

- Cranial strain patterns.
- Cranial bone sutural (articular) restrictions.
- Dural strain.
- Sacral somatic dysfunction related to inherent cranial motion.

Cranial Strain Patterns

The entire cranium, because of articulations, dural connections, and its spherical shape, can become dysfunctional. Cranial strain patterns are referenced by the position of the sphenoid in relationship to the occiput at the sphenobasilar synchondrosis (SBS). Because the SBS is deeply situated in the cranium, the position of the SBS can be inferred by palpating the greater wings of the sphenoid and the lateral angles of the occiput. Physiological cranial strain patterns are: flexion/extension, R/L torsion, and side bending rotation. Nonphysiological cranial strain patterns are R/L lateral strain, superior/inferior vertical strain, and SBS compression.

Cranial Bone Sutural (Articular) Restrictions

Sometimes one bone of the cranium becomes dysfunctional at a suture, and the position of the SBS is not affected in such a way that a strain pattern is produced. Cranial sutures with somatic dysfunction are often named as a sutural restriction, implying that both bones of the suture are asymmetric in position and/or exhibit motion restrictions. An example is bilateral occipitomastoid suture restriction.

Dural Strain

The dura mater spans the cranium and spinal canal and is a specialized type of connective tissue. Because it is a continuous structure with numerous attachments in the cranium and one at the sacrum, it has been called a reciprocal tension membrane. Changes in tension can be appreciated with layer palpation, and the dura itself can become the focus for correction when performing OCMM techniques. Dural connectivity also dictates that an injury to the sacrum affects inherent cranial motion, and an injury to the head affects the inherent motion of the sacrum.

Sacral Somatic Dysfunction Related to Inherent Cranial Motion

Sacral motion is coordinated with the inherent motion of the cranium. The sacrum also articulates with and moves at the sacroiliac and lumbosacral joints. For this reason, it can be challenging to distinguish sacral somatic dysfunction related to inherent cranial motion versus that related to articular biomechanics. Sacral somatic dysfunctions related to inherent cranial motion are named by the position of the sacrum, flexion (counternutation) or extension (nutation), or the cranial strain pattern. Guided practice with experts who perform OCMM is recommended to distinguish inherent cranial motion of the sacrum from other sacral somatic dysfunctions.

Exam for Cranial Somatic Dysfunction

This exam is classically performed by palpation of the cranium using a vault or fronto-occipital contact. The cranium is assessed for symmetry and inherent motion. Range of motion testing for cranial strain patterns may be performed but has been omitted from this exam because it is an intermediate skill that requires close faculty observation and guidance.

Positioning and Preparation

▶ Patient: supine.
▶ Physician: sitting at the head of the table with forearms resting on the table.

Tissue Contact–Vault Contact

Use the right hand to contact the right side of the patient's head and the left hand to contact the left side (**Fig. 13.1**).

- Contact the greater wings of the sphenoid with the pads of the second fingers.
- Contact the squamous portion of the temporal bone with pads of the third fingers.
- Contact the mastoid portion (not process) of the temporal bone with the pads of the fourth fingers.
- Contact the lateral angles of the occiput with the pads of the fifth fingers.
- Allow the fingers to wrap to the contour of the cranium. Do not leave space between your hands and the cranium.

Palpation for Asymmetry and Inherent Motion

- Allow the forearms to rest on the edge of the table. Release all pressure in the fingers and keep them relaxed, so they can be pushed by the inherent motion of the cranial bones.
- Gently layer palpate to the external periosteum.

- First observe the position of the finger contacts for symmetry. Positional asymmetry is a clue of underlying cranial somatic dysfunction.
- With fingertips relaxed, allow the inherent cranial motion to push against your fingers. When palpated, follow this motion with your fingers. Do not guide the bones.
- Observe cycles of flexion and extension, noting the rate and amplitude.
  - Note that in cases of SBS compression, no motion is palpable, or the motion is discordant.
- Gently layer palpate to the dural layer, then centrally to the SBS. Identify whether or not a strain pattern may be present.
  - Passive range of motion testing can be performed by moving the hands very slightly so as to "spring" the cranium into the directions of each strain pattern at the beginning of a flexion cycle, noting motion ease and motion restriction. Do not hold the hands in this position.
- Observe the cranial rhythmic impulse for a few cycles.
- Release the hand contacts at the beginning of a flexion cycle.

Fronto-Occipital Contact

An alternate hold is the fronto-occipital hold (**Fig. 13.2**). It can be used to diagnose SBS strain patterns, but it is particularly useful when attempting techniques to correct vertical and lateral strains.

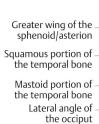
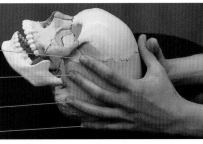

Greater wing of the sphenoid/asterion
Squamous portion of the temporal bone
Mastoid portion of the temporal bone
Lateral angle of the occiput

Fig. 13.1 Vault contact.

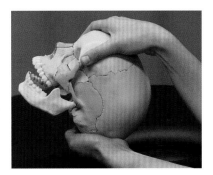

Fig. 13.2 Fronto-occipital contact.

Movements, Barriers, and Forces: Cranial Techniques

Balanced membranous techniques (BMTs) are a mainstay approach for performing OCMM (**Fig. 13.3**). BMT is the point of balanced membranous tension that is created when the cranial bones and membranes (dura) are positioned such that the body's inherent healing forces correct the somatic dysfunction. The tensions in the tissues are balanced around a fulcrum. There are four methods by which the point of balanced membranous tension can be reached: indirect, direct, disengagement, and opposing physiological motion.

- Indirect: a bone at a suture or a joint is moved toward the physiological barrier (the indirect method of BMT is very similar to indirect technique).
- Direct: a bone at a suture or a joint is moved toward the restrictive barrier.
- Disengagement: a suture is disengaged with compression or traction.
- Opposing physiological motion: one bone at a suture or joint is moved toward the restrictive barrier while the other bone is moved toward the physiological barrier.

Molding is another type of cranial technique that specifically addresses intraosseous strain, either on the immature bones of newborns or after a head injury. It is a way to "mold" or reshape cranial bones themselves, not correct sutural or dural restrictions.

Fluid techniques are yet another category of cranial techniques. These techniques most directly affect and use the fluid mechanics of the cerebrospinal fluid and are performed in the compression of the fourth ventricle (CV-4) technique.

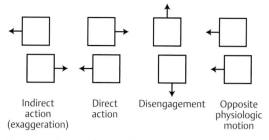

Indirect action (exaggeration) Direct action Disengagement Opposite physiologic motion

Fig. 13.3 Osteopathic cranial manipulative medicine technique principles.

Positioning and Preparation

▶ Patient: supine.
▶ Physician: sitting in an ergonomic, upright posture at all times.

Tissue Contact

Both hands are almost always used to perform cranial techniques. Tissue contact should be light enough to palpate motion but firm enough to actually guide the cranial bones and underlying dura.

Retest for Effectiveness

After performing an OCMM technique, the entire cranium should be assessed for changes in inherent motion and symmetry. Patients should be asked to remain still on the table for a few moments, then to rise slowly. Commonly, patients report feelings of relaxation and general well-being after OCMM techniques are performed. Some other common responses include lightheadedness and subtle changes in vision, energy levels, cognition, or emotional state. These responses are generally positive and related to shifts in bony positions and thereby function (e.g., shifts in the orbital bones affect vision), and improvements in vascular and cerebrospinal fluid circulation. Ask patients about symptoms of vertigo or dizziness, and, if present, the patient's cranium should be reassessed.

Head, Occipitoatlantal Joint Decompression

Method: Direct

Different from other techniques for the occipitoatlantal (OA) joint, this technique is focused on the inherent flexion and extension motions of the occiput and cranial dural attachments along with passive range of motion restrictions (**Fig. 13.4**). This technique is especially useful in newborns. It may also be incorporated as an additional step in the OCMM: venous sinus drainage technique.

Key Elements

- Somatic dysfunction corrected: any OA joint somatic dysfunction, including restriction of condylar passive range of motion.
- End goal: to restore normal occipital condylar position and inherent cranial motion of the occipital bone.

> **WATCH ▷ ▶ ▷**
>
> ▶ *Video 13.1 OA Joint Decompression—Narrated*
>
> *Example Somatic Dysfunction: Bilateral decreased condylar passive range of motion*

Positioning and Preparation

- ▶ Patient: supine.
- ▶ Physician: sitting at the head of the table with forearms resting on the table.

Tissue Contact

Both hands perform the technique.

- Performing hands: contact the occiput near the condyles with the pads of the second and/or third fingers. The fingers should point in the plane of the condyles. Allow the patient's head to rest on your hands.

Movements, Barriers, and Forces

Use both hands to do the following:

- Palpate and observe for inherent cranial motion.
- Apply gentle posterior and superior traction forces, guiding the condyles along the articular surfaces until the tissue tightens at the restrictive barriers.
  - Do this by approximating the wrists and pulling the arms posteriorly. Use your forearms for leverage by keeping your wrists relatively stiff and leaning your body weight forward onto your arms.
- Hold these forces.
- When release is palpated, or after ~ 2 minutes, release forces but not tissue contacts.
- Retest the OA joint for changes in position and passive range of motion.
- Retest the cranium for changes in inherent motion.

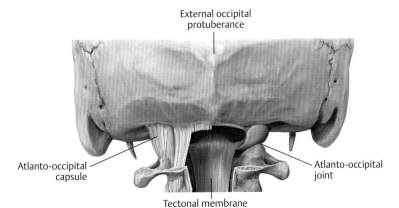

Fig. 13.4   Occipitoatlantal joint.

External occipital protuberance

Atlanto-occipital capsule

Atlanto-occipital joint

Tectonal membrane

Lumbar/Sacrum: Lumbosacral Joint Decompression

Method: Indirect

In this technique, the lumbosacral joint is "decompressed," or disengaged, to better access and correct both L5 and sacral somatic dysfunction (**Fig. 13.5**). Recall that the spinal dura is continuous with the cranial dura. In cases where cranial somatic dysfunction is not resolving adequately, consider assessing and correcting the sacrum with this technique, then return to the cranium. This technique is also commonly used in two-person osteopathic manipulative treatment, where one physician contacts the cranium and the other the sacrum. This is a powerful approach, especially for treatment of whole-body trauma, whereby two physicians can correct cranial and sacral somatic dysfunctions concurrently.

Key Elements

- Somatic dysfunction corrected: sacral nutation/counternutation, sacral somatic dysfunction related to dural strain, any somatic dysfunction of L5.
- End goal: to restore cranial motion and mechanics of the sacrum.

WATCH ▷ ▶ ▷

▶ *Video 13.2 Lumbosacral Joint Decompression—Narrated*

Example Somatic Dysfunction: Sacral nutation somatic dysfunction

---

Positioning and Preparation

► Patient: supine, with knees bent and feet on the table.

► Physician: sitting at the side of the table at the level of the patient's pelvis, facing the patient's head.

Tissue Contact

- Both hands disengage and position L5 and the sacrum at the lumbosacral joint. Use the hand nearer the patient to contact the sacrum and the other hand to contact L5.
- Sacral contact: with the pads of the second, third, and fourth fingers, contact the sacral base. Allow the palm of your hand to contact the rest of the sacrum, with the inferior lateral angles of the sacrum near or on the palm of your hand. Avoid putting pressure directly on the sensitive coccyx.
  - Detailed suggestion: ask the patient to lift the hips off the table. Locate the posterior superior iliac spine nearer you and place the pad of your fourth digit medial to it and your second digit medial to the other posterior superior iliac spine. Ask the patient to return the hips onto the table and onto your hand.
  - Be sure the patient allows her weight to rest on your hand.
- L5 contact: contact the spinous process with the pad of the second and/or third fingers.

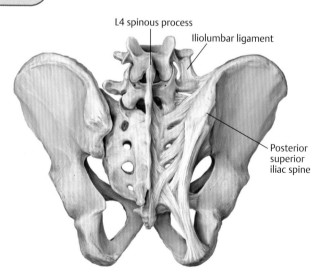

L4 spinous process

Iliolumbar ligament

Posterior superior iliac spine

Fig. 13.5 Lumbosacral joint.

Movements, Barriers, and Forces

- With the sacral contact, layer palpate to the dural layer. Observe for motion associated with thoracoabdominal breathing and for inherent cranial motion.
- With both hands, apply anteriorly directed forces to disengage the lumbosacral joint.
- With the L5 contact, move L5 in the directions of somatic dysfunction, or in the directions that loosen the tissues.

- With the sacral contact, move the sacral base in the directions of somatic dysfunction until the tissues loosen further.
- Hold positions until release occurs, or for up to 2 minutes.
- Release forces.
- Retest L5 and the sacrum for changes in position and inherent cranial motion.

Head, Sphenobasilar Synchondrosis

Method: Indirect

Use this technique to address cranial strains at the SBS. Unlike other indirect techniques, the use of disengagement forces is omitted to avoid excessive compression or distraction forces at the SBS.

Key Elements

- Somatic dysfunction corrected: SBS: R/L torsion, side bending rotation, lateral strain, and inferior/superior vertical strain.
- End goal: to restore normal position and inherent cranial motion at the sphenobasilar synchondrosis (SBS).

Note: This technique does not have an accompanying video because the hand contact is the familiar vault hold, and any motions made would be an exaggeration of the actual technique.

Positioning and Preparation

▶ Patient: supine.
▶ Physician: sitting at the head of the table.

Tissue Contact

- Both hands perform the technique.
- Performing hands: contact the cranium using the vault or fronto-occipital contact.

Movements, Barriers, and Forces

Use both hands to do the following:

- Palpate and observe the inherent motion of the cranium.
- Layer palpate (through the dura) to the SBS.
- Move the SBS by moving the greater wings of the sphenoid and the lateral angles of the occiput as levers in the directions of the cranial strain pattern/somatic dysfunction.
  - Note that the movements of the greater wings and lateral angles are not always in the same directions as the movement at the SBS.
- Hold positions until release occurs, or for up to 2 minutes.
  - Cranial inherent motion will continue. Avoid limiting or accentuating this motion.
- Release forces.
- Retest the cranium for changes in bone positions and inherent motion.

Head, Parietal Bone Disengagement

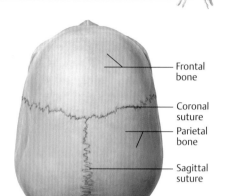

Method: Disengagement

Classically called the parietal lift, this technique is especially useful for treating newborns and infants, as well as patients suffering injuries to the top of the head (**Fig. 13.6**). Be sure to allow the parietal bones to return to neutral position after lifting.

Key Elements

- Somatic dysfunction corrected: internally or externally rotated parietal bone(s), and related sutural restrictions at the parieto-temporal, parieto-occipital, sphenoparietal, coronal, and sagittal sutures.
  - The parietal bones externally and internally rotate around an anterior to posterior axis such that, during external rotation, the lateral edges flare outward (laterally) while the medial edges move inward and downward slightly. During internal rotation, the medial edge raises and the lateral edges flare inward (medially).
- End goal: to disengage the parietal bones to release sutural and dural restrictions.

WATCH ▷ ▶ ▷

▶ *Video 13.3 Parietal Bones Disengagement—Narrated*

Example Somatic Dysfunction: Bilateral parietal bones internally rotated

---

Positioning and Preparation

▶ Patient: supine.

▶ Physician: sitting at the head of the table.

Tissue Contact

Use your right fingers to contact the right parietal bone and left to contact the left.

- Contact the anterior, inferior angles of each parietal bone with the second fingers and the parietomastoid angles with the fifth fingers. The third and fourth fingers are placed in between.
  - To be sure you are only contacting the parietal bones, palpate for the coronal, lambdoidal, and temporoparietal sutures.

Fig. 13.6 Parietal bones, superior view.

- Cross the thumbs and contact the opposite parietal bone lateral to the sagittal suture.

Movements, Barriers, and Forces

Movements are coordinated with the cranial rhythmic impulse (cranial flexion/external rotation and extension/internal rotation).

Use both hands to do the following:

- Palpate and observe the inherent motion of the parietal bones.
- During the extension/internal rotation phase, apply gentle medial force with the finger pads to disengage the parietal bone from the sphenoid and temporal bones.
  - This exaggerates the normal internal rotation of the parietal bones.
- Hold this position.
- Apply gentle superiorly directed forces to lift the parietal bones. Hold this force.
- During a flexion/external rotation phase, apply gentle pressure with the thumbs to exaggerate normal external rotation of the parietal bones.
- Hold these forces until release, or for up to 2 minutes.
- When tissue release is palpated, gently and slowly allow the parietal bones to return to normal position, guiding them back.
- Retest the cranium and parietal bones for position and inherent motion.

Head, Frontal Bone Disengagement

Method: Disengagement

Classically called the frontal "lift," this technique is especially useful for treating injuries to the forehead. It is also useful to help drain the sphenoidal and ethmoid sinuses in cases of sinusitis and seasonal allergies through normalizing tensions of the falx, which attaches at the crista galli. Be sure to allow the frontal bone to return back to neutral position after lifting (**Fig. 13.7**).

Key Elements

- Somatic dysfunction corrected: frontal bone internal or external rotation somatic dysfunction. Dural strain (falx cerebri) at the ethmoid notch.
  - The frontal bone develops as two bones that typically fuse at the metopic suture. Therefore, the frontal bone has motion similar to other paired bones. The frontal bone externally and internally rotates around two anterior to posterior axes such that, during external rotation, the lateral edges flare outward (laterally). During internal rotation, the lateral edges flare inward (medially).
- End goal: to reposition the frontal bone and restore normal dural tensions at the ethmoid notch.

> **WATCH ▷ ▶ ▷**
>
> ▶ **Video 13.4 Frontal Bones Disengagement—Narrated**
>
> **Example Somatic Dysfunction: Coronal suture restriction**

Positioning and Preparation

- ▶ Patient: supine.
- ▶ Physician: sitting at the head of the table.

Tissue Contact

- Both hands perform the technique.
- Performing hands: contact both lateral angles of the frontal bone with the heels of the hands. Interlace the fingers.
  - To be sure you are contacting only the frontal bone, palpate for the coronal and sphenofrontal sutures.

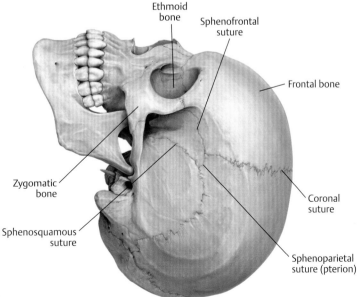

Fig. 13.7 Frontal bone, lateral view.

Movements, Barriers, and Forces

Movements are coordinated with the cranial rhythmic impulse (cranial flexion/external rotation and extension/internal rotation).

- Palpate and observe the inherent motion of the frontal bone.
- During the extension/internal rotation phase, apply gentle medial force with the heels of both hands to disengage the frontal bone from the parietal and sphenoid bones.
  - Create a fulcrum at the point where the fingers interlace at the palm, so the heels of the hands approximate. Focus efforts on lifting the fingertips rather than squeezing the frontal bone.
    - This exaggerates the normal internal rotation of the frontal bone.
- Hold this position.
- Apply gentle anteriorly directed forces to lift the frontal bone.
- Hold these forces until release, or for up to 2 minutes.
- When tissue release is palpated, gently and slowly allow the frontal bone to return to a normal position, guiding it back.
- Retest the frontal bone and cranium for position and inherent motion.

Head, Venous Sinus Drainage

Method: Direct, Disengagement

This technique releases dural tensions and improves drainage of the venous sinuses (**Fig. 13.8**). Impaired venous drainage in the cranium can manifest in a variety of ways: as dark circles under the eyes, mental "fogginess," and headache, among others. Although this technique specifically addresses venous blood drainage, it is a global treatment and can also improve circulation and congestion in the paranasal sinuses and nasopharynx.

This technique requires palpation through the bone with forces directed at the dura, which house the venous blood. Release is often felt as warmth due to increase in venous blood flow.

Before performing this technique, it is a good idea to be sure that the OA joint and thoracic inlet are free from restriction to ensure that venous blood returns to central circulation.

Key Elements

- Somatic dysfunction corrected: dural restrictions in the confluence of sinuses, occipital sinus, transverse sinus, and sagittal sinus.
- End goal: to resolve dural tensions in the cranial venous sinuses to increase venous drainage.

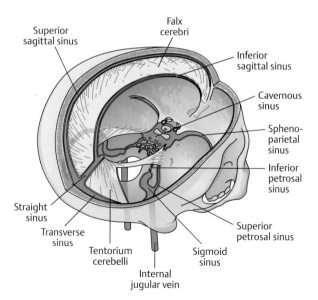

Fig. 13.8 Cranial venous sinuses.

WATCH ▷ ▶ ▷

▶ *Video 13.5 Venous Sinus Drainage—Narrated*

Positioning and Preparation

▶ Patient: supine.

▶ Physician: seated at the head of the table.

The four parts of this technique are presented sequentially.

Part 1: Confluence of Sinuses

Tissue Contact

- Contact the external occipital protuberance with the pad of one third finger. Place the pad of the other third finger underneath this finger.

Movements, Barriers, and Forces

- Layer palpate to the dura.
- Allow the weight of the patient's head to create the corrective force. If needed, create additional superiorly directed force with both contacting fingers.
- Hold until softening or warmth is perceived, or ~ 15 seconds.
- Release forces but not tissue contact.

Part 2: Occipital Sinus

Tissue Contact

- Move the finger pads inferiorly on the occiput, about a centimeter in an average adult.

Movements, Barriers, and Forces

- Layer palpate to the dura.
- Allow the weight of the patient's head to create the corrective force. If needed, create additional superiorly directed force with both contacting fingers.
- Hold until softening or warmth is perceived, or ~ 15 seconds.
- Release forces and tissue contact.

Optional: OA joint decompression can be performed at this time.

Part 3: Transverse Sinus

Tissue Contact

- Contact the lateral aspect of the external occipital protuberance with the pads of the fourth fingers, one on each side. Place the pads of the second and third fingers alongside in a horizontal line to be posterior to the transverse sinus.

Movements, Barriers, and Forces

- Layer palpate to the dura.
- Allow the weight of the patient's head to create the corrective force. If needed, create additional superiorly directed force with all contacting fingers.
- Hold until softening or warmth is perceived, or ~ 15 seconds.
- Release forces and tissue contact.

Part 4: Sagittal Sinus

Tissue Contact and Movements, Barriers, and Forces

- Contact just lateral to the sagittal suture, just superior to the lambda with the pads of the thumbs, crossing them.
  - Contact the left parietal bone with the right thumb and the right parietal bone with the left thumb.
- Layer palpate to the bony layer.
- Apply gentle lateral forces with both thumbs, as if separating the sagittal suture.
- Hold forces until softening or warmth is perceived, or ~ 5 to 10 seconds.
- Move the thumbs superiorly along the sagittal suture and repeat along the entirety of the suture until the bregma is reached.
- Contact the lateral aspects of the metopic suture, or where it would be in cases where it is ossified, with the tips of the second, third, and fourth or fifth fingers.
- Layer palpate to the bony layer.
- Apply gentle lateral forces with all contacting fingers.
- Hold until softening or warmth is perceived, or ~ 5 to 10 seconds.
- Release forces and tissue contact.
- Retest the cranium for changes in inherent motion.

Head, Compression of the Fourth Ventricle

The methods described here are disengagement, opposing physiological motion, and fluid technique.

The compression of the fourth ventricle (CV-4) is an attempt to affect the physiology in and around the fourth ventricle of the brain (**Fig. 13.9**). It does not actually compress the fourth ventricle; however, by compressing the occiput to disengage it at the occipitomastoid sutures, and holding it in a cupped position, the fluctuation of the cerebrospinal fluid is affected along with the autonomic ganglia located in the brain stem. It is commonly performed and promoted by Dr. Sutherland as the technique to perform when one does not know where to begin cranial techniques. It is especially useful for patients with chronic conditions or SBS compressions. However mysterious this technique may appear, literature suggests that this technique does indeed affect autonomic functioning.

Different from other OCMM techniques because the occiput is held motionless, it is common to feel discordant inherent cranial motion. The discordant motion eventually stops and settles into what is referred to as a still point. After this still point, the motion becomes coordinated, and the technique is complete. If a still point is not appreciated, hold the occiput in position for 3 minutes, which is the time that is commonly used in research studies. However, it can take up to 20 minutes for a still point to occur, so use clinical judgment.

Key Elements

- Somatic dysfunction corrected: performed empirically to affect brainstem autonomic function.
- End goal: to affect brainstem autonomic function.

WATCH ▷▶▷

▶ *Video 13.6 Compression of the Fourth Ventricle (CV-4)—Narrated*

Example Somatic Dysfunction: Decreased CRI rate and amplitude

Positioning and Preparation

▶ Patient: supine.

▶ Physician: sitting at the head of the table.

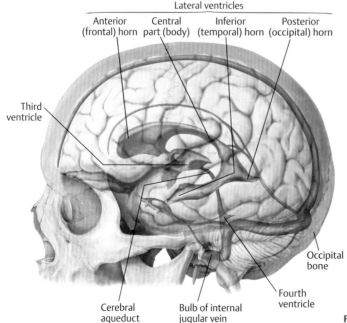

Lateral ventricles

Anterior (frontal) horn   Central part (body)   Inferior (temporal) horn   Posterior (occipital) horn

Third ventricle

Occipital bone

Cerebral aqueduct   Bulb of internal jugular vein   Fourth ventricle

Fig. 13.9 Cranial ventricles.

Tissue Contact

- Both hands create the corrective forces and perform the technique simultaneously.
- Performing hands: contact the occiput with both thenar eminences. The thumbs and fingers may be interlaced. The patient's head will rise off the table slightly but do not allow the neck to extend.
  - Do not contact or cross the occipitomastoid sutures.

Movements, Barriers, and Forces

Use both hands to do the following:

- Layer palpate to the occipital bone.
- Apply gentle medially directed forces with the heels of both hands at the lateral angles of the occiput to disengage the occiput from the temporal bones.
- Move the occiput posteriorly and superiorly just slightly, in the direction of cranial extension.
- Hold these forces and hand positions until a still point, softening, warmth in the tissues, or a release is palpated. In the event that a still point is not perceived, hold for 3 minutes.
  - Sometimes a chaotic pulsation or fluid movement is palpated. If this occurs, wait for the motion to stop. When it stops, it is referred to as a still point. Motion will recur, then the technique can be stopped.
- Allow the lateral angles of the occiput to return to neutral position.
- Slowly remove your hands, returning the patient's head to the table.
- Retest the cranium for changes in position and inherent motion.

Note: If the patient is rising from the table immediately after performing this technique, ask the patient to do so very slowly.

Chapter Summary

Gentle and powerful, osteopathic cranial manipulative medicine techniques are unique and fundamental to osteopathic medicine. This chapter offers the basics of cranial dysfunction diagnosis, followed by cranial techniques that should be accessible to every osteopathic medical student learner.

Review Questions

Q1. In which of the following patients is performing cranial manipulation contraindicated?

A. A 27-year-old woman who sustained a closed head injury in a car accident 2 years ago.

B. A 65-year-old woman with rheumatoid arthritis.

C. A 72-year-old man with an acute intracranial bleed.

D. A newborn baby boy with difficulty breast feeding.

E. An 18-year-old man 2 days after wisdom tooth extraction.

Q2. A 2-month-old baby girl presents with torticollis. Physical exam reveals that her head is shaped like a parallelogram. Which cranial strain pattern is most likely present in this patient?

A. Lateral strain.

B. Side bending rotation.

C. Sphenobasilar synchondrosis compression.

D. Torsion.

E. Vertical strain.

Q3. A 33-year-old man presents with acute sinusitis. As part of his treatment, you decided to release his cranial venous sinuses. To release the sagittal sinus, you start at this landmark:

A. Bregma.

B. Lambda.

C. Nasion.

D. Opisthion.

E. Pterion.

Q4. Which of the following is true about the frontal and parietal lifts?

A. Both lifts are initiated during the internal rotation phase.

B. Both lifts are initiated during the external rotation phase.

C. The frontal lift is initiated during internal rotation, and the parietal lift is initiated during external rotation.

D. The frontal lift is initiated during external rotation, and the parietal lift is initiated during internal rotation.

E. Internal and external rotation of the cranial bones is not relevant in these techniques.

Answers to Review Questions

Q1. The correct answer is **C**. All the other answers are indications.

Q2. The correct answer is **A**. All the other answers are incorrect.

Q3. The correct answer is **B**. All the other answers are incorrect.

Q4. The correct answer is **A**. Both the parietal lift and the frontal lift are initiated during internal rotation of their respective bones.

References

1. Sutherland WG. The cranial bowl: A treatise relating to cranial articular mobility, cranial articular lesions and cranial technic. 1939
2. Osteopathic Cranial Academy. Research bibliography. http://cranialacademy.org/research/bibliography
3. Magoun HI, Sutherland WG. Osteopathy in the Cranial Field. Sutherland Cranial Teaching Foundation; 1951

Suggested Reading

Sutherland WG. Teachings in the science of osteopathy. In: Wales AL, ed. Sutherland Cranial Teaching Foundation; 1990

Sutherland WG. Contributions of Thought: The Collected Writings of William Garner Sutherland, DO, Pertaining to the Art and Science of Osteopathy Including the Cranial Concept in Osteopathy Covering the Years 1914–1954. In: Sutherland AS, Wales AL, eds. Sutherland Cranial Teaching Foundation; 1998

Visceral Techniques

LEARNING OBJECTIVES

1. Explain the goals of performing visceral techniques.
2. Identify the clinical considerations, including indications, contraindications, and precautions for performing visceral techniques.
3. Compare and contrast the styles of visceral techniques.
4. Outline the general movements, barriers, and forces used to perform visceral techniques.
5. Identify the end goal for performing each visceral technique.
6. Visualize, verbalize, and identify the preparation, positioning, tissue contact, movements, barriers, and forces for each visceral technique.
7. Perform visceral techniques using appropriate visceral dysfunction diagnosis, preparation, positioning, tissue contact, movements, barriers, forces, retest for effectiveness, communication, and safe tissue handling.

Visceral Techniques Introduction

Visceral organs are suspended by connective tissues and ligaments that permit mobility or movement to accommodate gross body motions, including motions associated with thoracoabdominal respiration. Visceral structures are also regulated by constant nervous system activity that also influences organ movement, or motility, such as peristalsis. When visceral attachments are strained or nervous system activity becomes aberrant, visceral dysfunction can occur. Visceral dysfunction is impaired mobility and/ or motility of visceral organs, and can be corrected with visceral osteopathic manipulative techniques.

Visceral techniques may be used as a primary treatment, such as correcting large intestine dysfunction for functional constipation, or as an adjunct treatment. As a primary treatment, osteopathic manipulative treatment (OMT) can provide relief in cases where no known "organic" causative agent is found in imaging or laboratory studies, and when other treatments, such as medications, have failed. Adjunct treatment includes the use of OMT to influence the autonomic nervous system, which then affects organ function, such as peristalsis.

In general, osteopathic techniques performed on visceral organs and their fascial attachments can:

- Increase local arterial, venous, and lymphatic circulation.
- Improve organ mobility and motility.
- Normalize autonomic tone.
- Assist in restoration of normal organ function.

This chapter presents a small sample of abdominal visceral techniques that are easiest to perform. They can be used either as primary or adjunct treatments of common clinical conditions. However, every visceral organ that can be palpated can be diagnosed for dysfunction and treated with OMT.

Background

The osteopathic approach and osteopathic techniques were intended to treat all diseases, including visceral diseases. Some of the earliest visceral techniques were performed with the patient in a knee-to-chest or crawling position to suspend the visceral organs by their ligamentous attachments. Today, most modern techniques are performed with the patient in a supine, lateral recumbent, or seated position because the knee-to-chest position is often difficult for the patient to obtain.

Dr. Still also emphasized treatment of the spine to affect autonomic nervous system tone and improve fluid circulation to and from a diseased organ. Some techniques in this manual that most directly affect autonomic nervous system tone include soft tissue (ST): suboccipital inhibitory pressure; ST: thoracic/lumbar inhibitory pressure; articulatory (ART): costal; and ART: sacrum. An additional technique, visceral (VIS): ganglion inhibitory pressure, is presented in this chapter.

In the 1920s Frank Chapman, DO, added a unique perspective to the treatment of visceral diseases using OMT. He found and described distinct nodules that map to each organ when the organ is diseased. Colloquially called Chapman reflexes, this manual refers to them as neurolymphatic reflexes. *Neuro* implies that the nervous system is involved. The term *lymphatic* is used because the reflexes are purported to be areas of local lymphatic congestion due to the ganglion-formed or fusiform contracture of a sympathetic nerve that leads to the distinct nodule. Dr. Chapman's approach also emphasized the importance of pelvic biomechanics and endocrine function, which was only beginning to be scientifically understood at the time. Dr. Chapman's brother-in-law, Charles Owen, DO, wrote a book about his discoveries, *An Endocrine Interpretation of Chapman's Reflexes by the Interpreter*.[1] Today, neurolymphatic reflexes are used clinically as a diagnostic aid, and OMT can be performed on these reflexes as a component of comprehensive patient care.

Research

Scientific investigation of the viscerosomatic and somatovisceral reflexes was performed very early in the history of osteopathic medicine. Louisa Burns, DO, Stedman Denslow, DO, and Irvin Korr, PhD, are among the group of researchers who first established scientific connections between manual diagnosis, OMT, and the effects on a biological system (animals or humans). A short research bibliography that includes some of these seminal works, along with more recent literature, including clinical studies, is presented at the end of this chapter.

Clinical Considerations

Some common clinical things to consider for VIS techniques are listed in Table 14.1.

Visceral dysfunction should be differentiated from other visceral pathology, such as inflamma-

Table 14.1 Clinical considerations		
Indications	**Contraindications**	**Precautions**
Gastroesophageal reflux disease	Organ rupture	Partial bowel obstruction
Irritable bowel syndrome	Abdominal abscess	Pregnancy: exercise caution when
Constipation	Hemorrhage near or at visceral	performing techniques directly
Postoperative ileus	organs	on, or in close proximity to the
Generalized abdominal pain	Moderate–severe inflammation/	uterus.
Pleurisy	infection	
Visceroptosis	Postoperative less than 6 weeks	
Functional gastrointestinal	after visceral organ surgery	
disorders	Local implanted medical device	
Ganglia techniques: to affect	(drain, wire mesh)	
sympathetic tone		

tion, infection, rupture. Medical diagnosis cannot be overemphasized because any visceral disease must be accurately diagnosed and treated. Determining when OMT is an adjunctive or a primary treatment in cases of visceral disease requires clinical discernment. Always acquire adequate data in the form of an appropriate history, a thorough physical exam, and relevant diagnostic tests to exercise best clinical judgment before performing OMT.

Before performing OMT to a visceral organ, consider assessing and performing OMT on the paraspinal musculature, linea alba, and thoracoabdominal and pelvic diaphragms. These techniques ease tensions in the surrounding abdominal wall, making access to the organs easier.

Somatic and Visceral Dysfunction Corrected

Visceral dysfunction is defined as "impaired or altered mobility or motility of the visceral system and related fascial, neurological, vascular, skeletal, and lymphatic elements."[2] It is different from somatic dysfunction only in that the impairment in somatic dysfunction is in the somatic system, whereas visceral dysfunction involves impairment in visceral organs

Visceral Dysfunction Diagnosis

Impaired organ mobility, or the gross motions of an organ, can be diagnosed and corrected in a fashion similar to myofascial release (MFR) or indirect (IND) techniques. As in MFR and IND techniques for the somatic system, tissue texture abnormalities and/or specific range of motion directions are identified immediately before performance of a visceral technique. For this reason, visceral dysfunction diagnosis instructions are included in each Movements, Barriers, and Forces section of MFR and IND techniques.

As a caveat, it is common to substitute the term *somatic* for *visceral* when naming visceral dysfunctions, especially for medical billing purposes. For example, visceral dysfunction of the liver can also be named with the more general term *somatic dysfunction of the abdomen (liver)*.

Neurolymphatic Reflex Diagnosis

Neurolymphatic reflexes are diagnosed by the palpation of ganglion-formed or fusiform contracture, which meets the following criteria:

- Tissue layer: superficial and/or deep fascias.
- Description.
  - Small (~ 2–5 mm).
  - Firm.
  - Discrete.
  - Smooth.
  - The texture is similar to a tapioca pearl or grain of cooked rice.
- Tenderness: light palpation produces nonradiating tenderness.
- Location.
  - The location of the reflex does not change and is mapped onto the body.
  - Each reflex has an anterior and a posterior body location.
  - Some reflexes are bilateral and some are unilateral.
  - Tables with locations of common points can be found in section 14.6 VIS: Neurolymphatic Reflex Technique.

Positioning and Preparation

- Patient: the patient is often supine with the knees bent. Bent knees release tension in the anterior abdominal wall, which permits easier contact of the deeper organs. For techniques that are performed with the patient seated, a slumped position helps to decrease the tension in the abdominal wall.
- Physician: the physician stands or sits to best contact the organ.

Tissue Contact

One or both hands perform the techniques. The fingertips, finger pads, thumb pads, and heel of the hand can all be used. Because the visceral organs are palpated beneath the abdominal wall musculature, direct organ contact can be challenging. Tissue layer palpation and three-dimensional anatomical knowledge are therefore key to effective tissue contact.

Movements, Barriers, and Forces

There are three "styles" of visceral techniques in this manual:

- Myofascial release: single direction, direct method.
- Indirect.
- Soft tissue: sustained and rotatory inhibitory pressure.

The word *style* is used to infer that the principles (somatic dysfunction diagnosis and movements, barriers, and forces) of the technique are applied to visceral organs with recognition that there remain some slight differences between OMT performed on visceral versus somatic structures.

Myofascial Release: Single Direction, Direct Method

MFR techniques performed on the viscera resolve abnormal tensions of organ fascial attachments and ligaments. Any MFR method can be applied, but for simplicity, MFR: single direction, direct method has been selected for this chapter.

Indirect

IND techniques correct positional asymmetry and restrictions of the normal gliding motion between adjacent organs. The organ itself is assessed for passive range of motion restrictions and principles of IND technique are applied.

Soft Tissue: Sustained and Rotatory Inhibitory Pressure

Viscerosomatic reflexes that are sympathetically mediated produce palpable tissue texture changes in the paraspinal musculature between T1 and L2, and around the abdominal sympathetic ganglia. The principles of ST: sustained inhibitory pressure techniques can be applied to correct tissue texture changes in the fascias around the abdominal ganglia to help normalize sympathetic tone.

Neurolymphatic Reflexes

Neurolymphatic reflexes are corrected with the use of a slight inhibitory pressure directly over the reflex with the addition of small repetitive rotatory forces, or very small circular motions.

Retest for Effectiveness

After performing MFR-style techniques, retest the fascia for changes in tension. After performing IND-style techniques, retest the organ for improvements in passive range of motion. Techniques performed on neurolymphatic reflexes should result in immediate dissipation of the reflex, and techniques performed on the abdominal ganglia should yield decrease in tissue texture changes. However, performing a technique on a viscerosomatic or neurolymphatic reflex area does not constitute treatment of the underlying visceral disease. Neurolymphatic reflexes and tissue texture changes due to autonomic nervous system activity will return if the causative or underlying visceral pathology is not resolved.

Patients may not immediately sense changes in organ position or fascial tensions. Instead, patients may experience changes in organ function, such as increased intestinal motion (peristalsis), mild transient intestinal cramping, or a change in appetite. Sometimes after performing techniques on or around the liver, a patient may feel slight malaise or a headache due to the increased circulation and release of liver metabolites. Be sure to inform the patient of these possibilities and adjust diet and fluid intake accordingly (usually increased fluid if not contraindicated).

Summary steps for each technique can be found in the corresponding chapter in the technique introduction section and are not included in this chapter.

Abdomen, Gastroesophageal Junction

Style: MFR: Single Direction, Direct Method

Use this technique as adjunct treatment for gastroesophageal reflux disease (**Fig. 14.1** and **Fig. 14.2**). Be sure to assess and perform OMT on the thoracoabdominal diaphragm first to remove any restrictions around the esophageal hiatus.

Key Elements

- Somatic/visceral dysfunction corrected: fascial tightness of the phrenoesophageal ligament.
- End goal: to restore normal position of the gastroesophageal junction in relationship to the esophageal hiatus of the thoracoabdominal diaphragm.

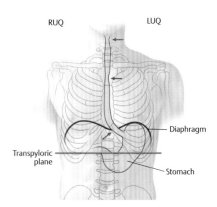

Fig. 14.1 Esophagus and stomach. Arrows indicate areas of possible esophageal constrictions.

> **WATCH** ▷ ▶ ▷
>
> ▶ *Video 14.1 Abdomen, Gastroesophageal Junction—Narrated*
>
> *Example Somatic Dysfunction: Fascial tightness of the phrenoesophageal ligament*

Positioning and Preparation

- ▶ Patient: seated.
- ▶ Physician: standing behind the patient.

Tissue Contact

- Both hands create the corrective stretching forces.
- Performing hands: contact the gastroesophageal junction with the pads of the thumbs, inferior to the xiphoid process and in between the medial costal margins. Do not contact the xiphoid process.

- After tissue contact, ask the patient to lean back onto your abdomen and slouch forward slightly. Place a pillow between the patient and your abdomen if necessary.

Movements, Barriers, and Forces

Use both hands to do the following:

- Layer palpate to the lower esophageal junction.
  - Skin → superficial fascia → abdominal musculature → gastroesophageal junction/phrenoesophageal ligament.
- Apply inferior traction force until a restrictive barrier is felt.
  - Slight movements to the right or left can be added to tighten the tissues further.
  - Ask the patient to rotate toward one side to loosen the diaphragm and decrease tension around the esophageal hiatus to permit more inferior traction forces.
- Monitor fascias until release or for ~ 2 minutes.
  - Optional: add fascial unwinding and/or respiratory cooperation.
- Release forces and return the tissues and patient to a neutral position.
- Retest the phrenoesophageal ligament for changes in tension.

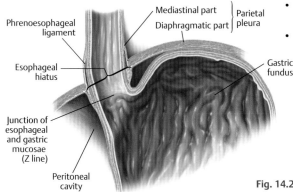

Fig. 14.2 Gastroesophageal junction.

Abdomen, Liver

Style: IND

Liver visceral dysfunction should be suspected when there is persistent dysfunction of the right thoracoabdominal hemi diaphragm, as the bare area of the liver is prone to restriction as it contacts the diaphragm. This technique also improves circulation to and from the liver, liberating metabolites (**Fig. 14.3** and **Fig. 14.4**). Because of this, be sure to inform the patient that transient nausea, headache, or malaise may be experienced after this technique is performed. Use caution in patients with significant liver disease.

Key Elements

- Somatic/visceral dysfunction corrected: passive range of motion restrictions in the liver.
- End goal: to restore normal mobility and motility of the liver by removing fascial restrictions around and fluid congestion within the liver.

WATCH ▷ ▶ ▷

▶ *Video 14.2 Abdomen, Liver—Narrated*

Example Somatic Dysfunction: Inferior, side bending right, rotation right

Positioning and Preparation

- ▶ Patient: supine.
- ▶ Physician: sitting or standing at the right side of the patient, near the liver.

Tissue Contact

- Both hands position the liver. Use one hand to contact the patient's posterior and lateral aspects of the liver, the other to contact the anterior and lateral margins.
- Anterior performing hand: Contact the liver with the entire palmar surface of the hand so that the heel of the hand is on the lateral edge and the fingers are inferior to the costal margin.
- Posterior performing hand: Contact the liver with the entire palmar surface of the hand and fingers with fingertips near the 12th rib.

Movements, Barriers, and Forces

Use both hands to do the following:

- Layer palpate to the liver.
  - Skin → superficial fascia → muscle/bone → deep fascia/musculature → liver.
- Test for passive range of motion with both hands in three directions:
  - Superior/inferior: move the liver superiorly, then inferiorly.
  - Translation: move the liver to the right, then to the left.
  - Side bending: move the liver into left side bending by pointing the fingers at an angle inferiorly, toward the patient's opposite hip. Reverse directions to test right side bending toward you.
- Position the liver in all directions of motion ease.
- Hold all forces and positions until the tissues release or for up to 2 minutes.
  - Optional: add respiratory cooperation.
- Release forces.
- Retest the liver for changes in passive range of motion.

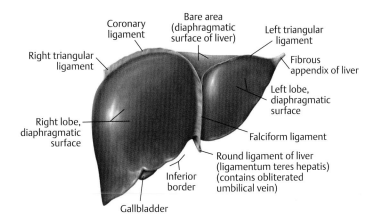

Fig. 14.3   Liver.

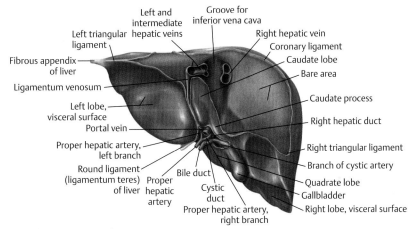

Fig. 14.4   Liver surface, posterior.

Abdomen, Mesenteries

Style: MFR: Single Direction, Direct Method

Traditionally called a mesenteric lift, this technique is useful for cases of constipation, intestinal discomfort due to food intolerances or sensitivities, colic in newborns, and to promote lymph circulation (**Fig. 14.5** and **Fig. 14.6**). The intestinal mesenteries package, protect, and provide passageways for the intestinal vasculature. This technique has two parts, and they are best performed sequentially. The transverse mesocolon is not addressed in this technique.

Key Elements

- Somatic/visceral dysfunction corrected: mesenteric fascial tightness (this technique can also be performed empirically in appropriate clinical conditions).
- End goal: to release tension in the intestinal mesenteries.

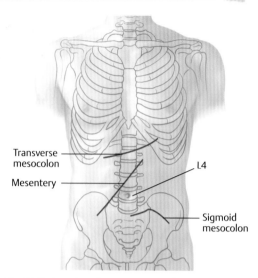

Fig. 14.5   Location of mesenteric attachments.

WATCH ▷ ▶ ▷

▶ *Video 14.3 Abdomen, Mesenteries— Narrated*

Example Somatic/Visceral Dysfunction Corrected: Mesenteric fascial tightness, sigmoid mesocolon fascial tightness

---

Positioning and Preparation

▶ Patient: supine, with legs bent and feet on the table.

▶ Physician: standing at the right side of the patient.

Tissue Contact

Performing hand: one hand creates the corrective stretching forces.

- Part 1: mesenteric root (mesentery).
  - Contact the inferior margin of the mesentery near the attachment, left lower quadrant of the abdomen.
- Part 2: sigmoid mesocolon.
  - Contact the lateral margin of the mesentery near its attachment on the posterior abdominal wall. The heel of hand is near the left anterior superior iliac spine (ASIS) and just superior to the left inguinal ligament.

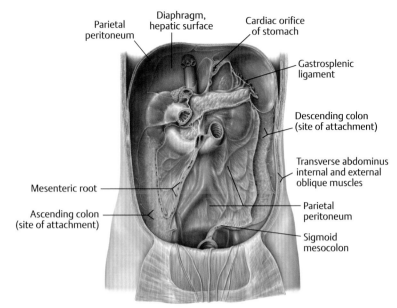

Fig. 14.6 Mesenteric attachments.

Movements, Barriers, and Forces

Use the performing hand to do the following:

Part 1: Mesenteric Root

- Layer palpate to the desired mesentery.
  - Skin → superficial fascia/adipose → abdominal musculature → omentum → small intestines.
- Curl the fingertips and gently scoop the loops of small intestine diagonally toward the right shoulder until resistance is felt in the deeper mesenteric root.
- Hold this force.
- Monitor tissues until release or for ~ 2 minutes.
  - Optional: add respiratory cooperation.
- Release the forces and return the tissues to a neutral position.
- Retest the mesentery for changes in tension.

Part 2: Sigmoid Mesocolon

- Layer palpate to the sigmoid.
  - Skin → superficial fascia/adipose → abdominal musculature → sigmoid colon.
- Curl the fingertips and gently scoop the sigmoid colon diagonally toward the right shoulder until resistance is felt in the deeper sigmoid mesocolon.
- Hold this force.
- Monitor tissues until release or for ~ 2 minutes.
  - Optional: add respiratory cooperation.
- Release the forces and return the tissues to a neutral position.
- Retest the sigmoid mesocolon for changes in tension.

Abdomen, Large Intestines

Style: MFR: Single Direction, Direct Method

This technique is specifically intended to decongest the tissues around the large intestines, effectively promoting peristalsis (**Fig. 14.7** and **Fig. 14.8**). It is therefore applicable in cases of functional constipation. This technique has three parts that are performed sequentially from distal to proximal, or from the sigmoid colon to the ileocecal valve. However, the technique may be performed in reverse order, especially when colonic stimulation is intended.

Key Elements

- Somatic/visceral dysfunction corrected: tightness in the fascial attachments of the large intestine.
- End goal: to release fascial tensions around the large intestine to improve intestinal function.

> **WATCH** ▷ ► ▷
>
> ► *Video 14.4 Abdomen, Large Intestines— Narrated*
>
> *Example Somatic Dysfunction: Large intestine fascial tightness*

Positioning and Preparation

- ► Patient: supine with bent knees.
- ► Physician: standing at either side of the patient.

Tissue Contact

This technique has three parts. One or both hands perform the technique.

- Performing hand(s)
  - Part 1: descending colon: contact the left side of the abdomen, about at the level of the anterior axillary line.
  - Part 2: ascending colon: contact the right side of the abdomen, about at the level of the anterior axillary line.
  - Part 3: iliocecal region: contact the right side of the abdomen, superiorly and medially to the anterior superior iliac spine.

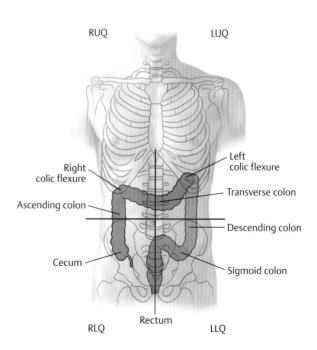

Fig. 14.7 Location of large intestine.

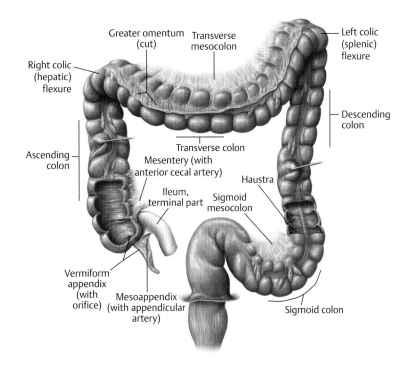

Fig. 14.8 Large intestine.

Movements, Barriers, and Forces

One or both hands perform the three-part technique.

Part 1: Descending Colon

- Layer palpate to the large intestine.
  - Skin → superficial fascia/adipose → abdominal musculature → large intestines.
- Curl the fingertips and gently scoop the large intestine medially until resistance is felt in the intestines.
- Hold this force.
- Monitor tissues until release or for ~ 2 minutes.
  - Optional: add respiratory cooperation.
- Release the forces and return the tissues to a neutral position.
- Retest the descending colon for changes in fascial tension.

Part 2: Ascending Colon

- Layer palpate to the large intestine
  - Skin→ superficial fascia/adipose → abdominal musculature→ large intestines.

- Curl the fingertips and gently scoop the large intestine medially until resistance is felt in the intestines.
- Hold this force.
- Monitor tissues until release or for ~ 2 minutes.
  - Optional: add respiratory cooperation.
- Release the forces and return the tissues to a neutral position.
- Retest the ascending colon for changes in fascial tension.

Part 3: Iliocecal Region

- Layer palpate to the large intestine.
  - Skin→ superficial fascia/adipose → abdominal musculature→ large intestines.
- Curl the fingertips and gently scoop the large intestine superiorly and slightly medially until resistance is felt in the intestines.
- Hold this force.
- Monitor tissues until release or for ~ 2 minutes.
  - Optional: add respiratory cooperation.
- Release the forces and return the tissues to a neutral position.
- Retest the iliocecal region for changes in fascial tension.

Abdomen, Ganglion Inhibitory Pressure

Style: ST: Sustained Inhibitory Pressure

This is a variation of soft tissue inhibitory pressure technique, in that inhibitory forces are directed at the ganglia themselves (**Fig. 14.9**). Use this technique to affect sympathetic tone of the organs the ganlion innervates. Recall spinal innervation levels: celiac ganglion: T5–T9, superior mesenteric ganglion: T10–T11, and superior mesenteric ganglion: T12–L2.

Key Elements

- Somatic/visceral dysfunction corrected: performed empirically for normalization of sympathetic nervous system tone.
- End goal: to normalize the tensions around and affect the tone of the sympathetic ganglia that innervate the gastrointestinal tract and related vasculature.

WATCH ▷ ▶ ▷

▶ *Video 14.5 Abdomen, Ganglion Inhibitory Pressure—Narrated*

Example Somatic Dysfunction: Superior mesenteric ganglion facilitation

Positioning and Preparation

- ▶ Patient: supine with knees bent and feet on the table.
- ▶ Physician: standing at one side of the patient.

Tissue Contact

- Perform on one ganglion at a time. One hand is used to perform the technique.
- Ganglion locations (in an average adult):
  - Celiac ganglion: about an inch inferior to the xiphoid process.
  - Superior mesenteric ganglion: halfway between xiphoid process and umbilicus.
  - Inferior mesenteric ganglion: about an inch superior to the umbilicus.
- Performing hand: contact the fascias anterior to the affected sympathetic ganglion with the tip of the second and/or third finger(s).

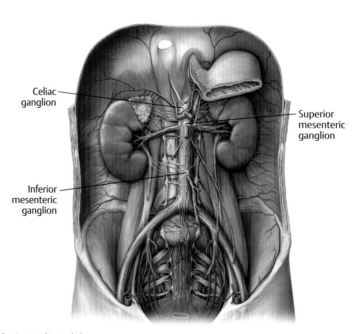

Celiac ganglion

Superior mesenteric ganglion

Inferior mesenteric ganglion

Fig. 14.9 Sympathetic ganglia in abdomen.

Movements, Barriers, and Forces

Use the performing hand to do the following:

- Layer palpate to the affected ganglion and related fascias.
  - Skin → superficial fascia → adipose→ linea alba → omentum→ visceral organs→ ganglion.
- When resistance is felt, hold the forces.
  - If and when the abdominal aorta is palpated, stop just when it is palpable and decrease the forces so you remain anterior to it.

- Monitor fascial tensions around the ganglion until release or for ~ 2 minutes.
  - Optional: add fascial unwinding and/or respiratory cooperation.
  - Often, the pulsation of the aorta becomes prominent, indicating release of tissues around the ganglion.
- Release forces and tissue contact.
- Retest is not necessary.

Neurolymphatic Reflex Technique

Style: ST: Rotatory Pressure

Patients can be easily taught to perform this technique on themselves at home. For example, patients with irritable bowel syndrome can perform the technique regularly on any present reflex points during a flare-up.

Key Elements

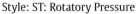

- Somatic/visceral dysfunction corrected: a neurolymphatic reflex.
- End goal: to affect autonomic tone to and stimulate lymphatic drainage of an affected visceral organ.

WATCH ▷ ▶ ▷

▶ *Video 14.6 Neurolymphatic Reflex Technique—Narrated*

Example Somatic Dysfunction: Appendix neuro-lymphatic reflex

Positioning and Preparation

▶ Patient: supine or prone.
▶ Physician: standing or sitting.

Tissue Contact

- One hand creates the activating, rotatory forces.
- Performing hand: contact the neurolymphatic reflex with the pad of one finger or thumb.

Movements, Barriers, and Forces

Use the performing hand to do the following:

- Layer palpate to the fascial layer where the neurolymphatic reflex is located (**Fig. 14.10** and **Fig. 14.11**); (Table 14.2).
- Apply a very slight force, directed perpendicularly into the neurolymphatic reflex, until the edges of the reflex are palpated. Hold this force.
- Create repetitive rotatory forces, or very small circular motions in any direction, until the reflex is no longer palpable or for ~ 10 to 20 seconds.
- Release the forces and tissue contact.
- Retest for the presence of the neurolymphatic reflex.

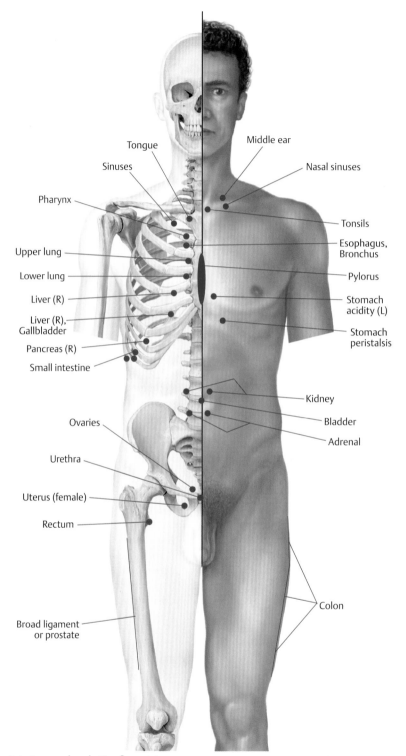

Fig. 14.10 Anterior neurolymphatic reflex points.

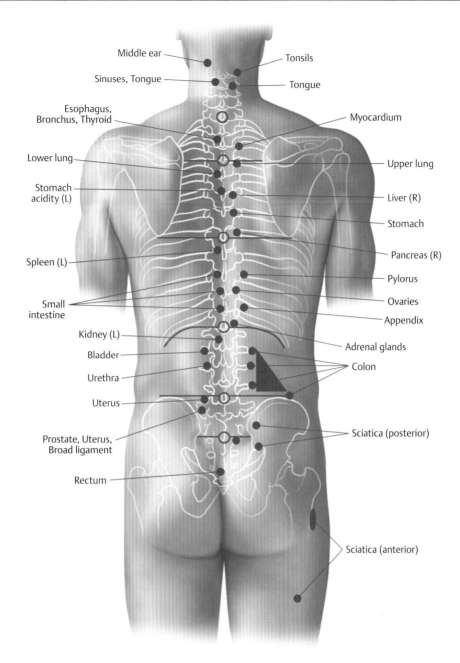

Fig. 14.11 Posterior neurolymphatic reflex points.

Neurolymphatic reflex[a]	Anterior location	Posterior location
Table 14.2 Neurolymphatic reflex points, anterior and posterior[3,4]		
Adrenal glands	2–2.5 inches superior and lateral to the umbilicus (side specific)	Either side of the spinous process of T11 or T12 (side specific)
Appendix	The tip of the right 12th rib	Between the right lateral edges of the transverse process of T11 and T12
Bladder	Periumbilical (in a radius of ~ 1 cm around the umbilicus)	Superior edge of the L2 transverse processes
Colon	Multiple points along the anterior lateral femur from the greater trochanter to the distal lateral condyle. These are more anterior to the iliotibial I band than the prostate or broad ligament reflexes	Multiple points at the tips of the transverse processes of L2, L3, L4, and in a triangular area made between those and the most superior point of the iliac crest
Esophagus, bronchus, thyroid	Between ribs 1 and 2, near the sternum	Midline on the T2 transverse process
Myocardium	Between ribs 1 and 2, near the sternum	Between the spinous and transverse processes of T2 and T3
Kidneys	2–2.5 inches superior and lateral to the umbilicus (side specific)	Between the spinous and transverse processes of L1 and L2 (side specific)
Pharynx	Between the clavicle and rib 1 about an inch from the sternum	Between the spinous and transverse processes of C2
Gallbladder	Between ribs 6 and 7 on the right, midclavicular line	Between the spinous and transverse processes of T6 and T7 on the right
Liver	Between the right ribs 5 and 6 and 6 and 7 on the right, midclavicular line	Between the spinous and transverse processes of T5 and T6 and T6 and T7 on the right
Lower lung	Between ribs 4 and 5, near the sternum	Between the spinous and transverse processes of T4 and T5
Middle ear	Superior edge of clavicle, sternal end	Superior margin of the transverse process of C1
Nasal sinuses	Costomanubrial junction	Inferior tip of the transverse process of C1 (inferior to angle of jaw)
Ovaries	Superior margin of the pubic symphysis	Between the transverse processes of T10 and T11
Pancreas	Between right ribs 7 and 8, near cartilage	Between the spinous and transverse processes of T7 and T8 on the right
Pylorus	Anywhere in the midline of the body of the sternum	Costovertebral joint of T10 on the right
Rectum	Lesser trochanter of femur	Sacrum, lower end of sacroiliac joint
Sinuses	Upper edge 2nd rib and 1st intercostal, 3.5 inches from sternum	Upper edge of the middle of the transverse process of C2
Small intestine	Multiple locations, between ribs 8 and 9, 9 and 10, and/or 10 and 11, near costal cartilage junction	Multiple locations, between the spinous processes and transverse processes of T8 and T9, T9 and T19, T0 and T11
Spleen	Between ribs 7 and 8 on the left	Between the spinous and left transverse processes of T7 and T8
Stomach acidity (L)	Between ribs 5 and 6 on left, between sternum and mid clavicular line	Between the spinous and left transverse processes of T5 and T6
Stomach peristalsis (R)	Between ribs 6 and 7 on left, between sternum and midclavicular line	Between the spinous and left transverse processes of T6 and T7
Tongue	Cartilage of rib 2, about an inch lateral to the sternum	Upper edge of the middle of the transverse process of C2
Tonsils	Between ribs 1 and 2, near the sternum	Midline of the transverse processes of C1
Upper lung	Between ribs 3 and 4, near the sternum	Between the spinous and transverse processes of T3 and T4
Urethra	Superior and medial aspect of the pubic symphysis	Superior edge of the transverse processes of L3
Uterus	Superior edge of the union of the pubic ramus and ischium	Iliolumbar ligament
Sciatica	Multiple points on the posterior lateral aspect of the femur	Posterior superior iliac spine and inferior lateral angle of the sacrum
Broad ligament or prostate	Multiple points on the lateral anterior femur between the greater trochanter and lateral condyle. These are more posterior to the IT band than the colon points.	Iliolumbar ligament

[a] Note: Reflexes are located bilaterally unless indicated otherwise.

Chapter Summary

This chapter offers straightforward osteopathic techniques that can be performed on visceral organs as either a primary or an adjunct treatment for common maladies. Primary visceral techniques offer relief to patients with mechanical visceral dysfunction. Adjunct visceral techniques can reduce medication usage and provide comfort for the patient while the body is healing. Three types of techniques are presented in this chapter: those that focus on the surrounding fascial and ligamentous structures, those that address the organs themselves, and those that address viscerosomatic and somatovisceral reflexes.

Clinical Cases and Review Questions

Case 1

A 42-year-old man presents to the clinic with epigastric burning pain that is worse after meals. He has tried over-the-counter antacids with only symptomatic relief, and he wishes to avoid daily medication. On exam, bowel sounds are present in all four quadrants, and the abdomen is soft without guarding. Mild tenderness is present in the epigastric region to deep palpation. Tissue texture changes are found in the T5–T9 paraspinal and suboccipital regions.

Q1. You perform a visceral technique to address biomechanical alterations directly related to his clinical condition. Which structure do you contact?
   A. Left thoracoabdominal diaphragm fascias.
   B. Phrenoesophageal ligament.
   C. Gastrophrenic ligament.
   D. Phrenopericardial ligament.
   E. Linea alba.

Case 2

A 28-year-old woman presents with constipation since returning to graduate school 2 months ago. She has a bowel movement every 2 to 3 days with some straining. She denies blood in her stool as well as changes in stool pattern or caliber. She has no family history of colon cancer. She has a typical omnivorous diet but has been consuming fast foods five to seven times per week for the past few months. Abdominal exam reveals active bowel sounds, and mild tenderness in the left lower quadrant without rebound or guarding.

Q2. What region on the abdomen should you contact to perform OMT to most directly improve her condition?
   A. Inferior to the xiphoid process.
   B. Periumbilical.
   C. Midline, halfway between the xiphoid process and the umbilicus.
   D. Just superior to the inguinal ligament on the left.
   E. Suprapubic.

Q3. What are the goals of performing OMT on this patient's mesenteries?
   A. Increased sympathetic tone to the intestines.
   B. Increased parasympathetic tone to the intestines.
   C. Decreased intestinal motility.
   D. Repositioning of the small intestines.
   E. Increased venous and lymph circulation to the intestines.

Q4. Where should you contact the abdomen to treat the ganglion that would help normalize autonomic tone to the sigmoid colon?
   A. Just inferior to the xiphoid process.
   B. Halfway between the xiphoid process and the umbilicus.
   C. Just superior to the umbilicus.
   D. Halfway between the umbilicus and the pubic bone.
   E. Just superior to the pubic bone.

Q5. A 50-year-old woman presents with irritable bowel syndrome, diagnosed in her 20s. Physical exam is positive for diffuse mild abdominal tenderness, bilateral paraspinal muscular tightness (T10–L2), and the presence of a few discrete, small, nodules in the fascia of her left iliotibial band near the proximal femur. Appropriate corrective force to address this nodule using OMT is to:
   A. Gently move fluid around the nodule toward the terminal drainage site.
   B. Hold a sustained force directed medially into the nodule.
   C. Perform oscillatory movements on the legs.
   D. Stretch the iliotibial band laterally.
   E. Use a rotatory force over the nodule.

Answers to Review Questions

Q1. The correct answer is **B**: Phrenoesophageal ligament. This ligament connects the diaphragm to the esophagus and directly influences mechanical tension around the lower esophageal sphincter.

A is incorrect. The right diaphragmatic crura makes up a large part of the lower esophageal sphincter, but the left crura is less related.

C is incorrect. The gastrophrenic ligament connects the stomach to the diaphragm, but not to the gastroesophageal junction, so it does not influence lower esophageal sphincter tone directly.

D is incorrect. The phrenopericardial ligament connects the diaphragm to the pericardium and would not influence lower esophageal sphincter tone directly.

E is incorrect. The linea alba is not directly connected to the esophagus.

Q2. The correct answer is **D**: The left lower quadrant just superior to the inguinal ligament.

A is incorrect. The xiphoid process is the contact for treating the gastroesophageal junction.

B is incorrect. The periumbilical is the region for Chapman's reflexes related to the bladder.

C is incorrect. Halfway between the xiphoid process and the umbilicus is the location for the superior mesenteric ganglion.

E is incorrect. The suprapubic is the location to affect the bladder and bladder fascias.

Q3. The correct answer is **E**: Increase venous and lymph circulation to the intestines. Improved fluid mechanics of the vasculature and lymph are a primary goal of mesenteric release in the abdomen.

A is incorrect. The technique to increase sympathetic tone to the intestines is directed at the mesenteries and not at the autonomic tone.

B is incorrect. The technique to increase parasympathetic tone to the intestines is directed at the mesenteries and not at the autonomic tone.

C is incorrect. Decreased intestinal motility would worsen symptoms of constipation.

D is incorrect. The technique to reposition the small intestines treats the sigmoid colon and directly stretches the mesenteric attachments.

Q4. The correct answer is **C**: Just superior to the umbilicus. This is where the inferior mesenteric ganglion lies and this ganglion innervates the distal colon.

A is incorrect. Just beneath the xiphoid process is the location of the celiac ganglion that innervates the stomach and proximal duodenum.

B is incorrect. Halfway between the xiphoid process and the umbilicus is the location of the superior mesenteric ganglion that innervates the small intestines and proximal large intestine.

D is incorrect. Halfway between the umbilicus and pubic bone is not the location of a ganglion that innervates the sigmoid colon.

E is incorrect. Just superior to the pubic bone is not the location of a ganglion that innervates the sigmoid colon.

Q5. The correct answer is **E**. It is a description of treatment of neurolymphatic reflex (Chapman's reflex point).

A is incorrect. It is a description of effleurage.

B is incorrect. It describes inhibitory pressure, soft tissue technique.

C is incorrect. It is a description of a pedal pump.

D is incorrect. It is a description of lateral stretching, soft tissue technique.

References

1. Owens C, Chapman F. An Endocrine Interpretation of Chapman's Reflexes. Academy for Applied Osteopathy; 1963
2. Glossary Review Committee for the Educational Council on Osteopathic Principles and the American Association of Colleges of Osteopathic Medicine. Glossary of Osteopathic Terminology;2002
3. Capobianco JC. American Academy of Osteopathy Annual Convocation, 2001 presentation and personal communication
4. Chila AG, ed.; American Osteopathic Association. Foundations of Osteopathic Medicine. Baltimore, MD: Lippincott Williams & Wilkins; 2010

Bibliography: Historic

Beal MC, ed. Selected Papers of John Stedman Denslow, DO. American Academy of Osteopathy, 1993

Burns L. Viscero-somatic and somato-visceral spinal reflexes. 1907. J Am Osteopath Assoc 2000;100(4):249–258

Korr IM. The Collected Papers of Irvin M. Korr. Newark, OH: American Academy of Osteopathy; 1979

Korr IM. Somatic dysfunction, osteopathic manipulative treatment, and the nervous system: a few facts, some theories, many questions. J Am Osteopath Assoc 1986;86(2):109–114

Bibliography: Modern: Viscerosomatic Reflexes

Giles PD, Hensel KL, Pacchia CF, Smith ML. Suboccipital decompression enhances heart rate variability indices of cardiac control in healthy subjects. J Altern Complement Med 2013;19(2):92–96

Gwirtz PA, Dickey J, Vick D, Williams MA, Foresman B. Viscerosomatic interaction induced by myocardial ischemia in conscious dogs. J Appl Physiol (1985) 2007;103(2):511–517

Henderson AT, Fisher JF, Blair J, Shea C, Li TS, Bridges KG. Effects of rib raising on the autonomic nervous system: a pilot study using noninvasive biomarkers. J Am Osteopath Assoc 2010;110(6):324–330

Ruffini N, D'Alessandro G, Mariani N, Pollastrelli A, Cardinali L, Cerritelli F. Variations of high frequency parameter of heart rate variability following osteopathic manipulative treatment in healthy subjects compared to control group and sham therapy: randomized controlled trial. Front Neurosci 2015;9:272

Bibliography: Modern: Visceral Techniques

Caso ML. Evaluation of Chapman's neurolymphatic reflexes via applied kinesiology: a case report of low back pain and congenital intestinal abnormality. J Manipulative Physiol Ther 2004;27(1):66–72

Chapelle SL, Bove GM. Visceral massage reduces postoperative ileus in a rat model. J Bodyw Mov Ther 2013;17(1):83–88

Collebrusco L, Lombardini R. What about OMT and nutrition for managing the irritable bowel syndrome? An overview and treatment plan. Explore (NY) 2014;10(5):309–318

Heineman K. Osteopathic manipulative treatment in the management of biliary dyskinesia. J Am Osteopath Assoc 2014;114(2):129–133

Lalonde F. The runner's kidney: A case report. Int J Osteopath Med 2014;17(3):206–210

Mirocha NJ, Parker JD. Successful treatment of refractory functional dyspepsia with osteopathic manipulative treatment. Osteopathic Family Physician. 2012;4(6):193–196

Shadiack DO, et al. Osteopathic Manipulative Techniques Alter Gastric Myoelectrical Activity in Healthy Subjects;2016

Smilowicz A. An osteopathic approach to gastrointestinal disease: somatic clues for diagnosis and clinical challenges associated with Helicobacter pylori antibiotic resistance. J Am Osteopath Assoc 2013;113(5):404–416

Thomas CW, Gorodinsky L. Does osteopathic manipulative treatment (OMT) improves outcomes in patients who develop postoperative ileus: A retrospective chart review. Int J Osteopath Med 2009;12(1):32–37

Washington K, Mosiello R, Venditto M, et al. Presence of Chapman reflex points in hospitalized patients with pneumonia. J Am Osteopath Assoc 2003;103(10):479–483

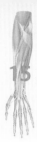

Counterstrain Techniques

LEARNING OBJECTIVES

1. Explain the goals of performing counterstrain techniques.
2. Identify the clinical considerations, including indications, contraindications, and precautions for performing counterstrain techniques.
3. Outline the general movements, barriers, and forces used to perform counterstrain techniques.
4. Identify the end goal for performing each counterstrain technique.
5. Visualize, verbalize, and identify the preparation, positioning, tissue contact, movements, barriers, and forces for each counterstrain technique.
6. Perform counterstrain techniques using appropriate somatic dysfunction diagnosis, preparation, positioning, tissue contact, movements, barriers, forces, retest for effectiveness, communication, and safe tissue handling.
7. Define a counterstrain tender point.

Counterstrain Techniques Introduction

Counterstrain (CS) technique is deceptively simple to perform and among the gentlest of techniques. Performing CS techniques can bring immediate and lasting relief to patients. A unique set of tender points has been mapped in relation to joint somatic dysfunction. These tender points are easy to find, and they resolve within 90 seconds after proper positioning of the patient.

Specificity in diagnosis and patient positioning, and awareness of related somatic dysfunctions are essential to the successful performance of this technique. The physician should avoid "chasing a patient's pain" by searching for tender points only. Each patient should be examined clinically, including osteopathic screening exams as well as focused exams for somatic dysfunction, to make an accurate clinical diagnosis and treatment plan. CS techniques are used by osteopathic physicians as well as manual therapists, owing to its ease of performance, safety, and efficacy.

CS techniques can achieve the following:

- Decrease pain.
- Restore muscular tension and tone.
- Improve joint motion.
- Improve arterial, venous, and lymph circulation.

Background

Counterstrain is a relatively modern osteopathic technique with a unique history. It was discovered and developed by Lawrence Jones, DO, in the 1950s. Dr. Jones initially discovered a system of resolving somatic dysfunction by finding tender areas, then positioning patients so that the tenderness resolved. Thus it was initially called spontaneous release by positioning. However, the name was changed to Jones strain-counterstrain because this better reflected what is believed to be the underlying physiological mechanism for the development and resolution of the tenderness of a tender point.[1] Dr. Jones correlated and named tender points to bones, joints, or nerves. Paul Rennie, DO, FAAO, correlated some tender points with muscles, and renamed them accordingly in his counterstrain manual.[2] This manual uses the names of muscles when appropriate and references Dr. Jones's original name.

Research

A short research bibliography is located at the end of this chapter. One study that may be of interest to novice students, in particular, is "Frequency of Counterstrain Tender Points in Osteopathic Medical Students" by Karen Snider, DO, who has also published a counterstrain manual.[3,4]

Clinical Considerations

Some common, clinical things to consider for CS technique are listed in Table 15.1. Always acquire adequate data in the form of an appropriate history, a thorough physical exam that includes an exam for somatic dysfunction, and relevant diagnostic tests to exercise best clinical judgment before performing osteopathic manipulative treatment.

Somatic Dysfunction Corrected: Tender Points

CS techniques rely on the use of a unique somatic dysfunction diagnosis: a tender point. Tender points are specific points on the body, ~ 0.5 cm in diameter, that are tender when local muscles, ligaments, or joints have somatic dysfunction. They are generated by aberrant nervous system activity due to abnormal tissue tensions and joint positions related to somatic dysfunction. Specifically, nociceptor and gamma efferent neuronal activity is increased, which causes pain and muscle contraction. Note that normal tissues will not manifest a tender point. As a general rule, tender points can be found in a few different locations: (1) the tendinous insertion of a muscle, (2) the belly of a muscle, (3) the periosteum, (4) a ligament, and (5) the anterior trunk wall. Those in the anterior trunk wall are correlated to posterior spinal tender points, which correlate to vertebral segmental somatic dysfunction.

To determine if a tender point is present, a gentle force should be applied with the finger pad into the tissues that are deep to the superficially mapped tender point location. Enough pressure should be used so that the physician's fingernail blanches, but not so much as to cause pain in the absence of somatic dysfunction. The same force is

Table 15.1	Clinical considerations		
Indications	**Contraindications**	**Precautions**
Acute minor musculoskeletal injuries Mechanical neck and back pain Temporomandibular joint pain Headache Muscle strains Muscle spasm Chronic pain conditions	Fracture or suspected fracture	This technique may be difficult to perform on patients who are unable to remain still, such as infants and children.

to be used during the technique performance to rate the tenderness of the tender point. The location of the tender point as well as the directional force to use for diagnosis and rating are found in each technique description.

In clinical practice, it is common that groups of tender points in one region are assessed to identify the most tender of tender points. For example, when a patient has neck pain, bilateral anterior and posterior cervical tender points should be assessed. Then the most tender of tender points is corrected first. The clinical recommendation is to perform a CS technique on three or fewer tender points in one region during a treatment session to avoid overtreatment. Clinical judgment is warranted.

- Somatic dysfunction diagnosis: indicate the location of the tender point. Commonly used abbreviations are listed by each tender point name.
  - Examples: right masseter tender point (TP), left PC7 TP.

Positioning and Preparation

▶ Patient: the patient must be comfortable and remain relaxed for the duration of the technique. CS techniques can be performed with the patient seated, supine, prone, or laterally recumbent. Occasionally, the patient may be asked to assist in creating the initial position. The patient must relax after any active positioning.

▶ Physician: the physician must be comfortable and positioned to ensure safety, using the best ergonomic posture and movements possible.

Tissue Contact

- Rating and monitoring hand: the pad of a finger should be used to rate the tender point for tenderness and to maintain contact with it throughout the duration of the technique.
  - If necessary for the physician's or patient's safety, the physician may stop monitoring the tender point.
- Performing hand: this contact is used to grossly position the patient. When the position of ease is found, the patient is held still for the duration of the technique. Recommended positions are in tables in each technique description. Positions should be adjusted to ensure proper ergonomics, while maintaining the position for at least 90 seconds without moving.

Movements, Barriers, and Forces

CS techniques are indirect, passive techniques that require patients to remain in a relaxed state. The end goal is to eliminate tenderness of a tender point, so as to resolve associated joint, fascial, and/or muscular somatic dysfunction. Significant reduction or elimination of tenderness is an indicator that abnormal activity in nociceptors and gamma motor fibers has been normalized.

CS techniques begin by asking the patient to "rate the tenderness of the tender point." This is done using the same direction(s) and forces used to identify the tender point. It is best to first present a rating system for the patient to use. Two suggestions are offered in Table 15.2.

Physician movements are created to place the patient into a position that reduces the tender-

Table 15.2	Suggested counterstrain tender point tenderness rating systems	
Rating by the patient	**Rating: numerical scale**	**Rating: percentage**
Initial: Before positioning, ask the patient to remember the initial tenderness as a maximum rating	"Rate this tenderness as a 10 out of 10 on a pain scale from 0 to 10."	"Rate this tenderness as 100% tender."
Retesting: After positioning, ask the patient to re-rate the tenderness.	"The initial tenderness was a 10 out of 10. What is it now?"	"The initial tenderness was at 100%. What percentage is the tenderness now?"
Appropriate positioning is achieved and the technique is effective when:	The patient reports a 3 or lower on the pain scale.	The patient reports that the tenderness is 30% or less.

ness of the tender point by 70%, although complete elimination of tenderness is ideal. This position is called the position of ease. At 70% reduction of tenderness, neuronal activity has been sufficiently affected. To determine if the tenderness has been reduced, the physician presses into the tender point and asks the patient to rate the tenderness. If the tenderness has not decreased by at least 70%, then the physician should make small adjustments to the patient's position, in one direction at a time, until at least a 70% reduction of the initial tenderness is achieved. At each adjustment, the tender point should be retested for tenderness. For example, when positioning the neck to resolve an anterior C4 tender point on the right, the initial position is flexion, left side bending and left rotation. If after initial positioning the tenderness is reduced by 50%, the physician can increase the amount of flexion and retest for tenderness. If the tenderness is still not reduced, the head should be returned back to the initial position, and the amount of side bending increased, again retesting for tenderness. This cycle of positioning and retesting for tenderness continues until at least 70% reduction is obtained. The degree and directions of movement to create to find the position of ease are somewhat arbitrary but often within the recommended positions. It is possible, but not common, that the required positioning is entirely different from the recommended positioning. This is especially true in cases of trauma where the body was subjected to excessive forces in multiple directions.

After the position of ease is found, the patient is held in this position until a tissue release is palpated with the monitoring hand, or for about 90 seconds.[1] Ninety seconds is approximately the time it takes for the gamma motor neurons to "reset" to normal activity, and for the tissues to release. Tissue release can be palpated as softening, sometimes accompanied by a pulsation from the resultant improvement in fluid circulation. Even when the physician is unable to palpate a tissue release, assuming proper diagnosis and positioning, the tissues should still release after about 90 seconds.

Both the physician and the patient should remain still to avoid activation of the musculature and the nervous system. If the patient or physician moves before a release occurs, or before 90 seconds have elapsed, the physician should retest the tender point for tenderness. If the tenderness is not increased from the initial positioning, the position may be held for the remainder of the 90 seconds. If the tenderness is increased, the patient must be repositioned into a position of ease and held for another 90 seconds.

When a release is palpated, or after 90 seconds, the physician returns the patient, who must remain relaxed, to a neutral position. The patient must remain relaxed to avoid sudden neuronal activation or contraction of the tissues that just released. It is important to clearly communicate this to the patient. Finally, when the patient has been returned to a neutral position, the tenderness of the tender point is retested using the same rating system.

Communicating a Rating Scale for Tenderness of a Tender Point

A tender point is subjective and must be rated for the amount of tenderness by the patient. A numerical or percentage rating system may be used and customized by the physician. Two examples are provided in Table 15.2. To rate the tenderness, the same direction and amount of force are used as when diagnosing the tender point.

Retest for Effectiveness

Complete resolution of tenderness or at least 70% reduction in tenderness of the tender point, indicates that the technique was effective. The underlying somatic dysfunction is also likely corrected. If the tenderness of the tender point does not resolve by 70% or more, it is possible that the tender point is not due to dysfunction within the soma. For example, tenderness due to an inflamed appendix at McBurney's point, which is very close to the iliopsoas tender point, will not resolve with CS technique. It is also possible that there are associated joint, fascial, or viscerosomatic reflexes. Therefore, a thorough examination is warranted.

- Retest documentation: indicate if the tenderness is resolved, improved, or unchanged with the CS technique.

Counterstrain Technique Summary Steps

Each technique lists the summary steps, along with a table of the tender point locations and the recommended patient positioning.

CS Technique Summary Steps

- Identify a tender counterstrain tender point.
- With the monitoring hand, ask the patient to rate the tenderness of the tender point.

- Be sure that the patient is passive and remains relaxed throughout the duration of the technique.
- With the performing hand, move the patient into the recommended position(s).
- With the monitoring hand, ask the patient to rate the tender point for tenderness.
- Move the patient as necessary until the patient reports a reduction of tenderness of 70% or more.
  - Retest the tender point for tenderness with each position change.
- Hold the patient in this position until the tissues release or for 90 seconds.
- Slowly return the patient to a neutral position. The patient should remain relaxed.
- Retest the tender point for tenderness using the initial rating system.

Learner Tip

The phrase "find it, fold, it and hold it" can help students remember the basic steps of performing CS techniques.

- Find it: find the tender point (step 1).
- Fold it: fold the body region around the tender point until the tenderness reduces/is eliminated (steps 3–5).
- Hold it: hold that position for 90 seconds (step 6).

Note: Videos are not performed in real time, but instead demonstrate the location, palpation, and monitoring of the tender point; patient positioning; return to neutral; and retesting of the tenderness of the tender point. When the tender point positions are similar, there is only one video example. The positions are not held for 90 seconds.

Head: Medial Pterygoid, Masseter

These techniques are useful for cases of bruxism and pain related to temporomandibular joint dysfunction (**Fig. 15.1**). Because the jaw is being moved, consider asking these patients to raise a hand to let you know when the tenderness of the tender point is reduced by 70%.

Key Elements

- Somatic dysfunction corrected: right/left: masseter, medial pterygoid tender points (Table 15.3).
  - Directional force to diagnose and rate the tender point for tenderness.
    - Masseter: apply perpendicularly directed force into the muscle belly.
    - Medial pterygoid: apply anteriorly directed force onto the mandible.
- End goal: to resolve local somatic dysfunction by significant reduction or elimination of the tenderness of the associated tender point(s) by positioning the jaw.

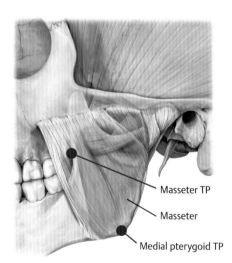

Fig. 15.1 Counterstrain tender points: medial pterygoid, masseter.

Table 15.3	Counterstrain: head: medial pterygoid, masseter tender points	
Tender point (TP)	Locations: bilateral	Recommended patient positioning: jaw
Masseter	Belly of the masseter muscle, anterior to the ascending ramus of the mandible	*Right TP* Right translation with the jaw open
Medial pterygoid	Posterior, inferior aspect of the angle of the mandible	*Left TP* Left translation with the jaw open

WATCH ▷▶▷

▶ *Video 15.1 Head, Left Medial Pterygoid TP*

Positioning and Preparation

▶ Patient: supine.
▶ Physician: seated or standing at the head of the table.

Tissue Contact

- Monitoring and rating hand: contact the tender point with the pad of the second finger.
- Performing hand: contact the jaw with the fingertips and thumb to move it.

Movements, Barriers, and Forces

- With the monitoring hand, ask the patient to rate the tenderness of the tender point.
- Ask the patient to slightly open the jaw then relax it.
  - Be sure that the patient remains relaxed throughout the duration of the technique.
- With the performing hand, move the jaw into the recommended position.
- With the monitoring hand, ask the patient to rate the tender point for tenderness.
- Move the patient with increased or decreased jaw translation until the patient reports a reduction of tenderness of 70% or more.
  - Retest the tender point for tenderness with each position change.
- Hold the patient's jaw in this position until the tissues release or for 90 seconds.
- Slowly return the patient's jaw to a neutral position. The patient should remain relaxed.
- Retest the tender point for tenderness using the initial rating system.

Cervical, Anterior 1–8

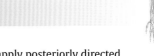

Cervical CS is an excellent technique for patients who have had whiplash injuries and those with acute neck pain (**Fig. 15.2**). In the case of whiplash injuries, examine both anterior and posterior tender points to determine which tender point is most tender. The tender points are numbered sequentially based on the exiting spinal nerve root.

Key Elements

- Somatic dysfunction corrected: right/left anterior cervical tender points 1–8 (AC1–8) (Table 15.4).
  - Directional force to use when rating for tenderness:
    - AC1: apply anteriorly directed force onto the periosteum of the mandible.
    - AC2–6: apply posteriorly and slightly medially directed force onto the periosteum of the tip of the transverse process.
    - AC7: apply posteriorly directed force onto the periosteum of the superior, medial edge of the clavicle at the clavicular attachment of the sternocleidomastoid muscle.
    - AC8: apply laterally directed force onto the periosteum of the medial edges of the clavicle at the sternal notch, at the sternal attachment of the sternocleidomastoid muscle.
- End goal: to resolve local somatic dysfunction by significant reduction or elimination of the tenderness of the associated tender point(s) by positioning the neck.

WATCH ▷▶▷

▶ *Video 15.2 Cervical, Left AC1 TP*
▶ *Video 15.3 Cervical, Left AC3 TP*

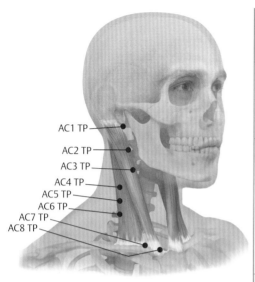

AC1 TP
AC2 TP
AC3 TP
AC4 TP
AC5 TP
AC6 TP
AC7 TP
AC8 TP

Fig. 15.2 Counterstrain tender points: AC1–AC8.

Table 15.4 Counterstrain: cervical, anterior 1–8 tender points[a]		
Tender point (TP)	**Locations: right and left**	**Recommended patient positioning: head and neck**
Anterior cervical 1 (AC1)	Ascending ramus of the mandible, posterior aspect near the middle of the ramus	*Right TP* Left rotation *Left TP* Right rotation Note: rotation is often ~ 90 degrees
Anterior cervical 2, 3, 4, 5, 6 (AC2, AC3, AC4, AC5, AC6)	Transverse process: anterolateral tip of the vertebra of the same name. Note: AC2–3 are located anterior to the sternocleidomastoid muscle, whereas AC4–6 are located posterior	*Right TPs* Flexion Left rotation Left side bending *Left TPs* Flexion Right rotation Right side bending
Anterior cervical 7 (AC7)	Clavicle, at the clavicular attachment of the sternocleidomastoid muscle	*Right TP* Flexion, marked Left rotation Right side bending *Left TP* Flexion, marked Right rotation Left side bending
Anterior cervical 8 (AC8)	Clavicle, at the sternal attachment of the sternocleidomastoid muscle	*Right TP* Flexion Left rotation Left side bending *Left TP* Flexion Right rotation Right side bending

Positioning and Preparation

▶ Patient: supine.
▶ Physician: seated or standing at the head of the table.

Tissue Contact

• Monitoring and rating hand: contact the tender point with the pad of the second finger.
• Performing hand: contact the posterior occiput and neck to move and hold it.

Movements, Barriers, and Forces

• With the monitoring hand, ask the patient to rate the tenderness of the tender point.
  – Be sure that the patient is passive and remains relaxed throughout the duration of the technique.

• With the performing hand, lift and move the patient's head and neck into the recommended initial position(s).
• With the monitoring hand, ask the patient to rate the tender point for tenderness.
• Move the patient's head and neck as necessary until the patient reports a reduction of tenderness of 70% or more.
  – Retest the tender point for tenderness with each position change.
• Hold the patient in this position until the tissues release or for 90 seconds.
• Slowly return the patient's head and neck to a neutral position. The patient should remain relaxed.
• Retest the tender point for tenderness using the initial rating system.

Cervical, Posterior 1–8

The tender points are numbered sequentially based on the exiting spinal nerve root (**Fig. 15.3**). Note that PC2 is on the superior aspect of the spinous process of C2, but PC3 is on the inferior aspect of the spinous process of C2.

Key Elements

- Somatic dysfunction corrected: right/left posterior cervical tender points 1–8 (PC1–8) (Table 15.5).
    - Directional force to diagnose and rate the tender point for tenderness:
        - PC1: apply anteriorly directed force into the occipital attachments of the trapezius and semispinalis capitis muscles.
        - PC2–8: apply anterior and medially directed force onto the side of the spinous process.
- End goal: to resolve local somatic dysfunction by significant reduction or elimination of the tenderness of the associated tender point(s) by positioning the neck.

WATCH ▷ ▶ ▷

- ▶ *Video 15.4 Cervical, Left PC1 TP*
- ▶ *Video 15.5 Cervical, Left PC5 TP*

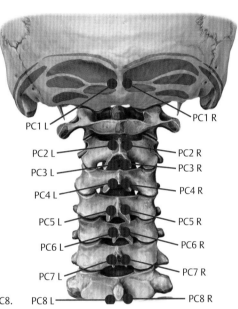

PC1 L PC1 R
PC2 L PC2 R
PC3 L PC3 R
PC4 L PC4 R
PC5 L PC5 R
PC6 L PC6 R
PC7 L PC7 R
PC8 L PC8 R

Fig. 15.3   Counterstrain tender points: PC1–PC8.

Table 15.5 Counterstrain: cervical, posterior 1–8 tender points		
Tender point (TP)	**Locations: right and left**	**Recommended patient positioning: head and neck**
Posterior cervical (PC1)	Occiput: a few centimeters lateral to the inion, below the nuchal line, in the trapezius and semispinalis capitis muscles	*Right or left TP* Extension (head only), with mild compression to shorten the musculature
PC2	Spinous process of C2: superolateral edges	*Right or Left TP* Extension (head and neck), with mild compression to shorten the musculature
PC3	Spinous process of C2: inferolateral edges	*Right TP* Flexion Left side bending Left rotation *Left TP* Flexion Left side bending Left rotation
PC4	Spinous process of C3: inferolateral edges	*Right TP* Extension Left rotation Left side bending *Left TP* Extension Right rotation Right side bending
PC5	Spinous process of C4: inferolateral edges	
PC6	Spinous process of C5: inferolateral edges	
PC7	Spinous process of C6: inferolateral edges	
PC8	Spinous process of C7: inferolateral edges	

Positioning and Preparation

▶ Patient: supine, with shoulders near the upper edge of the table.

    – Additional patient positioning: ask the patient to slide superiorly so the head falls off the table. As the head falls off, place your hand underneath to support it.

▶ Physician: seated at the head of the table.

    – During technique performance, consider placing your elbow on your thigh for additional support to hold the head and neck.

Tissue Contact

• Monitoring and rating hand: contact the tender point with the pad of the second finger.

• Performing hand: contact the posterior occiput and neck to move and hold it.

Movements, Barriers, and Forces

• With the monitoring hand, ask the patient to rate the tenderness of the tender point.

• With the performing hand, guide the patient's head into the recommended initial position(s).

    – Create only enough extension that the posterior cervical musculature relaxes. Do not hyperextend the neck.

• With the monitoring hand, ask the patient to rate the tender point for tenderness.

• Move the patient as necessary until the patient reports a reduction of tenderness of 70% or more.

    – Retest the tender point for tenderness with each position change.

• Hold the patient in this position until the tissues release or for 90 seconds.

• Slowly return the patient's head and neck to a neutral position. The patient should remain relaxed. Then ask the patient to slide inferiorly so the head can rest on the table.

• Retest the tender point for tenderness using the initial rating system.

Upper Extremity: Levator Scapulae, Supraspinatus, Infraspinatus

These techniques are excellent for treating minor rotator cuff strains or other mechanical shoulder pain (**Fig. 15.4**). The subscapularis tender point can be exquisitely tender, and a good tender point to know to help resolve cases of functional shoulder pain. Proceed cautiously when palpating this tender point, being sure to contact the subscapularis muscle, which is attached to the anterior scapular surface.

Key Elements

• Somatic dysfunction corrected: right/left: levator scapulae tender point, supraspinatus tender point, infraspinatus tender point (Table 15.6).

    – Directional force to diagnose and rate the tender point for tenderness: apply perpendicularly directed force into the musculature.

• End goal: to resolve local somatic dysfunction by significant reduction or elimination of the tenderness of the associated tender point(s) by positioning the upper extremity.

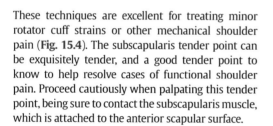

WATCH ▷ ▶ ▷

▶ *Video 15.6 Upper Extremity, Left Levator Scapulae TP*

▶ *Video 15.7 Upper Extremity, Left Supraspinatus TP*

▶ *Video 15.8 Upper Extremity, Left Infraspinatus TP*

Positioning and Preparation

▶ Patient: lateral recumbent, with the affected shoulder off the table.

    – Alternatively, the patient can be supine and close to the edge of the table on the side of the tender point.

▶ Physician: standing on the side of the table behind the patient at the level of the shoulder.

Fig. 15.4 Counterstrain tender points: levator scapulae, supraspinatus, infraspinatus.

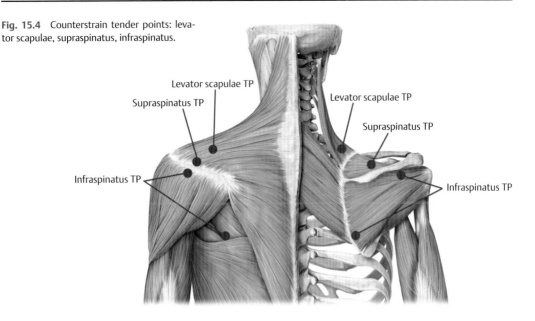

Tender point (TP)	Locations: right and left	Recommended patient positioning
Table 15.6 Counterstrain: upper extremity: levator scapulae, supraspinatus, infraspinatus tender points		
Levator scapulae	Levator scapula muscle, scapular attachment	Scapula elevation Optional: cervical side bending toward the side of the TP
Supraspinatus	Supraspinatus muscle belly	Arm and shoulder Flexion Abduction External rotation All positions are ~ 45 degrees
Infraspinatus	Infraspinatus muscle, belly or inferior attachment	Arm and shoulder Flexion, marked Abduction, ~ 45 degrees External rotation, ~ 45 degrees

[a]Note: The suggested degree of cervical flexion, rotation and side bending is ~ 45° unless otherwise indicated.

Tissue Contact

- Monitoring and rating hand: contact the tender point with the pad of the second finger.
- Performing hand: contact the arm on the side of the tender point with the palm and fingers so as to grasp it. It may be helpful to bend the patient's elbow and hold the arm at the elbow.

Movements, Barriers, and Forces

- With the monitoring hand, ask the patient to rate the tenderness of the tender point.
- With the performing hand, move the patient's shoulder and arm into the recommended positions.

- With the monitoring hand, ask the patient to rate the tender point for tenderness.
- Move the patient's shoulder/arm as necessary until the patient reports a reduction of tenderness of 70% or more.
  - Retest the tender point for tenderness with each position change.
- Hold the patient in this position until the tissues release or for 90 seconds.
- Slowly return the patient's shoulder/arm to a neutral position. The patient should remain relaxed.
- Retest the tender point for tenderness using the initial rating system.

Upper Extremity: Pectoralis Minor, Biceps Tendon, Subscapularis

The biceps and pectoralis tender points are often tender in cases of biceps tendonitis and acromioclavicular impingement (**Fig. 15.5** and **Fig. 15.6**). Look for a subscapularis tender point in cases of nonspecific musculoskeletal shoulder pain.

Key Elements

- Somatic dysfunction corrected: right/left: pectoralis minor tender point, biceps tendon tender point, subscapularis tender point (Table 15.7).
  - Directional force to diagnose and rate the tender point for tenderness: Apply perpendicularly directed force into the musculature (pectoralis minor and subscapularis) or tendon (biceps).
- End goal: to resolve local somatic dysfunction by significant reduction or elimination of the tenderness of the associated tender point(s) by positioning the upper extremity.

> ### WATCH ▷▶▷
>
> ▶ *Video 15.9 Upper Extremity, Left Pectoralis Minor TP*
>
> ▶ *Video 15.10 Upper Extremity, Left Biceps Tendon TP*
>
> ▶ *Video 15.11 Upper Extremity, Left Subscapularis TP*

Positioning and Preparation

- ▶ Patient: supine, with the affected shoulder near the edge of the table.
- ▶ Physician: seated or standing beside the table at the level of the patient's torso on the side of the tender point.

Fig. 15.6 Counterstrain tender point: subscapularis.

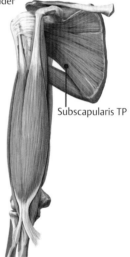

Subscapularis TP

Fig. 15.5 Counterstrain tender points: pectoralis minor, biceps tendon.

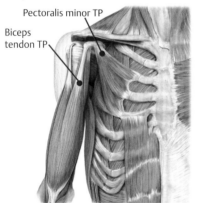

Pectoralis minor TP

Biceps tendon TP

Table 15.7	Counterstrain: upper extremity: pectoralis minor, biceps tendon, subscapularis tender points	
Tender point (TP)	**Locations: right and left**	**Recommended patient positioning**
Pectoralis minor	Pectoralis minor, attachment at the coracoid process	*Shoulder/arm:* Flexion, ~ 90 degrees Adduction, moderate Inferior traction, slight
Biceps	Biceps tendon, long head	*Shoulder:* Flexion, full Internal rotation, slight *Elbow:* Flexion, full *Forearm:* Supination, full
Subscapularis	Subscapularis muscle, inferior scapular attachment	*Shoulder/arm:* Extension, ~ 45 degrees Internal rotation, slight Abduction, slight

Tissue Contact

- Monitoring and rating hand: contact the tender point with the pad of the second finger.
- Performing hand: contact the arm on the side of the tender point with the palm and fingers so as to grasp it. It may be helpful to bend the patient's elbow and hold the arm at the elbow.

Movements, Barriers, and Forces

- With the monitoring hand, ask the patient to rate the tenderness of the tender point.
- With the performing hand, move the patient's shoulder and arm into the recommended positions.

- With the monitoring hand, ask the patient to rate the tender point for tenderness.
- Move the patient as necessary until the patient reports a reduction of tenderness of 70% or more.
  - Retest the tender point for tenderness with each position change.
- Hold the patient's shoulder and arm in this position until the tissues release or for 90 seconds.
- Slowly return the patient's shoulder and arm to a neutral position. The patient should remain relaxed.
- Retest the tender point for tenderness using the initial rating system.

Upper Extremity: Pronator, Supinator

The pronator tender point is often found in cases of medial epicondylitis and the supinator tender point is found in cases of lateral epicondylitis (**Fig. 15.7**).

Key Elements

- Somatic dysfunction corrected: right/left: pronator or supinator tender point (Table 15.8).
  - Directional force to diagnose and rate the tender point for tenderness: apply perpendicularly directed force into the musculature.
- End goal: to resolve local somatic dysfunction by significant reduction or elimination of the tenderness of the associated tender point(s) by positioning the arm.

> **WATCH** ▷ ▶ ▷
> ───────────────────────
> ▶ *Video 15.12 Upper Extremity, Left Pronator TP*
> ▶ *Video 15.13 Upper Extremity, Left Supinator TP*

Fig. 15.7 Counterstrain tender points: pronator, supinator.

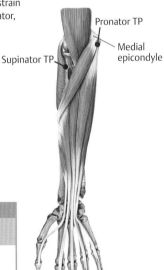

Pronator TP

Medial epicondyle

Supinator TP

Table 15.8	Counterstrain: upper extremity: pronator, supinator tender points	
Tender point (TP)	Locations: right and left	Recommended patient positioning
Pronator (also called medial epicondyle)	Pronator teres muscle: near attachment on medial epicondyle	*Elbow:* Flexion, ~ 90 degrees Adduction, moderate *Forearm:* Pronation, full
Supinator (also called radial head)	Supinator muscle: near attachment on the radial head	*Elbow:* Extension Abduction, moderate *Forearm:* supination, full

Positioning and Preparation

▶ Patient: supine.

▶ Physician: seated or standing beside the table near the arm with the tender tender point.

Tissue Contact

• Monitoring and rating hand: contact the tender point with the pad of the second finger.

• Performing hand: contact the wrist on the side of the tender point with the palm and fingers so as to grasp and move it.

Movements, Barriers, and Forces

• With the monitoring hand, ask the patient to rate the tenderness of the tender point.

• With the performing hand, move the patient's arm into the recommended positions.

• With the monitoring hand, ask the patient to rate the tender point for tenderness.

• Move the patient's arm as necessary until the patient reports a reduction of tenderness of 70% or more.

  – Retest the tender point for tenderness with each position change.

• Hold the patient in this position until the tissues release or for 90 seconds.

• Slowly return the patient's arm to a neutral position. The patient should remain relaxed.

• Retest the tender point for tenderness using the initial rating system.

Lumbar/Pelvis: Psoas, Iliacus

The iliacus and psoas tender points are excellent for cases of low back pain and of course, psoas syndrome (**Fig. 15.8**). They are found in the musculature that is deep in the abdomen.

Key Elements

• Somatic dysfunction corrected: right/left: psoas, iliacus tender points (Table 15.9).

  – Directional force to diagnose and rate the tender point for tenderness: apply posteriorly directed force into the musculature, using layer palpation to find the tender points: skin → superficial fascia → abdominal musculature → deep fascia → visceral organs → musculature.

• End goal: to resolve local somatic dysfunction by significant reduction or elimination of the tenderness of the associated tender point(s) by positioning the hip.

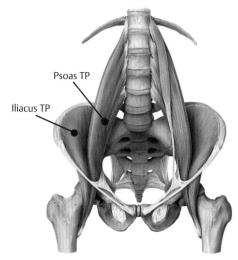

Fig. 15.8   Counterstrain tender points: psoas, iliacus.

Table 15.9	Counterstrain: lumbar/pelvis: psoas, iliacus tender points	
Tender point (TP)	**Locations: right and left**	**Recommended patient positioning**
Psoas	Psoas muscle: in the muscle belly, approximately at a point that is two-thirds of the distance from the anterior superior iliac spine to the midline of the abdomen	Bilateral hip flexion, 90 degrees Bilateral hip external rotation
Iliacus	Iliacus muscle: in the muscle belly in the iliac fossa, approximately at a point that is one-third of the distance from the anterior superior iliac spine to midline of the abdomen	Bilateral hip flexion, 90 degrees Bilateral hip external rotation, marked

WATCH ▷▶▷

▶ *Video 15.14 Lumbar/Pelvis, Right Psoas TP*

Positioning and Preparation

▶ Patient: supine.

▶ Physician: standing beside the table at the side of the tender tender point at the level of the patient's pelvis, facing the patient, with the table a few inches below the customary height.

▶ Additional patient positioning: ask the patient to bend the knees and place the feet on the table. Place your foot that is closer to the patient's feet flat on the table, bending your knee. Lift, or ask the patient to place, the ankles upon your bent knee. The patient's hips and knees should both be bent to ~ 90 degrees.

Tissue Contact

• Monitoring and rating hand: contact the tender point with the pad of the second finger.

• Performing contact: contact the patient's ankles and knees as necessary to move the ankles and knees in the technique steps. Use your knees to assist with this movement.

Movements, Barriers, and Forces

• With the monitoring hand, ask the patient to rate the tenderness of the tender point.

• Ask the patient to relax the legs. With the assisting contacts, move the patient's ankles and knees to move the hips into the recommended positions.
  – Move your thigh and body to do this.

• With the monitoring hand, ask the patient to rate tender point for tenderness.

• Move the patient's hips and knees as necessary until the patient reports a reduction of tenderness of 70% or more.
  – Retest the tender point for tenderness with each position change.

• Hold the patient in this position until the tissues release or for 90 seconds.

• Slowly return the patient to a neutral position. The patient should remain relaxed.

• Retest the tender point for tenderness using the initial rating system.

Lower Extremity: Piriformis, Gluteus Medius, Iliotibial Tract

Treatment of a piriformis tender point can be curative in cases of piriformis syndrome and sciatica (**Fig. 15.9** and **Fig. 15.10**). Runners and cyclists will benefit from treatment of the iliotibial tract tender point.

Key Elements

• Somatic dysfunction corrected: right/left: piriformis tender point, gluteus medius tender point, iliotibial tract tender point (Table 15.10).
  – Directional force to diagnose and rate the tender point for tenderness: apply perpendicularly directed force into the musculature.

• End goal: to resolve local somatic dysfunction by significant reduction or elimination of the tenderness of the associated tender point(s) by positioning the hips.

WATCH ▷▶▷

▶ *Video 15.15 Lower Extremity, Right Piriformis TP*

▶ *Video 15.16 Lower Extremity, Right Gluteus Medius TP*

Positioning and Preparation

▶ Patient: prone, with the side of the tender tender point near the edge of the table. For the piriformis tender point the patient may have to slide so the thigh can fall off the table.

▶ Physician:
  – Piriformis tender point: seated on the rolling stool at the level of the patient's knees. Hold the patient's thigh and move

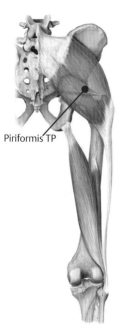

Fig. 15.9 Counterstrain tender point: piriformis.

Piriformis TP

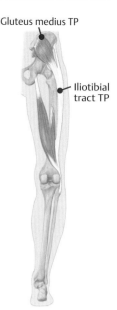

Gluteus medius TP

Iliotibial tract TP

Fig. 15.10 Counterstrain tender points: gluteus medius, iliotibial tract.

Table 15.10	Counterstrain: lower extremity: piriformis, gluteus medius, iliotibial tract tender points	
Tender point (TP)	**Locations: right and left**	**Recommended patient positioning: hip on the side of the tender point**
Piriformis	Piriformis muscle belly	Flexion, marked (> 90 degrees) Abduction, moderate External rotation, moderate
Gluteus medius	Gluteus medius muscle, near the lateral attachment on the iliac crest	Extension, moderate Abduction, slight External rotation, slight
Iliotibial tract (also called lateral trochanter)	Iliotibial tract, anywhere	Abduction, moderate

your entire body with the rolling chair to position the patient.

- – Gluteus medius tender point, iliotibial tract tender point: standing beside the table on the side of the tender tender point at the level of the patient's pelvis, facing the patient, with the table a few inches below the customary level.

▶ Alternate patient positioning: supine for correction of an iliotibial tract tender point.

Tissue Contact

- Monitoring and rating hand: contact the tender point with the pad of the second finger.
- Performing hand: contact the patient's thigh just superior to the patella to lift the thigh.

Movements, Barriers, and Forces

- With the monitoring hand, ask the patient to rate the tenderness of the tender point.
- Ask the patient to relax the leg that has the tender point. Lift and move the leg to position the hip into the recommended positions.
- With the monitoring hand, ask the patient to rate the tender point for tenderness.
- Move the patient if necessary, each time rating for tenderness, until the patient reports a reduction of 70% or more.
- Hold the patient in this position until the tissues release or for 90 seconds.
- Slowly return the patient's leg and hip to a neutral position. The patient should remain relaxed.
- Retest the tender point for tenderness using the initial rating system.

Lower Extremity: Popliteus, Gastrocnemius

The popliteus tender point is often present in cases of minor knee pain (**Fig. 15.11** and **Fig. 15.12**). The gastrocnemius tender points can be used as part of treatment for heel pain or plantar fasciitis.

Key Elements

- Somatic dysfunction corrected: right/left: popliteus tender point, gastrocnemius tender point (Table 15.11).
  - Directional force to diagnose and rate the tender point for tenderness: apply perpendicularly directed force into the musculature.
- End goal: to resolve local somatic dysfunction by significant reduction or elimination of the tenderness of the associated tender point(s) by positioning the lower extremity.

> **WATCH** ▷ ► ▷
> ---
> ► *Video 15.17 Lower Extremity, Right Popliteus TP*

Positioning and Preparation

▶ Patient: prone.
▶ Physician: standing beside the table at the level of the patient's knees, facing the patient.

Tissue Contact

- Monitoring and rating hand: contact the tender point with the pad of the second finger.
- Performing hand: contact the patient's ankle (popliteus) or calcaneus (gastrocnemius).

Movements, Barriers, and Forces

- With the monitoring hand, ask the patient to rate the tenderness of the tender point.
- Ask the patient to relax the leg that has the tender point. Flex the knee to ~ 90 degrees to position the tibia, ankle, and/or calcaneus into the recommended positions.
- With the monitoring hand, ask the patient to rate the tender point for tenderness.
- Move the patient's ankle as necessary until the patient reports a reduction of tenderness of 70% or more.
  - Retest the tender point for tenderness with each position change.
- Hold the patient in this position until the tissues release or for 90 seconds.
- Slowly return the patient's ankle and knee to a neutral position. The patient should remain relaxed.
- Retest the tender point for tenderness using the initial rating system.

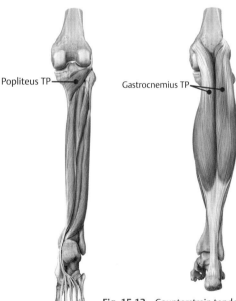

Fig. 15.11 Counterstrain tender point: popliteus.

Popliteus TP

Gastrocnemius TP

Fig. 15.12 Counterstrain tender points: gastrocnemius.

Table 15.11 Counterstrain: lower extremity: popliteus, gastrocnemius tender points		
Tender point (TP)	**Locations: right and left**	**Recommended patient positioning**
Popliteus	Popliteus muscle belly	Knee: flexion Tibia: internal rotation
Gastrocnemius (also called extension ankle)	There are two points in each gastrocnemius muscle: one in the medial and one in the lateral section	Knee: flexion Ankle: plantar flexion Compression: from the calcaneus into the knee

Lower Extremity: Peroneus Longus, Tibialis Anterior

The peroneus longus and tibialis anterior tender points may be associated with shin splints, foot drop, and nonarticular or nonspecific knee or ankle pain (**Fig. 15.13** and **Fig. 15.14**).

Key Elements

- Somatic dysfunction corrected: right/left: peroneus longus tender points, tibialis anterior tender point (Table 15.12).
  - Directional force to diagnose and rate the tender point for tenderness: apply perpendicularly directed force into the musculature.
- End goal: to resolve local somatic dysfunction by significant reduction or elimination of the tenderness of the associated tender point(s) by positioning the lower extremity.

> **WATCH** ▷▶▷
>
> ▶ **Video 15.18 Lower Extremity, Right Peroneus Longus TP**

Fig. 15.13 Counterstrain tender point: peroneus longus.

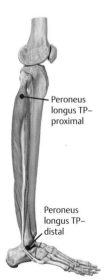

Peroneus longus TP– proximal

Peroneus longus TP– distal

Fig. 15.14 Counterstrain tender points: tibialis anterior.

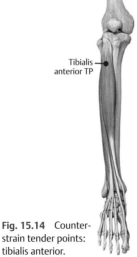

Tibialis anterior TP

Positioning and Preparation

- ▶ Patient: supine or prone.
- ▶ Physician: standing beside the table at the level of the patient's knees, facing the patient.

Tissue Contact

- Monitoring and rating hand: contact the tender point with the pad of the second finger.
- Performing hand: contact the patient's ankle.

Movements, Barriers, and Forces

- With the monitoring hand, ask the patient to rate the tenderness of the tender point.
- Ask the patient to relax the leg.
- With the performing hand, move the patient's foot and ankle into the recommended positions.
- With the monitoring hand, ask the patient to rate the tender point for tenderness.
- Move the patient if necessary, each time rating for tenderness, until the patient reports a reduction of 70% or more.
- Hold the patient in this position until the tissues release or for 90 seconds.
- Slowly return the patient's ankle and foot to a neutral position. The patient should remain relaxed.
- Retest the tender point for tenderness using the initial rating system.

Table 15.12 Counterstrain: lower extremity: peroneus longus, tibialis anterior tender points		
Tender point (TP)	**Locations: right and left**	**Recommended patient positioning**
Peroneus longus (also called lateral ankle)	There are two tender points: peroneus longus muscle: proximal and distal portions	Ankle: eversion Foot: plantar flexion
Tibialis anterior (also called medial ankle)	Tibialis anterior muscle belly	Ankle: inversion Foot: dorsiflexion

Chapter Summary

Counterstrain technique is a clinically effective method of osteopathic manipulation that is relatively simple for beginners. The novice learner must acquire skill in identifying tender point–specific anatomy and using precise patient communications. This chapter also highlights the need for proper ergonomics when supporting the full weight of a patient's head or extremity for 90 seconds.

Clinical Cases and Review Questions

Case 1

A 45-year-old man presents with right shoulder pain of 3 months' duration. He has tried stretching and ibuprofen with no significant relief. He has pain with shoulder abduction, which is limited in range of motion. Shoulder and arm muscle strength is intact. Examination also reveals a tender point in one of his right shoulder muscles. You suspect that the somatic dysfunction related to the tender point is contributing to his pain.

Q1. When performing counterstrain technique, positioning him by drawing the right scapula superiorly and side bending the cervical spine slightly to the right eliminates the tenderness of the tender point. The most likely tender point that is being corrected is the
   A. Levator scapulae.
   B. Supraspinatus.
   C. Infraspinatus.
   D. Pectoralis minor.
   E. Subscapularis.

Q2. For how long does the physician hold the patient in the position that eliminates the tenderness of his tender point?
   A. Five seconds.
   B. Thirty seconds.
   C. Sixty seconds.
   D. Ninety seconds.
   E. One hundred and twenty seconds.

Q3. This patient's tender point is
   A. An area of abnormal gamma efferent nerve activity.
   B. Caused by increased sympathetic tone from visceral disease.
   C. Generated from nerve compression.
   D. Indicative of micro-tears in the musculature.
   E. Referred pain from rotator cuff strain.

Case 2

A 66-year-old woman presents with neck pain for 1 week that began after she woke up in the morning. She denies trauma, and the pain does not radiate. The exam is positive for decreased cervical right rotation and diffuse right-sided paraspinal muscle tenderness. In addition, she has multiple tender points: right anterior cervical 3–5 and left posterior cervical 4–5. The right anterior fifth cervical tender point is rated as the worst.

Q4. Which tender point should be corrected first?
   A. AC3.
   B. AC5.
   C. AC6.
   D. PC4.
   E. PC5.

Q5. When performing counterstrain technique on any of her tender points, which of the following is the best indicator that her neck has been initially positioned correctly?
   A. The patient reports zero pain when the tender point is assessed for tenderness.
   B. The patient reports that the tenderness is reduced by 30% or less.
   C. The physician palpates tissue softening and loosening.
   D. The physician palpates tissue stretching and tightening.
   E. The physician positions the patient exactly in the described recommended initial positions.

Answers to Review Questions

Q1. The correct answer is **A**: Levator scapulae.

B is incorrect. The supraspinatus treatment position would be shoulder flexion, abduction, and external rotation (all to ~ 45 degrees).

C is incorrect. The infraspinatus treatment position would be shoulder flexion, abduction, and external rotation.

D is incorrect. The pectoralis minor treatment position would be flexion, adduction, and inferior traction.

E is incorrect. The subscapularis treatment position would be extension, abduction, and internal rotation.

Q2. The correct answer is **D**. Positioning for resolution of tender points is up to 90 seconds, with the exception of rib tender points. It is recommended that positioning to resolve a rib tender point lasts 120 seconds.

Q3. The correct answer is **A**: An area of abnormal gamma efferent nerve activity.

B is incorrect. Caused by increased sympathetic tone from visceral disease is the definition of a neurolymphatic reflex.

C–E are also incorrect.

Q4. The correct answer is **B**. The clinical recommendation is to perform the technique on the most tender tender point out of a group of tender points. AC5 is the only tender point that fits this criterion.

Q5. The correct answer is **A**. Zero pain reported when the tender point is assessed for tenderness is the only criterion for identifying the proper initial positioning when performing counterstrain.

B is incorrect. The correct percentage is 70% or more, not 30%.

C is incorrect. Tissue softening and loosening are not appropriate indicators.

D is incorrect. Tissue stretching and tightening are not appropriate indicators.

E is incorrect. Positioning the patient exactly in the described recommended initial positions is not an appropriate indicator.

References

1. Jones LH, Randall K, Edward G. Jones Strain-Counterstrain. ;1995
2. Rennie PR, Glover JC, Carvalho C, Kay, LS. Counterstrain and Exercise: An Integrated Approach. RennieMax; 2004
3. Snider KT, Glover JC, Rennie PR, Ferrill HP, Morris WF, Johnson JC. Frequency of counterstrain tender points in osteopathic medical students. J Am Osteopath Assoc 2013;113(9):690–702
4. Snider K, Glover J. Atlas of Common Counterstrain Tender Points: Version 1.1. Kirksville, MO: A.T. Still University; 2014

Research Bibliography

Ali MF, Selim MN, Elwardany SH, Elbehary NA, Helmy AM. Osteopathic manual therapy versus traditional exercises in the treatment of mechanical low back pain. Am J Med Med Sci 2015;5(2):63–72

Barnes PL, Laboy F III, Noto-Bell L, Ferencz V, Nelson J, Kuchera ML. A comparative study of cervical hysteresis characteristics after various osteopathic manipulative treatment (OMT) modalities. J Bodyw Mov Ther 2013;17(1):89–94

Collins CK, Masaracchio M, Cleland JA. The effectiveness of strain counterstrain in the treatment of patients with chronic ankle instability: A randomized clinical trial. J Manual Manip Ther 2014;22(3):119–128

Fryer G, Bird M, Robbins, B, Johnson JC. Electromyographic responses of deep thoracic transversospinalis muscles to osteopathic manipulative interventions. Int J Osteopath Med 2013;16(1):e3–e4

Klein R, Bareis A, Schneider A, Linde K. Strain-counterstrain to treat restrictions of the mobility of the cervical spine in patients with neck pain: a sham-controlled randomized trial. Complement Ther Med 2013;21(1):1–7

Liu Y, Palmer JL. Iliacus tender points in young adults: a pilot study. J Am Osteopath Assoc 2012;112(5):285–289

MacDonald R. The positional release phenomenon and the effects of Counterstrain manipulation: Reflections and implications. Int Muscul Med 2013;35(3):95–98

Wong CK. Strain counterstrain: current concepts and clinical evidence. Man Ther 2012;17(1):2–8

Wong CK, Abraham T, Karimi P, Ow-Wing C. Strain counterstrain technique to decrease tender point palpation pain compared to control conditions: a systematic review with meta-analysis. J Bodyw Mov Ther 2014;18(2):165–173

Wynne MM, Burns JM, Eland DC, Conatser RR, Howell JN. Effect of counterstrain on stretch reflexes, hoffmann reflexes, and clinical outcomes in subjects with plantar fasciitis. J Am Osteopath Assoc 2006;106(9):547–556

Index

Note: Page numbers followed by *f* and *t* indicate figures and tables, respectively.

A

AA joint. *See* atlantoaxial joint
abbreviation(s), 38*t*
abdomen
– palpation, 86
– somatic dysfunction, structures examined for, 84
– sympathetic ganglia in, 242, 242*f*. *See also* ganglion inhibitory pressure
– tenderness, assessment, 86
– tissue texture change, assessment, 86
abdominal aorta, 85*f*
abdominal organs, 85*f*
abdominal wall, anterior, myofascial release technique for, 113–114
abductor pollicis longus muscle, 74*f*
acetabular labrum, 78*f*
acetabulum, 78*f*, 145*f*
acromioclavicular joint, 70*f*, 146*f*
– active range of motion testing, 71
– palpation, 71
– passive range of motion testing, 71
– somatic dysfunction
–– diagnosis of, 71
–– exam for, 71
–– named, 71
acromioclavicular ligament, 70*f*, 146*f*
acromion, 70*f*, 72*f*, 73*f*, 158*f*
acromion process(es), 28, 29*f*
– observational assessment of, 71
active range of motion testing. *See also specific anatomical entity*
– grading rubric for, 13*t*
– in structural examination, 40
active techniques, 19
activity, after OMT, 6
acute-on-chronic changes, 38
adductor brevis muscle, 192*f*
adductor longus muscle, 192*f*
adductor magnus muscle, 59*f*, 192*f*
adductor minimus muscle, 192*f*
adhesive capsulitis, 163
adipose tissue, thoracolumbar, 41*f*
– palpation, 42
adrenal glands, neurolymphatic reflex locations, 244*f*, 245*f*, 246*t*
aftercare, 5–6
alar ligaments, 45*f*
American School of Osteopathy, 1
ankle(s)
– active range of motion testing, 83
– asymmetry, evaluation for, 83
– calcaneal angulation, 28, 29*f*
– passive range of motion testing, 83
– somatic dysfunction, 82

– sprain, 150
ankle mortise, 150*f*
anococcygeal ligament, 118*f*
anterior cervical effleurage, 129–130
anterior cervical region
– counterstrain tender points (AC1–AC8), 255–256, 256*f*, 256*t*
– muscular tissue texture changes in, 129*f*
– superficial fascial tissue texture changes in, 129*f*
anterior inferior iliac spine, 60*f*
anterior longitudinal ligament, 60*f*, 144*f*, 157*f*, 173*f*
anterior (ventral) ramus, 96*f*, 160*f*
anterior superior iliac spine, 58*f*, 59*f*, 60*f*, 144*f*
– distance from umbilicus, assessment, 63
– in indirect techniques
–– for pelvis, innominate positioning, 144, 144*t*
–– for sacrum positioning, 145–146
–– position assessment, 63
anterior superior iliac spine compression test, 62
aortic hiatus, 115*f*
apical lymph nodes, 119*f*
Apley scratch test, 72
appendix. *See also* mesoappendix; vermiform appendix
– neurolymphatic reflex locations, 244*f*, 245*f*, 246*t*
AROM. *See* active range of motion testing
articularis genus muscle, 189*f*
articular process(es), 50*f*
– inferior, 140*f*, 211*f*
articular process(s)
– superior, 64*f*, 140*f*, 211*f*
articulatory techniques, 154–167
– background, 155
– cervical C2–C7, 157–158
– *clinical cases,* 166
– clinical considerations, 154–155, 155*t*
– contraindications to, 155*t*
– costal, 232
–– rib 1, 158–159
–– ribs 2–12, 159–160
– direct method, 156
– disengagement, 156
– effects of, 154
– end goal of, 155–156
– indications for, 154, 155*t*
– indirect method, 156
– movements, barriers, and forces in, 155–156

– pelvis, innominate, 160–161
– positioning for, 155
– precautions with, 155*t*
– preparation for, 155
– research, 155
– retest for effectiveness, 156
– *review questions,* 166–167
– sacrum, 162–163, 232
– somatic dysfunction corrected, 155
– summary steps, 156
– tissue contact for, 155
– upper extremity
–– glenohumeral joint, 163–165
–– radiocarpal joint, 165
ascending colon, 239*f*, 240*f*, 241*f*
– visceral technique for, 240–241
ASIS. *See* anterior superior iliac spine
assessment
– competency-based, 7
– grade-focused, 7
– of OMT skills
–– levels in, 8, 9*t*, 10*t*, 11*t*
–– rubrics for, 7–14
–– strategies for, 7
assessment rubrics, competency-based, 7–14
assisting contact, 20
atlantoaxial articulation, 45*f*
atlantoaxial joint, 44*f*, 45*f*
– capsule, 45*f*
– high velocity low amplitude thrust technique for, 204
– muscle energy technique for, 180
– palpation: position assessment, 48
– passive range of motion testing, 48
– somatic dysfunction
–– diagnosis of, 49
–– exam for, 47–49
atlanto-occipital capsule, 221*f*
atlanto-occipital joint, 221*f*. *See also* occipitoatlantal joint
atlanto-occipital membrane
– anterior, 157*f*
– posterior, 157*f*
atlas (C1), 44*f*, 45*f*, 46*f*, 204*f*. *See also* atlantoaxial joint; occipitoatlantal joint
– transverse process of, 45*f*, 46*f*, 94*f*
autonomic nervous system, 232
autonomic reflex(es), 37–38
axillary lymph nodes, 133*f*
axis (C2), 45*f*, 46*f*, 140*f*. *See also* atlantoaxial joint
– spinous process of, 45*f*, 94*f*